Rural Nutrition in Monsoon Asia

Rural Nutrition in Monsoon Asia

Robert Orr Whyte

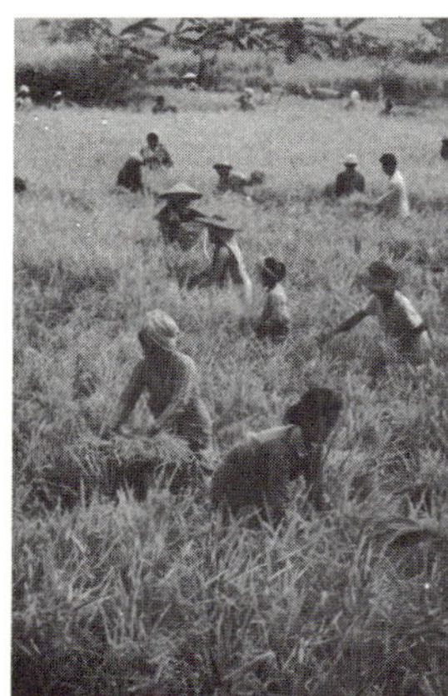
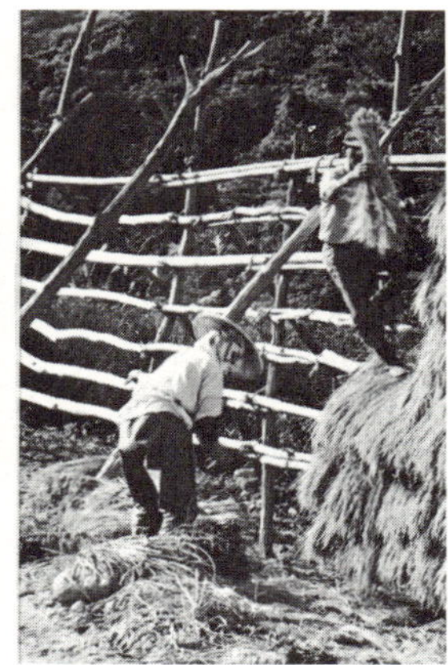
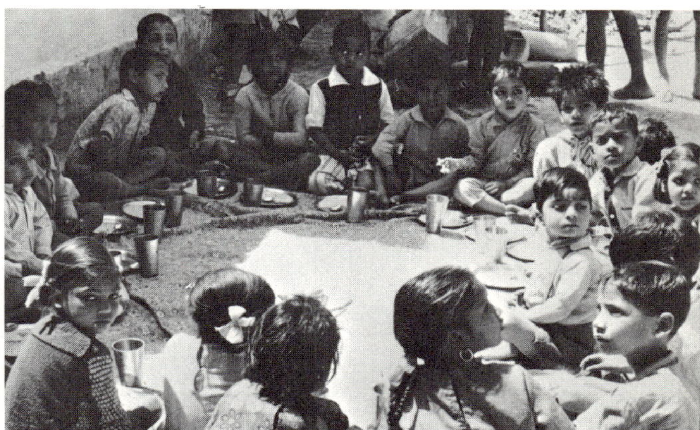
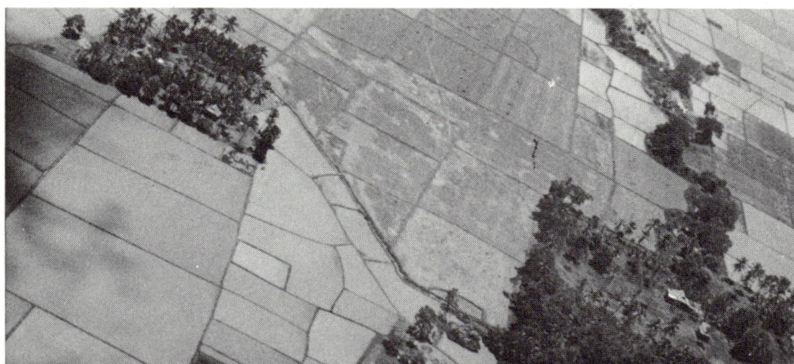
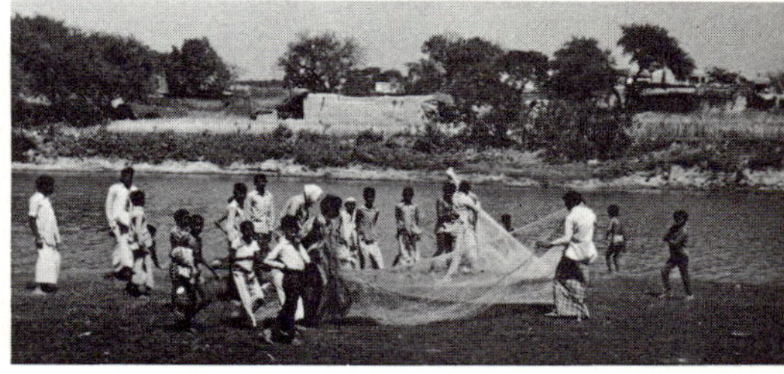
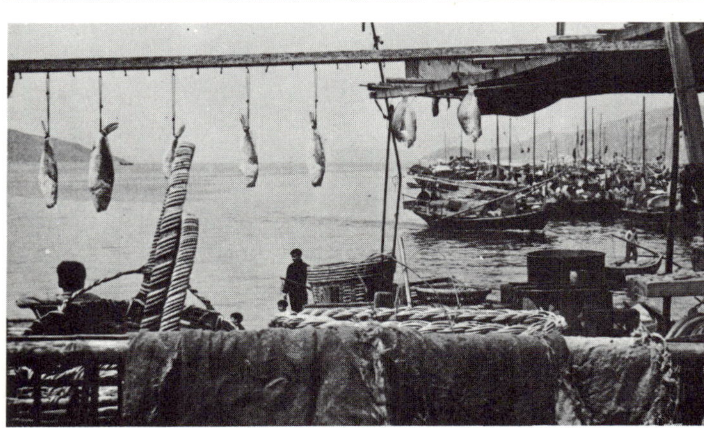
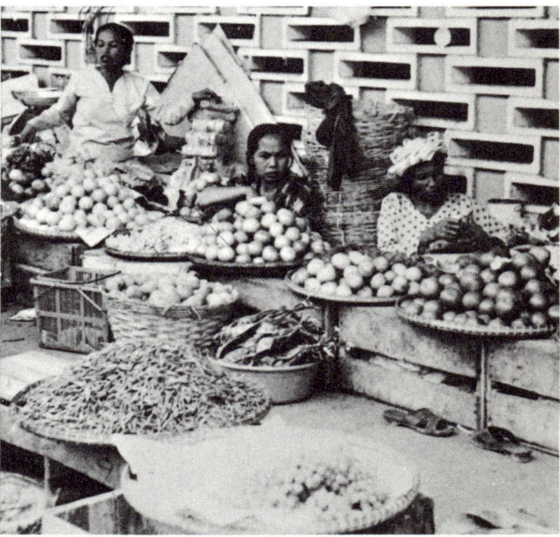

KUALA LUMPUR
OXFORD UNIVERSITY PRESS
LONDON   NEW YORK   MELBOURNE
1974

Oxford University Press, Ely House, London W.1
GLASGOW NEW YORK TORONTO MELBOURNE WELLINGTON
CAPE TOWN IBADAN NAIROBI DAR ES SALAAM LUSAKA ADDIS ABABA
DELHI BOMBAY CALCUTTA MADRAS KARACHI LAHORE DACCA
KUALA LUMPUR SINGAPORE JAKARTA HONG KONG TOKYO

Bangunan Loke Yew, Kuala Lumpur
● *Oxford University Press 1974*

Printed in Malaysia by
MUN SUN PRESS, KUALA LUMPUR

To the Memory
of
Robert Orr Whyte,
M.A., M.B., Ch.B. (Glasgow)

Preface

THIS study of the nutritional ecology of the rural Asians is designed to provide the essential background for those working, or preparing to work, on this fundamental aspect of rural life. It is hoped that the approach which has been adopted will indicate to the practitioners of each of the several disciplines involved how their knowledge and practical experience may contribute to an understanding of environmental processes.

Rural nutrition is a land science. Standards of rural nutrition are utterly dependent on the productivity of the farmer's own land—the food he can raise and the cash crops he can sell to buy food. Standards of urban nutrition are dependent upon family income and market availability, and are therefore the domain of the economist, the urban sociologist and the political scientist. It is within the rural areas, governed by environment, and the urban communities, governed by economics, that the dietary standards recommended by the nutritionist must be applied.

Planners and economists still know little of the present condition of the people on whom the fulfilment of their technological plans depends. The agriculturist who talks of food chains or webs, systems analyses and cost-benefit analyses is not, perhaps, paying sufficient attention to the factors of social ecology which govern the willingness and the capacity of the rural peoples to work harder and to produce more or different foods by improved methods; in other words, to accept change. The doctor, the nutritionist and the paediatrician are not always aware of the biological and economic limitations of the environment upon the production of the new foods they recommend. The anthropologist, who has the best knowledge of the attitudes and habits of the rural people he studies, does not always pay enough attention to human ecology, especially dietary practices. Only by a combination of all these disciplines, and by basing conclusions upon the study of the rural communities themselves, can viable national plans be evolved.

The future of Asia depends upon the physical strength of these people, on their enthusiasm for work in response to good incentives—or regimentation—and on their mental ability to accept new ideas and to learn new techniques. Apart from the rural traders, craftsmen and artisans, by far the majority of rural Asians are occupied in the production of food from the land and from the sea. They are responsible for feeding the urban communities and the non-food-producing rural people, and for providing cash crops for export. Yet their own standards of living and of nutrition are so pitifully low and so subject to marked seasonal variations that they are physically unable to respond to the claims for those increased efforts in production which are put upon them by national and international planning authorities.

The rural Asians depend almost entirely upon foods produced on their own land or in the vicinity of their villages. Thus dietary practices and standards are closely bound to the environment, and to the economic ecosystem which that environment has permitted to evolve. This interpretation of the applied ecologist brings him into conflict with those who support human determinism—economic or technological. These consider that man is captain of his fate and master of his environment, and that he needs only education and the necessary credit to be able to change the biological or economic ecosystems at his will.

In the environmental approach which has been adopted in this study, it is proposed that rural man is an essential part of the ecosystem in which he finds himself. His nutrition in particular is dictated by the food crops and domestic livestock which can be grown as the other economic components of that ecosystem. Environment dictates that the superior foodgrain, wheat, cannot be grown on most of the rice lands of Asia, and that the diet of the rice growers shall therefore be inferior in several respects. Over most of the region it is both unpractical and uneconomic to produce cheap animal protein on the scale that is required: the environment thus governs the use of this nutrient in the diet of the vulnerable groups.

Most of the rural people are living and farming on land which has been developed from its original natural condition in varying degree, and with a loss rather than a gain in the inherent soil fertility and productivity. Even with the maximum use of economic and technological inputs, each field, farm or catchment area has its own plateau of production ordained by its biological environment, and beyond which it is uneconomic to proceed. The present situation of under-nutrition and malnutrition throughout most of Monsoon Asia is an expression of chronic disequilibrium between rural man and his environment. It remains to be seen and proved under what conditions, with what inputs and at what a cost some semblance of a new equilibrium might be achieved, and in what period of time, in the face of the great increases in population and nutrition density per unit area which are occurring.

Hong Kong   R.O. WHYTE
January 1972

Contents

CONTENTS

List of Tables

List of Figures

Abbreviations

ANP	Applied Nutrition Program
ASEAN	Association of South-East Asian Nations
ASPAC	Asia and Pacific Council
CARE	Cooperative for American Relief Everywhere
CCTA	Commission de Coopération Technique en Afrique
CMA	Chinese Medical Association
ECAFE	Economic Commission for Asia and the Far East
FAO	Food and Agriculture Organization of the United Nations
FNRC	Food and Nutrition Research Council (Philippines)
IARI	Indian Agricultural Research Institute
ICAR	Indian Council of Agricultural Research
ICMR	Indian Council of Medical Research
ICNND	Interdepartmental Committee on Nutrition for National Defense (U.S.A.)
ILO	International Labour Office
IRRI	International Rice Research Institute
JCRR	Joint Commission for Rural Reconstruction (Taiwan)
PAG	Protein Advisory Group
UN	United Nations
UNDP	United Nations Development Program
UNESCO	United Nations Educational, Scientific and Cultural Organization
UNICEF	United Nations Children's Fund
UNSF	United Nations Special Fund
USAID	United States Agency for International Development
WHO	World Health Organization

Glossary

VERNACULAR TERMS

ande (Sri Lanka)	sharecropping leasehold
arhar (India)	*Cajanus cajan*
bajra (India)	*Pennisetum typhoides*
barrio (Philippines)	village
batti (India)	Baked dumplings made of wheat flour, dipped in hot ghee and eaten with dhal
belachan (Malaysia)	preserved paste of dried, ground shrimps and salt
bhares (India)	unidentified food plant from Himachal Pradesh
bhatoora (India)	fermented chapathi
bokkum (Korea)	roasted side dish without fluid, i.e. cabbage, pumpkin, leek
bonze	Buddhist monk
brinjal (India)	egg plant, *Solanum melongena*
broomcorn millet	*Panicum miliaceum*
carabao (Philippines)	buffalo
catty (translit. Chinese)	0.6 kg.
chapathi (Indian subcontinent)	unleavened bread in shape of pancake
chaulai (India)	*Amarantus gangeticus*
chiau (Laos)	fish sauce and pepper
cholam (India)	*Sorghum vulgare*
cholla (India)	buckwheat, *Fagopyrum esculentum*
cogon (Philippines)	*Imperata cylindrica*
congee (Far East and overseas Chinese communities)	rice gruel
crore (India)	ten million
cumbu (India)	*Pennisetum typhoides*
dhal (Indian subcontinent)	dehusked, split legumes
djengkol (Indonesia)	*Pithecolobium lobatum*
dola-duka (Indian subcontinent, Sri Lanka)	symptoms of pregnancy
foxtail millet	*Setaria italica*
gadung (Indonesia)	*Ipomoea* and *Dioscorea* spp.
gaplek (Indonesia)	dried cassava root
ghee (Indian subcontinent, Sri Lanka)	clarified butter

gram: Bengal gram	*Cicer arietinum*
black gram	*Phaseolus mungo, Ph. radiatus*
green gram	*Phaseolus aureus, Ph. radiatus*
horse gram	*Dolichos biflorus*
red gram	*Cajanus cajan*
gram sevak (India)	village extension worker
gulen (Indonesia)	vegetables cooked in coconut milk
gur (India)	unrefined sugar made from sugar-cane or palmyra sap
Hari Raya Puasa	day of celebration at the end of the fasting month of Ramadan
jaggery (India)	unrefined sugar made from sugar-cane or palmyra sap
jhangora (India)	*Echinochloa crusgalli*
jin (China)	0.6 kg.
jorim (Korea)	side-dish of hard-boiled food with salt, i.e. beef with soybean sauce
jowar (India)	*Sorghum vulgare*
kamote (Philippines)	sweet potato, *Ipomoea batatas*
kampong (Malaysia, Indonesia)	village
kankong (West and East Malaysia)	*Ipomoea reptans*
kaoliang (China)	*Sorghum vulgare*
karela (India)	bittergourd, *Momordica charantia*
kenaf	fibre plant, *Hibiscus cannabinus*
kerbau (Malaysia)	buffalo
kharif (India)	wet monsoon crop season, June-October
khesari (India)	*Lathyrus sativus*
khich (India)	husked bajra mixed with pulse in ratio of four to one, boiled thick in water
khichri (Indian subcontinent)	rice cooked with dhal, salt, turmeric and sometimes fat
kimchi (Korea)	pickled cabbage or radish
kodo (India)	*Paspalum scrobiculatum*
kodra (*koda*) (India)	*Paspalum scrobiculatum*
koori (India)	curry of husked gram flour, milk, sour curd or butter and leafy vegetables
kurthi (India)	*Dolichos biflorus*
kyat (Burma)	21 U.S. cents
lakh (India)	100,000
lapar biasa (Indonesia)	the usual hunger
Lembaga Sosial Desa (Indonesia)	Organization of Village Social Development
lauki (India)	bottlegourd leaves, *Lagenaria vulgaris*
mahua (India)	*Bassia latifolia*
malunggay (Philippines)	*Moringa oleifera*
mandua (India)	*Eleusine coracana*
masur (India)	*Lens esculenta*
matha (India)	*Pisum sativum*
miso (Japan)	paste of fermented soybean, wheat or rice and salt

mongo (Philippines)	*Phaseolus aureus, Ph. radiatus*
mou (China)	15 mou = 1 ha.
mung (India)	*Phaseolus aureus, Ph. radiatus*
nat (Burma)	predominantly anthropomorphic spirits
n.p. (India)	naye paise: one hundredth of a rupee
ngabyayei (Burma)	fish water
ngapi (Burma)	salted fish paste
nuoc nam (Vietnam)	fish sauce
padek (Laos)	fermented salted fish kept several months before use
panchayat (India)	village council
pantang (Malaysia)	denial: food restrictions
paratha (India)	pan-fried chapathi
pulses	grain legumes
rab (India)	flour diluted in buttermilk
rabi (India)	winter crop season, October–March
radbi (India)	boiled flour in buttermilk
ragi (India)	*Eleusine coracana*
Ramadan	9th month in Muslim calendar; fasting during daylight hours
rasam (India)	soup of red gram dhal, salt, spice, and either tamarind, lemon or tomato
roti (India)	unleavened bread made from foodgrain flour
rupee (Indian subcontinent)	unit of currency
sambar (India)	soup of red gram dhal, vegetables, tamarind juice, salt, spice, coconut paste and herbs.
sarson sag (India)	leaves of rape (*Brassica napus*)
sattu (India)	paste of mixed roasted foodgrain flour with gur and water
sawah (Indonesia)	padi, irrigated rice field
sedahan (Indonesia)	ecological unit around a major drainage (or catchment) area
sogar (India)	thick bread of bajra, baked hard
subak (Indonesia)	all rice terraces irrigated from a single dam and major canal. Also irrigation community based on it
tahu (Indonesia)	soybean curd
tairu (India)	unidentified edible root of Himalaya foothills
tchige (Korea)	boiled food, i.e. pumpkin, cabbage, white potato
tempe (Indonesia)	fermented soybean preparation
tempura (Japan)	fish, crustaceans or vegetables, deep-fried in batter, eaten with sauce
tic (Burma)	one hundredth of a viss; 0.0016 kg.
tidak apa (Malaysia)	'no need to worry'
toddy (India)	fermented coconut palm sap
tofu (China, Korea, Japan)	soybean curd
tonglad (Philippines)	*Cymbopogon citratus* (spice)
tuba (Philippines)	fermented coconut palm sap
ukas (Sri Lanka)	mortgage

urud (India)	*Phaseolus mungo*
varagu (India)	*Paspalum scrobiculatum*
variga (Indian subcontinent, Sri Lanka)	subcaste
viss (Burma)	1.6 kg.
yuan (China)	unit of currency

TECHNICAL TERMS

amino acids	chief structure or 'building blocks' of protein
angular stomatitis	ulceration of corners of mouth (riboflavine deficiency)
arginine	amino acid, possibly essential only for infants
ascorbic acid	vitamin C
Ayurvedic	Sanskrit *ayurveda*: the science of life. Indian system of medicine based on Hindu Scriptures or Vedas
B.V.: biological value	proportion of absorbed nitrogen in food retained in body
carotene	provitamin A
cystine	non-essential amino acid
E/T ratio	mg. essential amino acids per gm. total nitrogen
folic acid (folate)	B complex vitamin
galactagogue	substance promoting flow of milk
G.N.P.	gross national product
histidine	amino acid essential only for infants
isoleucine	essential amino acid
i.u.: international unit	expression of quantity of vitamin A. 1 i.u. vitamin A = 0.3 μg retinol or 0.6 μg carotene
kcal	kilocalorie = 1,000 calories
keratomalacia	softening and ulceration of the cornea, causing permanent blindness (severe vitamin A deficiency)
kwashiorkor	deficiency disease primarily due to inadequate protein, especially in children after weaning
lactase	enzyme which breaks down lactose during digestion into glucose and galactose
lactose	principal sugar in milk
lathyrism	crippling disease caused by neurotoxin in *Lathyrus sativus*, when eaten in large amounts

leucine	essential amino acid
lot viable (*Fr.*)	minimum area of cultivated land required to support a family
lysine	essential amino acid
marasmus	wasting deficiency disease due to grossly inadequate diet
methionine	essential amino acid
μg.	micromilligramme
NDpCals per cent	net dietary protein calories per cent: utilizable protein content of diet in terms of calories expressed as percentage of total metabolizable calories
niacin	nicotinic acid, member of vitamin B complex
N.P.U.	net dietary protein utilization: biological value plus digestibility
pellagra	deficiency disease due to inadequate niacin and/or tryptophan and excess of leucine in diet
phenylalanine	essential amino acid
Reference Man (*Woman*)	healthy adult whose height and weight are taken as standard
riboflavine	vitamin B_2
swidden	shifting or slash-and-burn method of cultivation
thiamine	vitamin B_1
threonine	essential amino acid
tryptophan	essential amino acid
tyrosine	non-essential amino acid
valine	essential amino acid
xerophthalmia	drying of the conjunctiva affecting the cornea, which becomes hazy (vitamin A deficiency)

Part I

THE ECOLOGY OF RURAL NUTRITION

1 The Significance of the Rural Asian

THE primary concern of this book is rural Asia. Here lives half the total world population, some 80 to 85 per cent of a total Asian population that must be around 2,000 million, increasing at some 50 to 60 million per year. The nutritional future of Asia depends in the final analysis on the energy and enthusiasm of the rural cultivators and their families. The productive energies of these peoples to produce food depends on their correct nutrition, on the creation of adequate incentives to give them the mental and physical energy so that they may produce more and better crops per unit area, to provide food for their own improved subsistence and also for export to urban and industrial centres, and cash crops for export to the developed world. From the increased efforts of the rural peoples as cultivators and animal husbandmen, industrial development, economic progress, greater national and regional self-sufficiency in food and freedom from food aid will be achieved.

The main requirements for improving the nutritional status of the rural people of Asia are both to produce more and better food, and to ensure that the rural people appreciate the merits of superior foods, correctly prepared. It was a nutritionist who said that 'a nutritional survey must be an exercise in ecology' (Dean, 1961). It would be presumptuous for an ecologist to deal at length with the sciences of human nutrition, reproduction and health. These aspects are therefore discussed rather briefly, as the background against which conclusions based on ecological assessment are reached. Studies of human nutrition, health and reproduction show that the indicators of undernutrition and malnutrition are widespread. A continuing and critical situation must surely be admitted if the findings of specialists in human nutrition and health are correct, that up to 80 per cent of the young children and adolescents in rural Asia are suffering from malnutrition in various clinically recognizable or latent forms, and that some 40 to 50 per cent of rural children die before reaching school age.

There are conflicts of opinion and interpretation as to the nature and seriousness of the situation. It is essential that these be reconciled quickly, at least among the scientific community. Such reliable facts as may be available must be carefully assessed to provide a basis for a scientific and agronomic blueprint, which is an essential precursor to an economic plan for the region and its component political units. This calls for a preliminary review, applying the principles of ecology to scientific disciplines relevant to the Asian environment.

The rural Asians are components of specific and complex economic ecosystems which they appreciate in their own way. Their knowledge of their monsoonal environment and its cyclic behaviour enables them to maintain their families up to a certain, albeit inadequate, level of subsistence.

... a poor peasant society, whatever it calls itself, is subject to the same cruel parameters of over-population, insufficient land, insufficient capital, insufficient education, and a technology that is limited by all these .... Circumstance, if sufficiently obdurate and compelling, leaves little opening for ideological preference (Galbraith, 1970).
... the only really significant social change in South Asia in the Independence era has been rapid population increase (Myrdal, 1968).

People living at this level cannot afford to take the slightest risk in introducing new techniques which have been proved in a central research station. They must themselves be convinced that success will be assured and that their lot will be improved. It is already late to contemplate modifying the approach of the rural agriculturists to change on the scale that is necessary. Yet it is only with their co-operation that the potentialities of new techniques will be

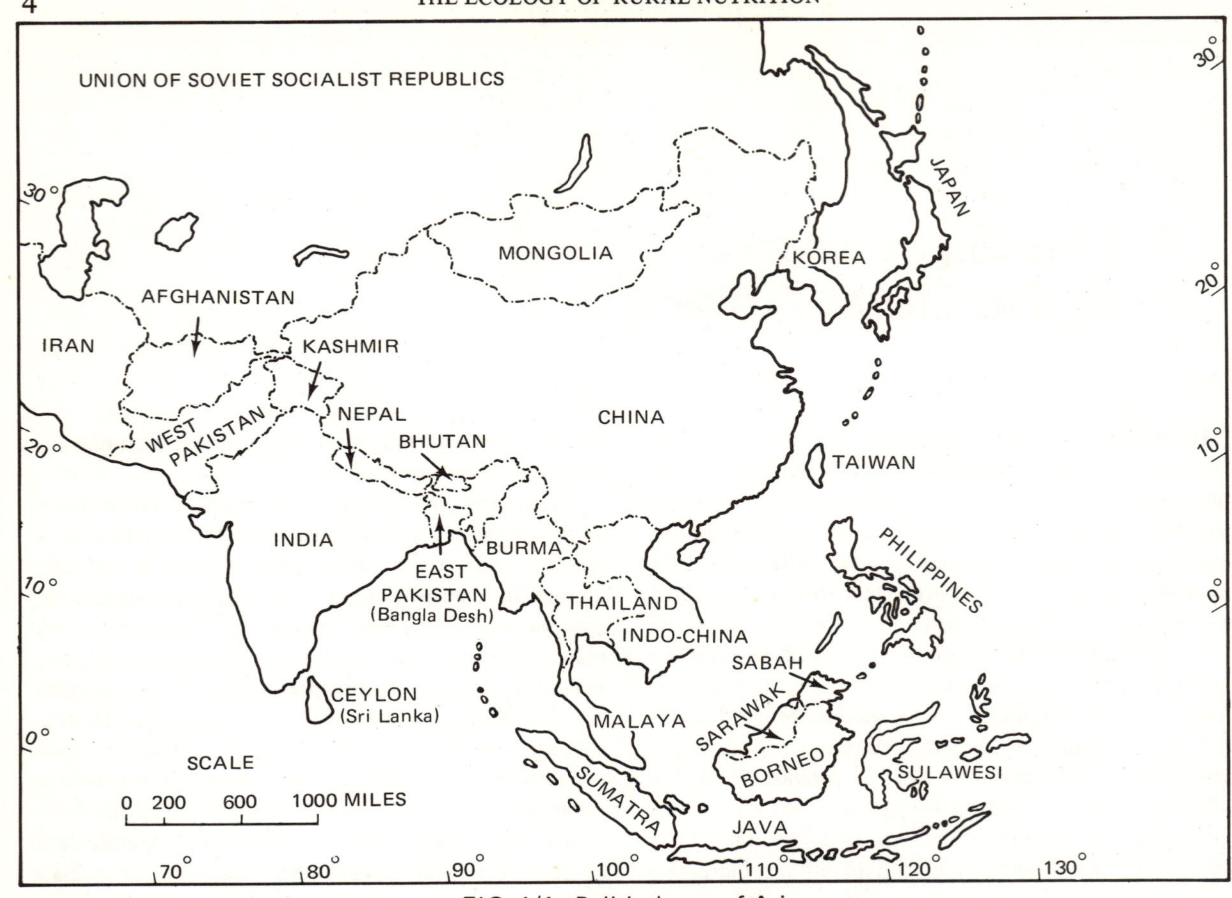

FIG. 1/1   Political map of Asia

achieved up to the biological maxima, within the limitations imposed by the environment.

If statistics cannot give a true picture, as Myrdal stresses repeatedly in *Asian Drama* (1968), how then can the Asian condition be understood and interpreted for the purpose of planning for improvement? The answer seems to lie in more field investigations. It is considered unwise to examine the problems of human nutrition in the rural areas — dietary standards and customs, conditions or diseases caused by nutritional deficiencies, or the physical and mental after-effects of a period of malnutrition during early growth — without at the same time considering what the land practitioners say may actually be produced.

Following the collection and collation of data, the geographers may map Monsoon Asia in terms of the environmental factors, e.g. rainfall, aridity, humidity, temperature, latitude, altitude, the characteristic and seasonal climatic rhythm and the frequency of its recurrent crises. Regional patterns may be recognized in respect of crop and livestock distribution, ethnic groups and dietary habits, incidence of malnutrition and related matters, even including lactose intolerance and addiction to betel chewing.

THE ECOLOGICAL APPROACH

Ecology as a scientific discipline hardly exists in Asia, applied ecology even less. Nevertheless, field practitioners such as agronomists, animal husbandmen, foresters and nutritionists have for long unconsciously applied in their daily work the principles and techniques of ecology in an empirical manner. As knowledge and reliable data in this new field of Asian science accumulate, students of the life sciences will become increasingly aware of the all-pervading influence of environment on plant, animal and human life in Asia.

Applied ecology involves the assembly for practical utilization of the available knowledge regarding the total environment. This is the environment in which man and his economic means of existence, his cultivated crops and domestic livestock, have to live and find their being and multiply, as the most important parts of a complex ecosystem. It comprises the geomorphology and geology as expressed primarily in topography, climate in its macro- and micro-manifestations, the soils and the water resources. Natural vegetation plays a dual role — assisting in maintaining an equable environment, and contributing in the form of forests and of grass and scrub cover to the requirements of the economic occupants. There must be a parallel study of the actual and potential reactions or adaptabilities of the economic occupants of the environment, man and his domestic animals and crop plants. It is the observation of the interactions between the economic occupants and the monsoonal environment, and of their reactions one to another, to be followed by the evolution of practical systems of management and improvement, that represent applied ecology in the Asian, as in any other context. And the most important, the most neglected aspect of applied ecology, is human ecology.

Geertz (1968) uses these criteria for the two important ecosystems in Indonesia: swidden or shifting cultivation, and sawah or wet rice cultivation:

> The ecological approach attempts to achieve a more exact specification of the relations between selected human activities, biological transactions and physical processes by including them within a single analytical system, an *ecosystem*. In ecology generally, an ecosystem consists of a biotic community of interrelated organisms together with their common habitat and can range in size, scope and durability from a drop of pond water together with the micro-organisms which live within it to the entire earth with all of its plant and animal inhabitants. The concept of an ecosystem thus emphasizes the material interdependencies among the group of organisms which form a community and the relevant physical features of the setting in which they are found, and the scientific task becomes one of investigating the internal dynamics of such systems and the ways in which they change.

The successful agricultural systems of the world have generally involved the progressive simplification of former ecosystems, with a corresponding loss in inherent stability. The study of the way in which complex ecosystems work is a major objective of the International Biological Programme. The functions involved must be put on a quantitative basis; the initial data to be obtained should relate to the primary production of the ecosystems — the production achieved by the green plants that are a starting point of all food webs. In this I.B.P. terminology, it appears somewhat strange to limit the scope of the term 'ecosystem' to biological systems. Surely the applied ecologist would use the term (whether ecological or economic system) for the whole succession of productive enterprises on the land, from the most primitive, extensive and still semi-biological to the most intensive (Table 3/1).

A degree of parallelism exists between type and intensity of land use and systems of crop and animal husbandry on the one hand, and the nutritional status of the rural peoples following these systems and practices on the other. It would be necessary to examine each local ecosystem (in the broad sense) to decide whether it could be economically and ecologically improved to a higher level of productivity, whether it were static but still viable as a secondary or intermediate land use system, or whether it were already on the downgrade, with reclamation being too costly. Surveys of the integrated type adopted by the C.S.I.R.O. Division of Land Research in Australia should ideally be carried to the stage at which one may define any given land system in terms of the adequacy of human diets in subsistence and/or shifting economies, and thus of the geography of the possible food deficiencies and the extent of under-nutrition or malnutrition.

It has been estimated that the land required to maintain the annual cropping sequence in the widespread system of shifting cultivation (swidden, slash-and-burn, fire-field and hoe, culture après brulis), may reach the figure of around 100 million hectares; the clearance of forest for shifting or permanent agriculture is still proceeding, particularly in Indonesia and the Philippines. Apart from estate agriculture, some 90 per cent of the cultivated land of the outer islands of Indonesia is under the shifting system. The nutrition of the peoples practising this system is a subject in itself, involving a trend away from the conditions of low population density and a relatively high intake of animal protein under a hunting and collecting economy, to conditions of high population density with undiversified, unbalanced diets and annual occurrence of 'the usual hunger' before the next grain crop becomes available.

Most of the 'natural' grasslands of Monsoon Asia, secondary communities in forest climaxes, are part of a belt of tropical covers in monsoonal bioclimates which extend from Senegal to Queensland (Whyte, 1968b). Their potential contribution to the improved nutrition of the Asian peoples is unfortunately low. In arid and semi-arid areas and at higher elevations which are not too wet, monsoonal grasslands can maintain breeds of sheep and goats kept primarily for wool and mohair production, and only incidentally for meat; they may also be used in the rearing of cattle for draught. Monsoonal grasslands, either in the natural state or improved by the reseeding of monsoonal species, are useless for productive dairy bovines, whether in milk or dry. The true potentialities of Asian grasslands for beef production in areas of high and low rainfall are not yet known, where this form of animal protein is acceptable in the diet.

The land ecologist and the human nutritionist have somewhat different interpretations of the term, 'land'. The nutritionist would accept the definition of land as representing the total environment, with particular reference to its capacity to provide an optimal standard of living for the rural people, and particularly for the maximum production of foods of plant and animal origin which will ensure the maintenance of the energy and physical and mental health of the family in both rural and the dependent urban communities. With the increasing gap between the food that the land can produce and the demand from increasing rural populations, the cultivation of crops, annual or perennial, for sale for cash will continue to be justifiable only if a good percentage of the proceeds can be used by rural cash-crop producers for the purchase of food imported from elsewhere.

The main objective of land studies would be to discover whether, while still meeting the criteria applied by the conservation specialists, the productivity of any particular ecosystem can be increased sufficiently and rapidly enough to provide all the food needed for consumption by human beings. Statistics relating to the area of land under permanent or shifting cultivation do not, however, give the breakdown necessary to assess the potentialities of any particular country, ecological region or local ecosystem.

This calls for classification of land for its optimal use, for forest, grazing, crop cultivation and conservation. On land classified for cultivation under irrigation, the intensification of agriculture is the objective. Land classification will inevitably indicate on what a small proportion of the total area it will be economic to apply the costly ingredients of intensification — more irrigation and better water management, greater use of fertilizers, improved cultivars and control of pests, diseases and weeds. These measures may be economically correct in specific areas, but the production of all items for a balanced diet demands that the intensification should also cater for maximum integration of crop husbandry with the more efficient forms of animal husbandry, on the same land (Table 3/1).

It is, however, unrealistic and uneconomic to propose application over a wide area of measures which would so dilute investment, equipment and technical staff as to make them ineffective. The question is: can we even keep pace with the foodgrain demands of the Asian population, increasing at more than 200 million every five years, merely by concentrating all efforts on land classified for maximum intensification? Can the populations, generally of lower density, on the far greater areas of secondary and tertiary lands be neglected in this way? Is it wise, either economically or politically?

THE STUDY OF RURAL LIFE

Governments do not always distinguish sufficiently between the one-fifth of their total population that may be called urban, and the four-fifths which comprise the peasant and tribal peoples in the rural areas. The United Nations has stated that a single definition is not applicable to all countries. It generally depends on the countries themselves to classify their own populations into urban and rural. The Food and Agriculture Organization also accepts the classification provided by countries, and considers agriculture to be the principal occupation of the rural population (FAO, 1969d). Criteria for a uniform classification of rural and urban populations may be found in the U.N. *Demographic Yearbook;* those adopted in India and China are given in Chapters 14 and 15.

Contributions to the ecology of rural nutrition have been made by those who conduct field studies of villages and other rural communities, and who cover in varying degree the dietary customs and health status, as well as the basic facts regarding land use and crop and animal husbandry. This group contains specialists in anthropology, rural sociology, demography, agriculture and animal husbandry, land development surveys, human nutrition, home economics, medicine, maternal and child welfare. Thus one has to consider the merits and demerits of interdisciplinary research. Different concepts and techniques are adopted by those working on individual aspects of this field of research — by the specialist, the interdisciplinary or cross-cultural practitioner, or the synthesizer of data from different disciplines into a coherent whole.

In his adoption of the ecological approach in cultural anthropology for the study of ecological change in Indonesia, Geertz (1968) hoped that he had established a fruitful interaction between the biological, social and historical sciences:

I am convinced that an adequate understanding of the new countries of the 'third world' demands that one pursue scientific quarry across any fenced-off academic fields into which it may appear to wander.... I hope that my effort will at least suggest the profits to be gained in such poaching expeditions.

From within this relatively discrete monsoonal region have arisen peoples of diverse ethnic origins; from outside the region have come other peoples and influences which have greatly affected the picture. This has led to a wide diversity of land economies, and thus of nutritional standards and practices, but in which a degree of common unity may be recognized within the regional framework.

Although recent effects of economic independence may be leading to increased homogeneity in the social, political and economic setting, great ethnic and social diversity still exists. A region characterized by such diversity presents great problems for administrators concerned with the organization of better social life in rural communities. The problem is how to create out of plural societies and primitive communities an integrated social and economic structure which can support and profit from the introduction of modern technology.

There is a far greater difference between urban and rural life in Asia than in the European or American worlds (Thuc, 1963):

The style of living of the present peasants of South-East Asia is almost identical with that of their ancestors 200 years ago. Even in the twentieth century, the peasants still continue to cultivate their lands with primitive ploughs drawn by water buffaloes, to irrigate their rice-fields with bamboo scoops, to carry their rice by means of baskets hung on the end of a flexible pole. They continue to do without electricity, running water, radio, telephone and newspapers. In sickness, they still have recourse to healers or sorcerers.
The influence of the West is virtually concentrated only within the narrow limits of the cities. It has never penetrated into the country, despite several centuries of European presence.
We can assert without exaggeration that the country areas of South-East Asia have become the domain of archaism, backwardness, and naturally, of pauperism. In fact, if the old techniques had assured the peasants of the pre-industrial era a relatively decent life, they no longer allow a population which has consistently increased to conserve the same real income. Compared with the increasing comfort of the cities, rural poverty becomes more and more profound.
Thus, while technical progress has liberated the peasants of the West from the servitudes which derive from the nature of agricultural activity, the same servitudes continue to impose themselves progressively on the peasants of South-East Asia.

THE RURAL ASIAN IN HIS ECOSYSTEM

The world of the sedentary rural Asian has until now been a small one. It includes the plot or plots on which he grows his agricultural and horticultural crops; the land over which he tends his animals; his village or other social unit; possibly a near-by village if it is the centre of his cult or religion; also the nearest town if he markets his surplus products direct, and where he may buy, throughout his life, the few consumer goods which he cannot purchase in his village. He may visit another village to collect his bride, and she will go back there with her children occasionally.

To the rural Asian, family takes precedence over all else in his endeavours. He knows that his wife will lose half or more of the children she bears, and hopes that the remainder will be able to look after their parents when they are old and can no longer carry out the heavy labour of the agricultural cycle. The home itself may be kept as clean as circumstances permit; the faecal contamination (by humans and animals) surrounding the dwelling and the village, and the lack of safe drinking water will cause parasitic infestation and recurrent illness. Intestinal, respiratory and other diseases transmitted by direct contact with the sick, by impure water, dust, rodents, snails, mosquitoes, flies, sandflies, lice, ticks, all exacerbate and are exacerbated by malnutrition and diminish the capacity to work. The rural family is likely to seek traditional practitioners to cure a serious illness or remedy the results of an accident, since modern medicine is rarely within reach, and is consequently unfamiliar.

The rural Asian would smile at the concept, if it were explained to him, that man is master of his environment. He knows only too well the extent to which he is subject to all the vagaries of climate and soil, and attacks by animal, bird, insect and pest. He is aware, if he is a swidden or settled dry-land farmer, that within a certain period of time, he will have one, two or more critical years in which the rains will fail or be insufficient in amount and distribution for his crops. For the farmer with irrigated land, such failure may affect the flow of water from higher up in the catchment, the supply of water from his wells, and so the supply into his irrigation channels. The cultivator usually knows when it is safe to plant his crops, but his guess may not always be correct. His first sowing may germinate on a false rain, and wither before the true rains begin. If he can get more seed, he faces deepening indebtedness, if not, hunger. He always stands the risk of having his crops flattened by a cyclonic storm before he can harvest them. Those in the delta lands live with the threat of devastation by flood. The true monsoonal environment is the most difficult in the world in which to farm without supplementary water. The tradition of his people and his own experience enable the Asian cultivator to do an excellent job in the circumstances. It cannot be wondered that he is conservative and suspicious of the advice of those who come from a world other than his own. These are the farmers who will be responsible for carrying out the national plans for increased food production.

The rural Asian is bound by tradition, which is influenced by his ethnic culture, his environment, the local social and economic customs, religion and the supernatural. He is not always ready to accept the well-meant advice he receives to improve his systems of using the land or of feeding his family. This is quite understandable. Any innovation in the foods he produces or in the methods which he adopts to produce them involves a certain amount of risk to himself and his family in partial or wholly subsistence economies. Hundreds of millions of rural Asians live on a razor's edge of existence. Because of their own poverty or the poverty of the environment in which they are born and still find themselves, they have come to endure continuous under-nutrition and periods of hunger and malnutrition. These are experiences which they realize must be avoided if at all possible; this means that they should continue to rely on the known rather than gamble with the unknown.

Rural people do not always welcome the advent of year-round irrigation to their land, because it involves them in long days, weeks and months of back-breaking toil in the heat of the noonday sun, in a season that was formerly one of essential rest and recuperation for themselves, their wives and the other working members of their families. Once it has been possible to raise the wet-season production sufficiently to provide reserves for the dry season, why do more, for the sake of the better nutrition of remote urban communities, or for the overall economic welfare of some abstract concept such as the nation?

2 The Origins of Food Production

To appreciate the rural dietary patterns of the present, one must know something about their history and evolution. This calls for a synthesis of a number of disciplines:

(a) ecology, as it relates to the definition and subdivision of the monsoonal and equatorial environments and to the reactions and interactions of human beings, animals and plants to those environments and to each other in the innumerable ecosystems — ecological and economic systems — which exist;

(b) history of climate;

(c) evolution of systems of land use, cropping systems, and methods of crop and animal husbandry;

(d) history of cultivation and domestication of plants, from discussion of their probable centres of origin, through the primitive cultivated forms, to the improved and high-yielding varieties (cultivars) of the present-day;

(e) principles and techniques of conservation of plant gene resources;

(f) history of domestication of animals of economic value to man;

(g) ethnology, the science of the human races, of their centres of origin, subsequent development, migration and intermingling;

(h) cultural anthropology, the science of human behaviour and practices, especially in relation to the nutritional potentialities of the environment.

The collection and analysis of archaeological and other records have not proceeded as far in Monsoon Asia as in other parts of the world. This situation is related in part to the high humidity and acid soils of the humid tropical part of the Asian environment. Although this brief review of the history of climate, the origin of land-use systems and the domestication of crops and domestic livestock must necessarily be speculative, it does show the types of information that are needed before any firm conclusions can be drawn.

HISTORY OF ASIAN CLIMATES

The degree and frequency of climatic change before and since world climates became stabilized at the end of the Pleistocene have had a profound effect on the evolving patterns of land use and so on the history of human nutrition. During the past million years there have been four periods of desiccation interrupted by three periods of relative abundance of rain. As these and shorter droughts would have generated from the heartland of Asia, they would have affected the whole of Monsoon Asia from the eastern mountain valleys of Afghanistan eastward and southward.

It was wind, during the long periods of desiccation that characterized the Pleistocene climate of north China, that transported the loess material from far and near and deposited it to create the 'classic' loess highlands. During the intervening rainy periods, widespread erosion would have caused the transport of loess material from the higher grounds to the low plains of north China.

Although the causes of the formation of the loess of the low plains are highly complex, much of the soil of this area is of alluvial and diluvial origins. In many localities in the low plains the soil contains a mixture of pebbles, gravels, and conglomerates. In contrast, the loess of the highland area, which is largely of aeolian origin, is texturally uniform, fine, pliable and porous, and hence offered much less resistance to primitive wooden digging sticks. This may have been one of the reasons why, in spite of more arid climatic conditions, the loess highland area was the cradle of Chinese Neolithic culture (Ho, 1969).

In relation to the subsequent history of crop ecology and land use systems, one may consider three other types and intensities of alterations in climate, each of which would vary greatly in their biological and economic significance (Whyte, 1963).

(i) changes which persist for 100 to 300 years;

(ii) variations or trends which are experienced for 10 to 50 years; and

(iii) changes induced by the action of man in 'destroying his landscape', which may be distinct from or may be interwoven with (i) and (ii).

A comprehensive review is needed to relate climatic history to biological and human history in Asia.

The conditions of aridity in western Rajasthan originated during geologically Recent and Sub-Recent time, consequent upon the rise of the Himalayan and Siwalik ranges (Raheja, 1965). In protohistoric and prehistoric times, the region was well-drained by mighty river systems (Seth, 1963). With the receding of the Tethys Sea and the gradual drying out of the river systems, desertic conditions set in over the west of the Indian subcontinent about 2,000 to 1,500 B.C. This process was hastened by the invasion of nomadic tribes from Central Asia. Precipitation is now steadily but slowly decreasing as the heat and moisture balance becomes more disturbed. Ho (1969) gives the present consensus of opinion on the Chinese loess:

despite the alternations between very dry and relatively wet periods during the entire Pleistocene epoch, the long-range climatic tendency has been one of periodic and probably progressive desiccation.

Frenzel (1968) has described the Pleistocene vegetation of northern Eurasia, including the significant border (see below) between steppe and forest in north China. Further south in the equatorial zone, the past and present distribution of plant genera and species in the botanical province of Malesia has been well-related to the influence of the last Ice Age (van Steenis, reviewed by Whyte, 1968b). This was accompanied by a general lowering of the level of the sea; the increase of land masses changed the wind regimes and the air humidity. With the post-glacial rise of sea-level, the conditions of the present day in Malesia became established.

The climatic history of Asia may be due as much to the occurrence outside the regions of those 'changes which persist for 100 to 300 years' as to smaller variations and trends within the region itself. A recurrence of a long period of excessive drought in the heartland of Asia would have repercussions far beyond its borders on the production of food crops and dietary patterns. The southward spread of aridity would probably have greater effect in China than in the Indian subcontinent, because of the difference in altitude between the Himalaya and the west/east ranges in China.

It is important to consider whether the outpourings of animal husbandmen from Central Asia at various times were caused by the desiccation of their grazing resources following the recession of the Tethys, or whether they may have been related to one of those long-term fluctuations in moisture availability proposed by Brooks (1949), Huntington (1907) and repeated by von Eickstedt (1944) and Wiens (1954). More recently Chappell (1970) reviewed climatic change, with special reference to the pulsations in the climatic history of Inner Asia. Although Russian workers did not formerly accept the concept of climatic change, it appears from recent geographical literature that the general opinion may have changed, from the economic determinism of Marxist theory to environmental determinism. In the standard Soviet monograph on the physical geography of Chinese Central Asia, Sinitsyn (1959) suggests that the desiccation of the Tarim Basin may be due to an increasing rain-shadow effect created by the continuing uplift of the Kun Lun and Himalayan systems (12 metres per century since the end of the Pleistocene). The Soviet climatologists have found a high correlation in the wheat lands of Kazakhstan between precipitation in June (the crucial month for summer wheat), and high sunspot numbers. Chappell (1970) concludes that both political and historical geography would benefit greatly from a renewed appreciation of climatic pulsations, considering also the two-dimensional concept of the 'pivot area' or heartland of Asia proposed by Mackinder (1904) with reference to the historic migrations of Inner Asian nomads.

The possible effect of these occurrences to the north on the so-called pressure pulsations in the population chambers of the settled valleys of China is discussed in Chapter 5. One of the two major historical movements in China around the middle of the first millennium B.C., that of the mounted nomads from the Central Asiatic Steppes (Phillips, 1965) may, however, have been partly due to a long-term deterioration of climate in their homeland, and partly again to the desiccation caused by the disappearing Tethys.

During long periods of normal or especially favourable climate, the animal husbandmen of the vast grazing lands of the heartlands of Asia would find good growth of grasses and other forage plants for their livestock. The percentage of stock losses characteristic of an arid or semi-environment would fall appreciably. Livestock populations would be built up far above the level which could be maintained during long periods of drought. Hence the pulsations would occur also in those grassland ecoclimates, with lasting effects on the history of migration and on the ethnic history of the lands to the south and west. Great

TABLE 2/1

China: number of droughts per century during different dynasties

DYNASTY	TANG	FIFTH DYNASTY AND NORTH SUNG	SOUTH SUNG	YUEN	MING	MANCHU
Christian Era	*618 - 907*	*908 - 1126*	*1127-1279*	*1280 - 1367*	*1368 - 1643*	*1644 - 1847 1861 - 1900*
Capital	*Chang-an Shensi*	*Kai-fung Honan*	*Hangchow Chekiang*	*Peking Chihli*	*Peking Chihli*	*Peking Chihli*
Honan	4.2	17.8	1.3	34.4	2.2	26.0
Chihli	2.1	6.9	3.9	25.3	1.8	43.7
Shensi	9.1	1.8	3.9	4.6	2.2	11.6
Shansi	0.7	2.3	–	4.6	7.3	12.3
Shantung	1.7	5.5	0.7	20.7	2.2	27.7
Kansu	0.3	1.8	1.3	5.7	–	8.3
Chekiang	1.4	1.4	17.8	4.6	4.0	22.7
Kiangsu	1.4	2.7	9.9	3.4 ·	1.5	43.8
Hupeh	0.3	0.9	4.6	4.6	0.7	26.2
Szechwan	0.7	–	2.6	–	1.1	2.9
Anhwei	0.7	3.7	5.9	4.6	–	36.3
Kiangsi	0.7	1.4	5.9	4.6	1.5	21.8
Hunan	–	1.4	–	3.4	1.1	20.6
Fukien	–	0.9	4.6	4.6	3.3	6.5
Kwangsi	–	0.5	–	1.2	0.7	1.6
Yunnan	–	–	–	–	6.9	2.5
Kweichow	–	–	–	–	–	2.5
Kwangtung	–	0.5	0.7	2.3	1.5	7.0

Source: Mallory, 1926·

TABLE 2/2

China: number of floods per century during different dynasties

DYNASTY	TANG	FIFTH DYNASTY AND NORTH SUNG	SOUTH SUNG	YUEN	MING	MANCHU
Christian Era	*618 - 907*	*908 - 1126*	*1127 - 1279*	*1280 - 1367*	*1368 - 1643*	*1644 - 1847 1861 - 1900*
Capital	*Chang-an Shensi*	*Kai-fung Honan*	*Hangchow Chekiang*	*Peking Chihli*	*Peking Chihli*	*Peking Chihli*
Honan	4.2	24.2	5.3	21.9	2.9	12.4
Chihli	2.1	9.1	9.9	29.9	5.1	26.9
Shensi	4.5	6.9	5.3	12.7	7.3	9.5
Shansi	4.5	2.3	5.3	19.6	13.8	7.3
Shantung	3.4	3.7	6.6	8.1	4.0	19.0
Kansu	0.4	1.4	0.7	5.8	0.7	7.0
Chekiang	3.1	4.1	15.2	6.9	16.7	13.9
Kiangsu	4.2	4.1	14.5	10.4	3.3	15.7
Hupeh	1.7	2.3	4.6	12.7	16.0	11.2
Szechwan	1.7	–	9.2	2.3	1.5	0.4
Anhwei	4.5	7.8	9.9	4.6	2.2	14.5
Kiangsi	1.7	0.9	6.6	3.5	4.4	13.6
Hunan	1.7	2.7	4.0	6.9	5.1	8.7
Fukien	1.4	1.4	5.9	4.6	7.6	3.7
Kwangsi	–	0.5	–	6.9	4.7	2.1
Yunnan	–	–	–	–	6.5	0.8
Kweichow	–	–	–	–	1.1	–
Kwangtung	–	–	1.3	4.6	2.9	0.8

Source: Mallory, 1926

droughts at the centre of a region would cause lesser droughts in contiguous areas, inducing further migration of peoples who had settled there during an earlier pulsation.

These considerations of climatic history provide a background to the present distribution of systems of crop and animal husbandry, and hence of the dietary patterns of peoples with these kinds of climatic origins. In more recent centuries, there is the history of floods and droughts in China presented by Mallory (1926): see Tables 2/1 and 2/2. It is not known whether a comparable study has been made for the Indian subcontinent. These impressions of imbalance in the hydrologic cycles are intensified by the ever-increasing impact of those changes of climate induced by the action of man (Pelzer, 1968). Bad grazing management on semi-arid land, the extension of crop cultivation into critical rainfall zones or up dangerous slopes, the clearing of forests to provide timber or fuel or more land for shifting cultivation, these and other types of misuse have transformed the Asian landscape. This has led to serious soil erosion and excessive run-off, to siltation and flooding in the lower valleys and deltas, and to increasing desiccation of the micro- and macro-climates in general.

POPULATION

The demographic history of the large and small ecosystems of Asia is relevant to a study of evolving nutrition. It is in this region that man has reproduced himself to such an extent, and particularly in recent decades, that an ever-increasing imbalance between human population and food resources has become the most critical problem.

It has been suggested that the basic subsistence groups and larger social groupings for Pleistocene hunters were around twenty-five persons. In their review of the global literature on food in antiquity, the Brothwells (1969) refer to the views of Coon (1959) on the possible size of breeding units of Pleistocene man. Modern breeding isolates among residual Stone Age communities generally contain no more than eighty to one-hundred breeding family units; such figures would seem to be applicable to most pre-Neolithic communities. Deevey (1960) suggests social and seasonal (environmental) restraint, and estimates that density during the Palaeolithic period did not exceed 0.04 human individuals per square kilometre. 'Palaeolithic man who stuck to business would have found enough food in two square kilometres, instead of twenty or 200. Social forces were probably more powerful than mere starvation in causing man to huddle in small bands.' Deevey believes that the total world population for early hominids of about a million years ago may have been much less than half a million. With larger amounts of flesh in the diet, it may have increased to over 3 million by the end of the Palaeolithic period. With the beginning of village farming of high-calorie cereals and of urban development about 7,000 years ago, populations may have increased rapidly within a period of 2,000 or 3,000 years to over 100 million (Deevey, 1960; and Brothwell, 1969).

It has been frequently stated that primitive hunting and gathering peoples had a miserable standard of living and nutrition. But a Symposium on *Man the Hunter* (Lee and De Vore, 1968) concluded that we cannot compare ancient hunting ecosystems with those of the present day, with their social structures affected by contact with modern civilization, and pushed on to marginal lands. Modern ethnographies have only limited applicability to the interpretation of archaeological material. Hunting by males was of less nutritional significance than the foraging by women for wild plants, roots and tubers for subsistence. Life and nutrition in the early hunting and collecting communities were not so precarious as is sometimes thought, on the evidence of modern communities in contact with adjacent cultivator societies, and disturbed by exposure to disease, the operations of missionaries and other factors.

One may ask whether the features of modern population increase are of equal significance in all rural communities. Would it be correct to say that, with many primitive groups, particularly the hunters and the most isolated communities practising shifting cultivation, poverty and hard conditions of life still do much to reduce the rate of population increase? In Chapter 3 it is suggested, however, that people living in more remote areas of shifting cultivation may have a reasonably balanced diet, if perhaps inadequate in quantity, because they still hunt for sources of animal protein and collect plant foods in adjacent forest to supplement the food from their plots. Thus animal ecology, and particularly the progressive extinction of edible forms of wildlife, is relevant to the present study. At the opposite extreme of land use, settled communities practising dry-land or irrigated (especially monocultural) systems of cropping are likely to lack the sources of diversity needed to provide balance in their diets. Thus, what may appear to be progress in land use practices, when combined with increasing pressure of population on the land, may lead to the calorie-protein deficiency so characteristic of the region (Table 3/1).

Most Asian rural societies have for long contained inbuilt, traditional systems for limiting population by applying during the critical phases of life the selective power of reduced nutrition on the mother and child — a procedure that has obviously done much to keep the number and therefore physical resistance of populations at a desired level. Nutritional taboos eliminate the weak and the sick who might become an economic burden. The mortality rate of children up to 5 years of age is as high as 50 per cent. To offset this, parents have regarded numerous offspring as essential, hoping that enough sons will remain alive to provide adequate family labour in the fields, insurance for the old age of their parents, and to perform the rites which are essential to carry them into the next life and ensure their subsequent comfort.

Western philosophy, developing in a favourable environment, has been able to favour the individual. On this basis, the West has brought its technology to Asia, where a more difficult environment has led to emphasis on the greater importance of the society, clan, tribe, kinship group or village. Western concepts of social progress have been introduced into the East in three stages, and these were successive, when they should have been simultaneous: preventive medicine; improved nutrition; and finally, only recently, birth control. This has led to increased populations but to a deterioration in the quality of life.

EVOLUTION OF SYSTEMS OF LAND USE

The evolving history of land use, from the primitive hunter collector ecosystems to the present day, must to a great extent explain the origin of the rural social unit, the types of crop and animal husbandry, and hence the dietary practices and standards of the rural people. Progress from one 'more primitive' stage to a higher, 'more advanced' stage (plateau) is possible only within the limits imposed by the environment, which in turn tends to deteriorate with more intensive, unscientific exploitation.

Archaeological research in China and South-East Asia has drawn attention to the emergence of food production (Triestman, 1970). It is possible to recognize a phase of sedentism still supported by the intensive collection of wild foodstuffs, and to study the ecological conditions surrounding the appearance of efficient agriculture:

The growing evidence of the existence of several early centers of civilization, in China and in South-East Asia, at once challenges any theories of grand-scale diffusion (either from the west or from northern China), and it stirs controversy in the formulation of general concepts about the growth of civilization.

The enormous task of providing the chronological skeleton of historical interpretation has not yet been achieved. Only a few clues exist, from palynology (pollen analysis) and carbon-14 dating.

A review of the history of development of rural social units may start with the earliest cultural stage of the northern Chinese farmers, the Yang-shao culture, or with the horticultural (with or without agriculture or fishing) communities of South-East Asia (Matthews, 1966) or with the earliest sites in the Indian subcontinent. Throughout the Yang-shao stage settlements were confined to the river valleys and small basins in the western highlands of north China (Chang, 1968 a and b). These early cultivators lived in villages. It appears that the village settlements shifted from one place to another after a short period of occupance, that certain favourable sites were repeatedly occupied, and that this shifting and repetitive settlement probably resulted from the slash and burn technique of cultivation. Chang's conclusions do not agree with those of Cheng Te K'un (1959), who considers that the Yang-shao villages were large, sedentary communities.

The developmental sequence which Chang (1968a) is able to demonstrate for the plains of the Hwang-ho has not yet been replicated (Triestman, 1970). There are now several thousand 'neolithic' sites in China. Some may represent a long reliance on intensive food collection supplemented by casual cereal cropping. Triestman quotes from field work in Taiwan (see also Chang, 1966) that the pattern of subsistence which relies upon utilization of diversified resources does not lead to the formation of dense villages (a response to specific marketing needs) but to a pattern of diffuse or scattered settlements with little or no centralization. On many rich, well-watered plains, however, there are village complexes which may be parallel to the development of the efficient agriculturist way of life in the nuclear area of the Hwang-ho. Triestman's conclusion is that, for all Asia, there is developing a picture of local cultures, each with its own unique history but each also participating in active intercalated exchange. In support of this, she quotes Solheim's 'very speculative' thesis (1967) that his South-East Asian centre in north-east Thailand, represented in its mature phase in the Funan State, had an important influence on the Chinese and on the greater Pacific area (see also Triestman, 1972).

It is usually said that the permanence of villages came with the Neolithic; Spencer (1966) would question the word 'permanence', and also the implications of a lack of sedentariness in earlier times, or for non-agricultural peoples. Would fishing communities with a permanent resource not have been rather sedentary, even in late Palaeolithic times, and therefore might not the initial cultivation and domestication of crops have occurred in and around such dual-purpose communities, on sea coasts, on lakesides, or along major rivers?

Spencer understands permanence as indicating continued occupance of the same general location for a matter of decades, as opposed to occupance of radically new locations selected annually for two or three years at a time. There is a relation between human nutrition and the type and intensity of shifting cultivation, together with its partial systems involving a varying degree of integration with established agriculture of a permanent nature — supplementary, incipient or opportunistic (Spencer, op. cit. Uhlig, 1969).

Groupings of camp-sites and home-sites may have increased in size towards village status with the advent of food production, but Spencer finds little evidence to support this with regard to the simple cropping systems. The tendency to social structuring inherent in an ethnic unit continued to determine the size of residential groupings long after crop growing had evolved a continuing pattern. The siting of villages, hamlets, housing clusters or homes is partly affected by the cropping system, but other criteria govern the siting of a residence: protection, domestic water, stream transport, exposure, material convenience, privacy. Considerations relating to cropping systems are important for the gross locational elements of residence among groups that live in permanent villages. Among peoples to whom village life is unimportant, considerations based on cropping system become predominant; housing tends to go where the crop site is located (Spencer, op. cit.).

Wolf (1966) has distinguished between primitive societies and peasants:

In primitive societies, producers control the means of production, including their own labour, and exchange their own labour and its products for equivalent goods and services among their own and other similar groups. In cultural evolution, these simple systems have been superseded by others in which control of means of production and disposition of human labour passed from the hands of the primary producers into the hands of groups that do not carry on the productive processes themselves . . . . Peasants are rural cultivators whose surpluses are transferred to a dominant group of rulers who use the surpluses both to underwrite their own standard of living, and to distribute the remainder to other groups that do not farm but must in turn be fed for their specific goods and services.

Moerman (1968) uses the term 'dependent incompleteness' to describe peasants, since they depend on the goods and actions of communities outside their own, and upon superior centres of control — markets, priests, capitals. Such clear-cut definitions are useful, but are difficult to apply to communities in transition from the primitive to the peasant, beginning to take on the characteristics of one group while retaining many of the old. This is perhaps particularly true of the hill peoples of mainland South-East Asia.

To what extent are the statements of Wilson (1967) regarding South-East Asia generally applicable?

. . . a reasonable generalization, adopted by most scholars who treat the region as a whole (a recent example is Burling, 1965) is that which distinguishes a tribally organized population inhabiting the upland regions and a politically dominant but socially amorphous peasant population living in the lowland areas. Not only is the lowland population politically dominant but its culture dominates the politically defined nation (as in Burma, Thailand and Vietnam) and is economically more sophisticated. Whereas the lowland population of each nation draws its cultural boundaries to coincide approximately with its political boundaries, the upland hill tribes straddle all national boundaries. Among the major problems in the development of South-East Asian nations are reconciling the highland and lowland populations, and hastening a political jell of the highland tribes.

Uhlig generalizes for the Himalaya (1970) and parts of South-East Asia which are dominated by forested hill slopes and intermontane basins (1969). The slopes are occupied by differentiated tribes, self-sufficient and belonging to a clan society, often with temporary settlement and cultivation. The irrigated basins offer favourable sites for rice culture and for permanent village societies which form the nuclei of territorial development. Uhlig makes the debatable statement that the rice basins are the older, the hills the younger settled areas (except in Sabah, where the order is reversed); (see also Spencer and Thomas, 1971).

In the densely populated irrigated lowlands of Java, former rural units have expanded and coalesced into blocks and strips of several square miles, alternating with uninterrupted areas of irrigated land. Village units have expanded far beyond the daily interaction groups, and vaguely defined neighbourhoods have evolved within the villages. Few villages lie more than ten to fifteen miles from an urban or semi-urban centre where agricultural produce is collected and retail goods and services distributed (Jay, 1956). Such a trend inevitably leads to greater imbalance in rural diet.

The origins of village structure and land-use patterns are a matter of debate among anthropologists and ecologists. Anthropologists traditionally consider that kinship and social structure of a rural community determine the way land is used and worked. The land ecologist believes that the environment dictates land-use patterns, and that these in turn have determined the evolution of social structures adapted to each individual ecosystem. It seems, however, that some anthropologists recognize the dominant significance of ecological factors and economic organization on social development.

Freedman (1965, 1966) has studied the relation between the extensive lineages of south-eastern and parts of central China, and land use. The extensive lineage is found in irrigated rice-growing areas, which allow dense populations to build up on small surfaces of land. The large settlement could continue to develop only when it was possible to reach the furthest fields within an economic time. Where ample cultivable land was not available in the immediate area of village, people would have to set up house near their new fields. In broken agricultural country, villages, and ultimately lineages must of necessity have been small. In the course of settlement, the early occupation of the best lands made it difficult for late-comers to build their villages into equally large units. Freedman quotes Skinner (1964) as suggesting that the lineage is likely to be centred in a catchment area around the lowest level of market town.

In support of Freedman's view that the home of the lineage is the home of double-cropped rice, Anderson (1970) states that, while lineage continues to be important in the New Territories of Hong Kong, it has never developed among the boat people:

The very dense, nucleated population of this land, in which each village is an economic and social unit, is a result of the wet rice ecosystem; and the vast power of the lineage seems to result in turn from this demographic fact and from the associated problems of social control and management. Once the keystone of the system — the rice paddy — is removed, the

system fails. When the more radical step of removing all land and agriculture is taken, the system disappears.

Economic organization, and particularly the way land is used, determines the organization of society. The hierarchical nature of Thai society has also been attributed to the organizational demands of wet rice agriculture. The great lineages in China were characterized by a strong sense of identity related to individual and collective ownership of specific areas of crop land. With the elimination of land ownership and the organization of cultivation in work teams, it is assumed that the traditional lineage group has not survived (Freedman, 1966).

In his study of land tenure and kinship in Ceylon (now Sri Lanka), (Leach, 1961) provided a critical test of the theory and method of contemporary British social anthropology:

This is a study of a small peasant community subsisting by the cultivation of rice in irrigated fields of fixed size and position. The emphasis is on the relevance of kinship and marriage for the practices relating to land holding and land use. Unilineal descent is not a factor in the situation. Although the ethnography has an extremely narrow range, the community has an ecology which has parallels in many parts of the world; for that reason some aspects of the analysis are of general significance . . .

But the Pul Eliya community does not only operate within an established framework of legal rules, it also exists within a particular man-made ecological environment. It is the inflexibility of topography — of water and land and climate — which most of all determines what people shall do. The interpretation of ideal legal rules is at all times limited by such crude nursery facts as that water evaporates and flows downhill. It is in this sense that I want to insist that the student of social structure must never forget that the constraints of economics are prior to the constraints of morality and law . . . .

Every anthropologist needs to start out by considering just how much of the culture with which he is faced can most readily be understood as a direct adaptation to the environmental context, including that part of the context which is man-made. Only when he has exhausted the possibility of explanation by way of normality should it be necessary to resort to metaphysical solutions whereby the peculiarities of custom are explained in terms of normative morality.

In Tihingan, Bali, Geertz (1967) noted that each major drainage or catchment, running lengthwise from the mountain towards the sea, is considered by the population to be a single, self-contained ecological unit. This long, narrow strip centred around a larger river is called a *sedahan;* each *sedahan* is broken down into a large number of *subak* (defined as all the rice terraces irrigated from a single dam and major canal), the fundamental elements of the whole system.

The term *subak* is commonly translated as 'irrigation society' because of the central role this institution plays in the regulation of water supply. But the *subak* is in fact very much more: an agricultural planning unit, an autonomous legal corporation, and a religious community. Aside from house gardening, virtually everything having to do with cultivation lies within its purview. Effective power with respect to agricultural matters lies and seems always to have lain in the *subak;* it is thus not a mere appendage of the larger order units, which as political entities are hardly more than tax districts. Theories of 'hydraulic despotism' to the contrary notwithstanding, water control in Bali is an overwhelmingly local and intensely democratic matter.

The creation of new land ecosystems in place of the old continues today in the name of 'planned development'. The last remaining resources of tropical rain forest are being cleared for the cultivation of perennial and other crops, not always for the benefit of the nutrition of the local people. It has yet to be seen what all these synthetic ecosystems will mean in terms of increased run-off and flooding and reduced efficiency of rainfall. Floods are reported with increasing frequency for Malaysia and Indonesia. China is trying to restore the hydrological balance with vast schemes of water conservancy and river control. The modern floods of Uttar Pradesh and Bihar are the result of the excessive clearance of vegetative cover, protective and water-retaining, in the belt of the Terai, and in the foothills of the Himalaya. For every hectare reclaimed in the Terai, a hundred hectares are placed under flood risk in the Gangetic plain proper.

Irrigation is being widely adopted to raise the land to the next plateau of production in this region of maldistribution and unreliability of rainfall. The injection of the Rajasthan Canal in western India and the belt of cultivated land which it will command from the Punjab border to Jaisalmer and Barmer will bring forth entirely new types of rural food-producing ecosystems. An incidental factor is causing great concern to entomologists. These new irrigated crops will provide a great new food resource for the insect pests that are at present in some kind of balance with the arid and semi-arid environment in which they exist. The environmental brake imposed upon their reproduction by starvation will thus be removed, and results may be disastrous over a wide area.

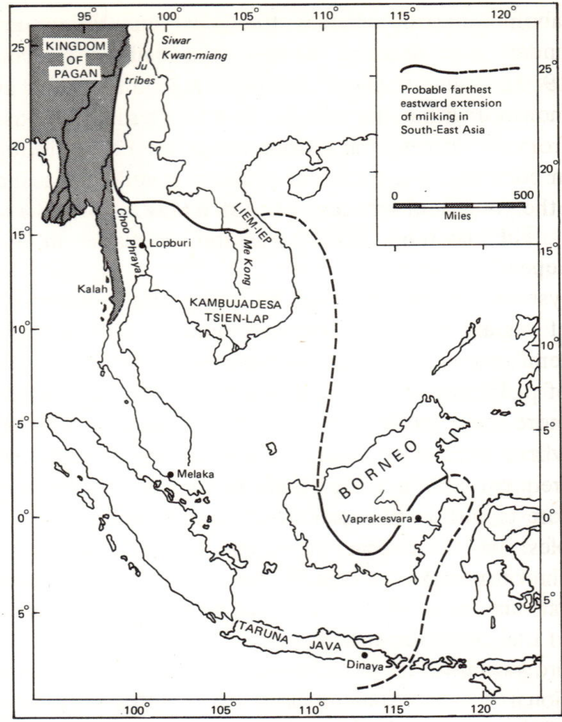

FIG. 2/1   The easternmost limits of the introduction of Zebu cattle from the Indian subcontinent during the first millenium A.D., to provide milk for immigrants from the same region
Source: Wheatley, 1965

DOMESTICATION OF ANIMALS

There is ample evidence to show that the rich fauna of Asia has until quite recently made a major contribution to the varied diet of the rural Asian. Although total food intakes may have been inadequate and subject to wide seasonal fluctuations, the many types of animals, large and small, provided a good balance in the diet. However, with increase in human population, an increased intensity of unplanned land use and destruction of protective habitats, a general ignorance of the significance to man of the wild fauna in the biological ecosystem, and the absence of any attempt at conservation, the wild fauna has progressively become extinct or greatly reduced in numbers and distribution. To replace them, man has had to turn to those few types which were amenable to herding or other simple forms of husbandry that might come within the meaning of the term domestication.

Some of the major domestic animals have been classified as mammals domesticated in the pre-agricultural phase, in the early agricultural phase, or as mammals domesticated primarily for transport and labour by agriculturists in the forest zone, or by secondary nomads and river valley civilizations (Zeuner, 1963). Most of the so-called domestic livestock of monsoon and equatorial Asia have not progressed far from the wild to the domesticated state, if efficiency in conversion of feeds and fodders into the food and other requirements of man is taken as the criterion.

The major groups of livestock (in numbers) are still dependent upon the factors of their biological ecosystem, the climate and the climax or secondary forms of vegetation — the sheep and goats on the arid and semi-arid grass and scrub ranges and in the dry forests of plain and mountain; the cattle in these and certain more mesophytic environments; the buffalo on lands where fibrous gramineous feeds and opportunity for frequent ablution are available; the pig in the wet forests and woodlands and wastelands and crop stubbles. Modern husbandry of cattle, buffaloes, pigs and chickens seeks to replace these environments with various methods of housing or penning for part or all of the day or year, combined with an artificial feeding programme designed to eliminate the seasonal nutritional swings of the natural environment. It is the cost of this creation of economic ecosystems on the scale required that puts the several sources of valuable animal protein beyond the purchasing power of most Asians.

If one adopts the practice of considering man as an integral part of his ecosystem, it is then found that the habits of man on the one hand and of certain animal species on the other made the appearance of domestication almost inevitable (Zeuner, 1963). A recent review of animal domestication will be found in Ucko and Dimbleby (1969), but apart from papers by Allchin on India (1969) and Watson on China (1969), there appears to be little progress in studies on animal domestication in Asia.

The early history of cattle has not yet been clearly defined. One of the offshoots of *Bos primigenius*, the wild long-horned cattle that roamed Asia and Europe from Pleistocene times, is thought to be *B. namadicus*, which inhabits southern Asia and the Arabian peninsula. The Zebu, *B. indicus*, first depicted in India more than 6,000 years ago, may be descended from *B. namadicus*, but the links in the chain are tenuous. Preliminary identification of bones from the Spirit Cave in north Thailand suggests a late Zebu connexion. In modern times the Indians moving down into South-East Asia brought with them the concept of the Zebu cow both as a milch and as a draught animal, but with little effect on diets other than their own. Most of the cattle of South-East Asia today are of mixed Zebu nondescript origin in which it is difficult to trace the original parentage. Were there any South-East Asian breeds of cattle?

There is not yet full agreement as to the origin and sequence of domestication of the Asian or Indian types of buffalo (Zeuner, 1963, Whyte and Mathur, 1966; Cockrill, 1966). The buffalo must have been indigenous to the rain forests of South-East Asia where, in the absence of grass, they must have subsisted on bamboo shoots, ground vegetation and on leaves of smaller shrubs and trees. One may postulate that wild or semi-tamed buffaloes were first used for sacrifice and consumed as meat. Although its use as a draught animal developed in South-East Asia, it was probably as an animal for sacrifice that it was introduced into India during the Neolithic. At a much later stage these animals would have met the high-protein leguminous fodder crops which were introduced into the irrigated lands of the Punjab from the Mediterranean. This higher plane of nutrition and husbandry would gradually have given rise to the Murrah and other types of milch buffalo, the major source of milk in the Indian subcontinent today.

Domesticated pigs are the descendants of a species group of wild pigs ranging from Europe to eastern Asia (Zeuner, 1963). The European representative is the wild pig, *Sus scrofa*, the eastern Asiatic is the banded *S. vittatus* (Sunda pig: Malay peninsula, Sunda Isles to Timor), with *S. cristatus* (the Indian wild pig: Indian subcontinent, Ceylon but not Malay peninsula). The Chinese pig is a descendent of *S. vittatus*. Zeuner states that in Asia the domesticated pig is associated with permanent post-Neolithic settlements only (it is not clear whether he includes communities of shifting cultivators).

The red jungle fowl (*Gallus gallus*) is considered to be the chief ancestor of the domestic fowl, and occurs from Kashmir to Tonkin, and on the peninsula south of the Godavari in India. One of the centres of domestication of the duck was China. When Zeuner wrote, archaeological evidence was lacking 'but the biological evidence points clearly to a great age of the domestic duck in the Far East'.

INTRODUCTION, CULTIVATION AND DOMESTICATION OF CEREALS

The history of human nutrition starts with the collection of foods provided by plants and with the hunting of animals in their biological ecosystems. On the plant side, the next step is the initial cultivation of wild plants found by experience to be superior and palatable — the cutting away of wild competitors around these wild plants, and the leading to them of small canals of water to extend their season of growth and to increase their productivity. Helbaek (1969) has defined the oft-misused terms, 'cultivation' and 'domestication':

the first word means particular and persistent interest in something. In plant husbandry, it means promotion of favourable growth conditions — changing the microbiology of the topsoil through hoeing and ploughing and, in many regions, by controlling water supply; further, by artificial dispersal of seeds and by keeping out competition from animals and plants that may infringe upon the maximum prosperity of the chosen species — in the hope that these endeavours will prove profitable also to the benefactor.

This does not necessarily mean that the cherished 'cultivated' species will die if the care of the cultivator comes to an end. Domestication, on the other hand, calls for a conscious effort in the way of selection, nursing and propagation of the crop plant, creating a reciprocal dependency or form of symbiosis between the plant and man. Once fully 'domesticated', a plant cannot exist in the absence of man. This, according to Helbaek's interpretation, applies equally to crop plants and to their accompanying weeds which have been exposed at the same time to spontaneous selection. On abandoned crop land and in the absence of other biotic factors, these weeds must ultimately be eliminated by the dominant ground cover of the original vegetation, if seed sources still exist.

The terms 'agriculture' and 'primitive farming' are also used in an imprecise manner. In the forested regions of greater South-East Asia (including south China) the clearing of vegetation first for shifting and then for settled agriculture could not have taken place on any significant scale until iron implements had come into general use. The earliest cultivation may thus have been in the valley bottoms, where, with great labour and given enough time, man (with stone and wood implements) might have removed a few shade trees and prepared a rough plot for stream or flood-water irrigation. He might even have been able to extend his cultivated land one or at the most two steps up the hillside, and so begin a primitive form of terracing. Scanty crops might also have been grown in the other ecological niches in the tropical rain forest.

The Origin of Asian Cereals

The history of the evolution of those Asian members of the Gramineae which now provide most of the world's foodgrains hinges upon the taxonomic, physiological and genetical distinction between annuals and perennials. The causes, dates and possible geographical locations of the creation of annual forms of Gramineae out of perennial are highly significant to world history; the availability of such forms contributed to the origins of crop agriculture, to the first major population explosion and hence to the early migrations of peoples (Whyte, 1972b).

It is generally accepted that our understanding of the underlying causes of the movements and cultural changes of which prehistory is composed must remain imperfect until a more complete picture of ecological change has been built up. One important event in this early history of man in his ecosystem was the appearance of the grains of annual forms of the Gramineae and the consequent origins of crop cultivation. Why did these annual forms become available to man over such a relatively short time-span in geobotanical history?

It is proposed that this was because there were no annual species/ecotypes/genotypes in Asia before the end of the Pleistocene, no annuals of *Triticum* nor of the genera which have contributed to the genomic structure of wheat (*Aegilops, Secale, Haynaldia, Agropyron* and *Elymus*), nor annuals of *Hordeum, Avena, Setaria, Panicum* or *Oryza*. The same interpretation may be applied to the domestication of annual cereal species of the genera *Brachiaria, Digitaria, Eleusine, Eragrostis, Pennisetum* and *Sorghum* in the lowland and highland zones south of the Sahara.

During the Neothermal, there occurred successive periods of fluctuating but increasing desiccation, combined with seasonally alternating low and high temperatures around the fringe of the continental anticyclonic area, 'the heartland of Asia'. This would not only have been a zone of vegetational transition, say between shrub-steppe and a grassland climax, where active hybridization and hence speciation might be expected to occur. The zone or zones of transition themselves would be moving under the influence of progressive climatic change. Thus would be provided conditions to which the ancient perennial species had not been exposed hitherto, and which promoted a slow, progressive change, probably over millenia, from perenniality to annuality among the wild perennial ancestors of the food cereal annuals, at a rate of evolution acceptable to geneticists. The taxonomy of the cultivated members of the Gramineae calls for less work in the herbarium, and more in the laboratory, the experimental field or in the centres of variability themselves.

Peoples of primitive hunting and collecting communities in the desert fringe lands of continental Asia who had been accustomed to hand-stripping the ripe heads of the perennials as one of their sources of plant food gradually began to note a new resource being 'handed to them on a platter', as it were, the large-grained annuals, in ever-increasing numbers and greater diversity. These new annual forms would have become established on the bare ground between the perennial species of a climax grassland that had become impoverished by desiccation and by overgrazing by the flocks and herds of the early pastoralists/ hunters/collectors. They would note that the annuals had the habit of seed-shattering, and would learn to push the seeds into the ground to protect them from marauding flocks of birds, so proceeding gradually to the digging stick and to the beginnings of dry-land cultivation.

Continuing and probably increasingly severe desiccation then caused the peoples themselves, with their thirsty and hungry animals, to move out of the desert fringes into regions less affected by drought, to the west and north-west, to the Anatolian Plateau, the Near East, the north-west of the Indian subcontinent and into China. They would take with them their new-found source of food which they had learned to cultivate in a primitive manner — the annual types of the Gramineae. These types, already highly variable because of their origin, were thus introduced into entirely new environments in which their perennial ancestors had not grown before. In passing, one may note that the perennial ancestors of wheat, barley and rye are primarily species of the Asian continental eco-climates, and that their annual descendants (cultivated and 'wild') which appeared in the Near East in particular, are of a secondary, or more correctly, intrusive ecological status in the Irano-Turanian and Mediterranean ecoclimates.

In the Near East, in particular, some of these non-indigenous annuals escaped from cultivation into the ecological niches which had formerly been occupied by local indigenous perennials, which had themselves been reduced or eliminated by overgrazing during earlier pastoral cultures, or by burning by hunters. The new annuals were already adapted to the seasonal droughts of these new environments, because of their drought-escaping character of annuality. Their original variability changed in character, in cultivation and in the wild, in a secondary explosion of diversity which represents the field material of the latter-day plant collector and conserver of genetic resources.

It is not necessary to attribute greater ingenuity to any people, race or culture in the introduction of these annual Gramineae into cultivation. The annual-creating conditions of desiccation and alternating high and low temperatures may have operated earlier, with greater severity and/or longer duration, in the west of the Asian continental desert fringes than in the east. If so, the *Triticum* and *Hordeum* annuals of Russia and the Near East evolved before the *Setaria* and *Panicum* of China.

Later, these factors of desiccation and seasonally fluctuating temperatures extended further, into the northern limits of distribution of the highly susceptible tropical and subtropical perennial species of *Oryza*. These occurred in a belt from north-east India (Bengal) to south-eastern China (Kwangsi, Kwangtung and Fukien). There is no need to postulate a primary centre in or around Assam and a secondary centre in China, involving a direction of movement which is quite contrary to that accepted by modern anthropologists. The evolution of annuals throughout these northern limits of the many perennial species of *Oryza* happened at the same time, producing the polyphyletic origin of cultivated rice and its many annual relatives which are incorrectly called 'wild rice'. Hitherto, wild perennial forms of *Oryza* could not grow in nature north of the present limits of double-crop rice in the southern and south-eastern provinces of China. With the appearance of annual forms within the perennial, it then became possible for the Lungshanoid cultivators to take this new crop north into less equable regions where the winters were too cold for rice. Cultivated annual rice was also carried south with movements of peoples (and iron tools) into the densely forested lands of South-East Asia, where until then only perennial rice had been cultivated or collected.

3 Environment, The Land and Nutrition

MONSOONAL AND EQUATORIAL ECOCLIMATES
WITHIN the region which the geographers call Monsoon Asia (l'Asie des moussons), to distinguish it from continental Asia, an annual, relatively brief season of rainfall, varying in amount from very light to very heavy, alternates with a dry season which varies considerably in duration and in the ambient temperatures. There are significant departures from the climatic pattern of the zone, which incorporates the other sub-regional groupings — the Indian subcontinent, South-East Asia, the Far East, the equatorial zone and the regions recognized by United Nations and its Specialized Agencies.

Monsoon Asia extends from the mountainous borders between Iran and Afghanistan (at the eastern limits of the Irano-Turanian region) and Pakistan, eastwards to Ussuri and Zee-Buryat provinces of Far-East U.S.S.R. The zone includes the southern and eastern provinces of mainland China, where some 70 per cent of that country's people lives. The insular nations of Japan (especially the lowland districts), Taiwan, the Philippines and Indonesia may also be included (Figs. 3/1, 3/2, 3/3), with the last two introducing the equatorial element (Spencer and Thomas, 1971).

The systems of land use and of crop and animal husbandry that are the basis of the nutritional ecology of the human occupants are governed partly by the amount and duration of the monsoonal rains, but perhaps even more by the nature of the other, generally dry season. There is a major difference, however, between western and eastern monsoon Asia. In the west, the hot, dry summer season of maximum temperatures (April-June) precedes the cooler, wet monsoon months (July-September). In eastern Asia, for example, on the Chinese mainland, the season of maximum temperatures and the wet season coincide. South of the Nanling, 60 to 90 per cent of the rainfall comes between May and October. In north China, 60—75 per cent falls between June and the end of August.

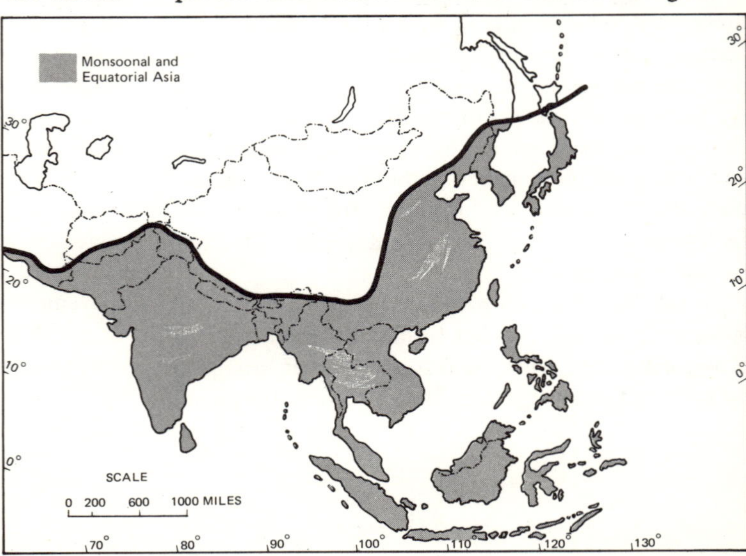

FIG. 3/1 Monsoonal and equatorial Asia

FIG. 3/2 Mean circulation in January

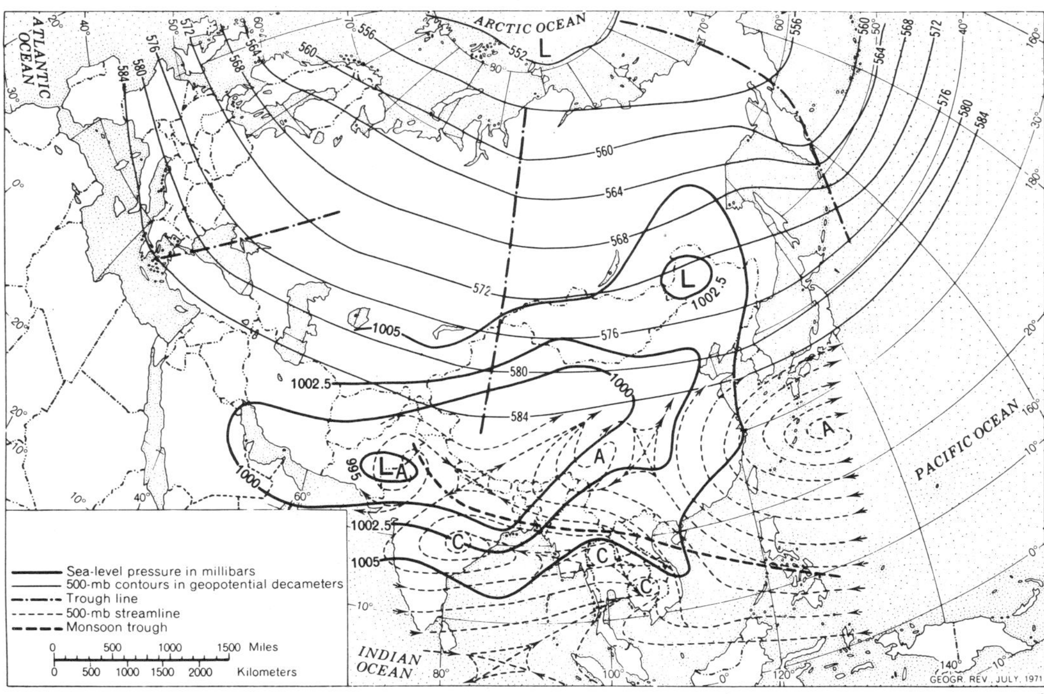

Source: Chang Jen-hu, 1971

FIG. 3/3 Mean circulation in July

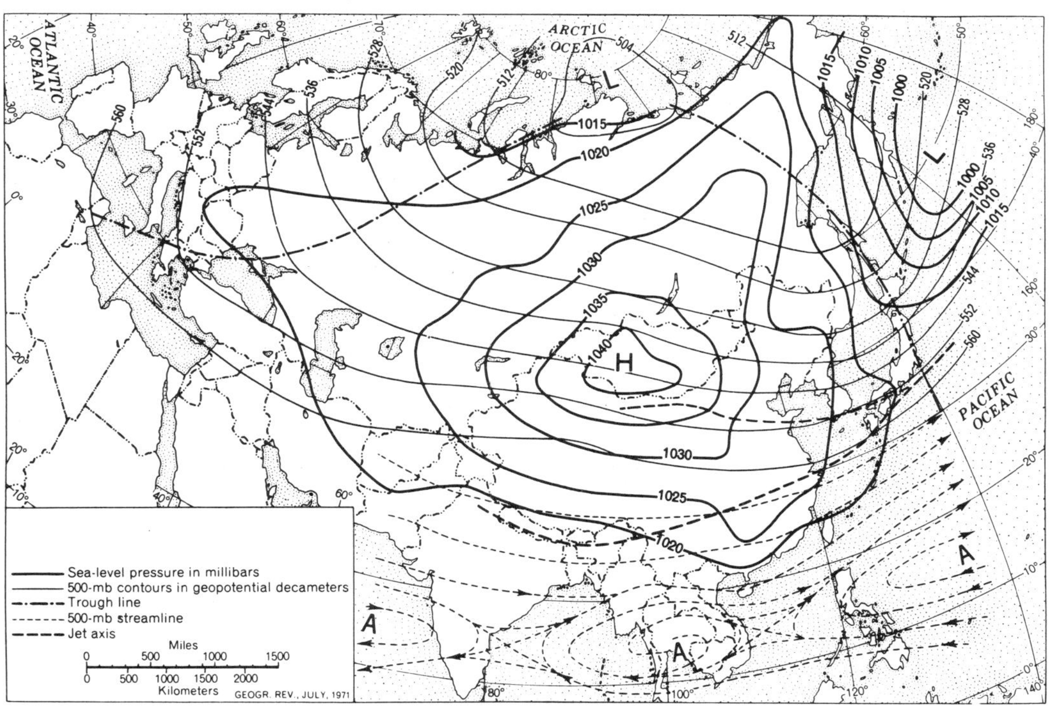

Source: Chang Jen-hu, 1971

At the eastern end of the zone, monsoonal summers coming up from the Pacific are associated with cool to temperate winters in the southern and central provinces of mainland China, Japan, Korea and the northern districts and mountains of Taiwan. This region is exposed to the Siberian air streams, unlike the Indian subcontinent, which is protected by the Himalayan range. In equatorial Indonesia, areas with a monsoonal sequence occur in what has been called a preponderantly 'everwet' zone.

In western Monsoon Asia, the long dry winters of the monsoonal ecoclimate are an annual occurrence. These dry periods have had a marked selective influence on the vegetation; perennial species are adapted to persist throughout the long, dry periods rather than to utilize fully the moisture available during the wet season. In less arid areas in Monsoon and equatorial Asia, the occurrence of dry years in a series with 'normal' years ('unexpected' in the absence of the necessary calculations and maps of rainfall expectancy) may cause surprise to planners and administrators, and be regarded as an erratic and anti-political act of a malevolent and unpredictable Nature. Extremes of drought may also cause severe hardship to the rural peoples, who are largely unprepared for these nevertheless, recurrent crises. In fact, the spasmodic droughts in the densely populated humid areas so common over Monsoon Asia are more disastrous in human terms than an annual period of drought among communities well adapted to that way of life.

La Peninsule Indochinoise et les îles de l'Insulinde sont des pays tropicaux soumis au régime des moussons. Malgre des variations d'une annee a l'autre qui peuvent être desastreuses pour la culture, il en resulte une alternance des saisons sèches et des saisons pluvieuses qui conditionne la vie des populations sédentaires (Coedès, 1964).

The methods now used for the assessment and presentation of climates, especially the extremes, are out of date. Smith has stated (1969).

Evidence suggests a kind of cyclic variation with varying time wave lengths, rather than fixed cycles of dry and wet. In any case, the climate odds can be stated and allowed for in any long-term planning. Averages are useless, it is frequency that is important. Climate summaries must be functional. With the necessary interpretation of climate into agricultural effects, contingency tables can be formulated in the nature of decision matrices which not only include the climate odds but also the economic consequences.

The terms ecoclimate, bioclimate and agroclimate are used somewhat loosely. It may perhaps be stated that ecoclimate is the climate of the total environment, that bioclimate is the climate in which all living things grow and reproduce themselves, and that agroclimate is the climate of that proportion of the land in which agriculture and animal husbandry are practised.

Climate defines the areas within which certain types of farming are possible. Within these areas the relative distribution of crops is still controlled by climate, although the general level of efficiency or intensity of production is influenced by economic and sociological factors. A rural cultivator is in a difficult position because he often has no alternative system of farming for his dry-land plot. He is always far more at the mercy of the weather; for subsistence farming, economics have a zero effect.

In advanced countries outside Asia, and in Japan, the rural people are only partially dependent upon the ecosystem in which they live, because they can obtain much of their food needs from elsewhere. Over most of rural Asia, however, the people depend almost entirely for their staples and other basic foods upon what they themselves grow, or on what is produced and is available locally. Only in the vicinity of large urban centres do the rural people have access to more exotic sources of supply. Their purchases from the urban markets or the itinerant traders are, however, not usually foods, but other commodities and consumer goods.

Thus, it is the agroclimate which largely governs whether the staple food of a particular community can be rice, wheat, sorghum or millets or other sources of carbohydrates. Crops and methods of crop husbandry have their own ecological succession. Irrigation and the provision of adequate fertilizers may change the environment considerably; this may make it possible to extend the range of economic production of rice into new agroclimates, but less so with wheat and barley (Figs. 3/4 to 3/7).

THE GEOGRAPHY OF RURAL NUTRITION

The question to be asked in reviewing the rural dietary patterns presented in the appendix is: taking monsoonal and equatorial Asia as the unit, is it possible to recognize and define regional or sub-regional patterns in the types and qualities of foods grown or consumed by the rural populations? The ecologist, concerned with the total environment — climate, land, plants, animals and human beings — claims that it is the environment above all that governs the types of foods that can be grown, and hence the nutritional

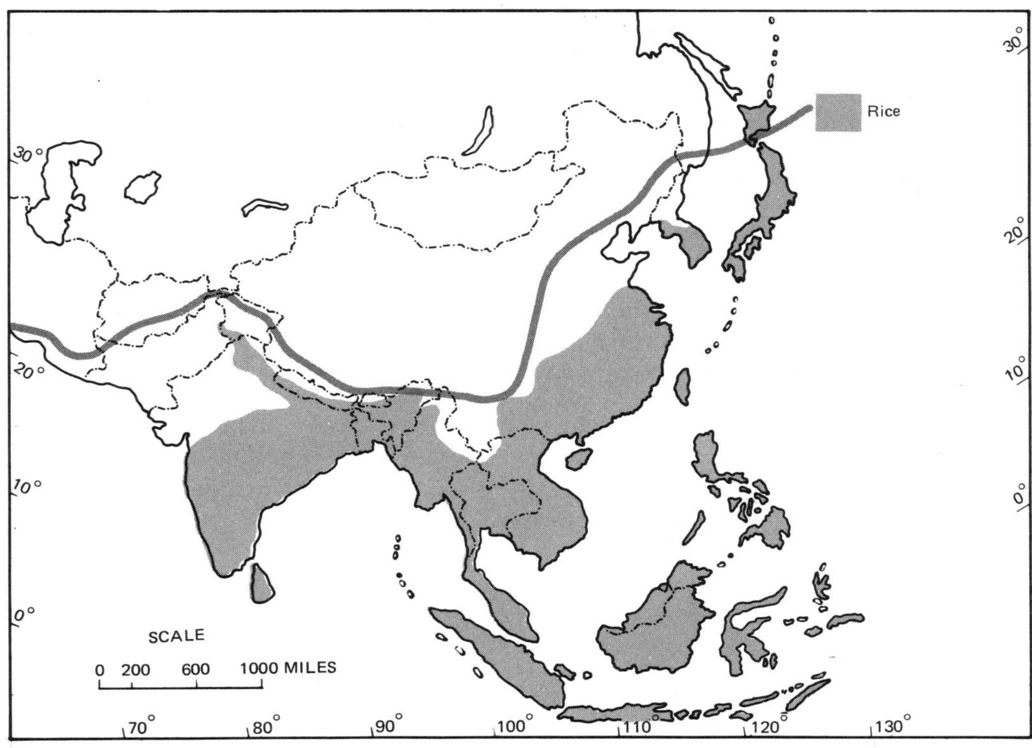

FIG. 3/4   The food cereals in agriculture and rural nutrition a. rice b. wheat and barley

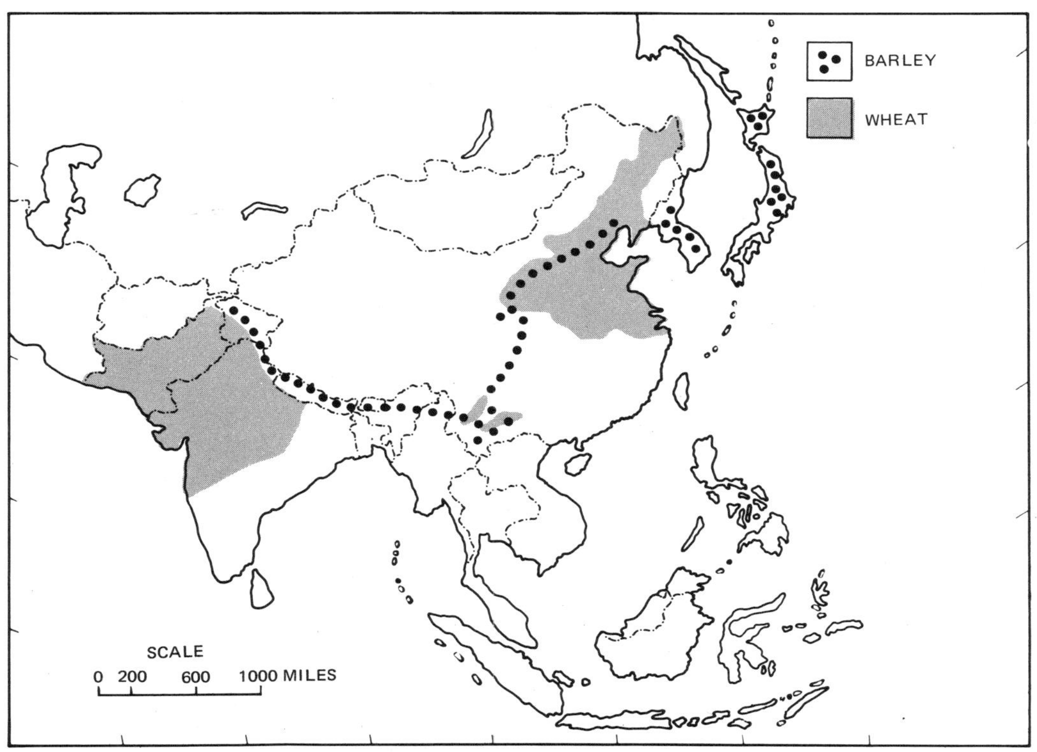

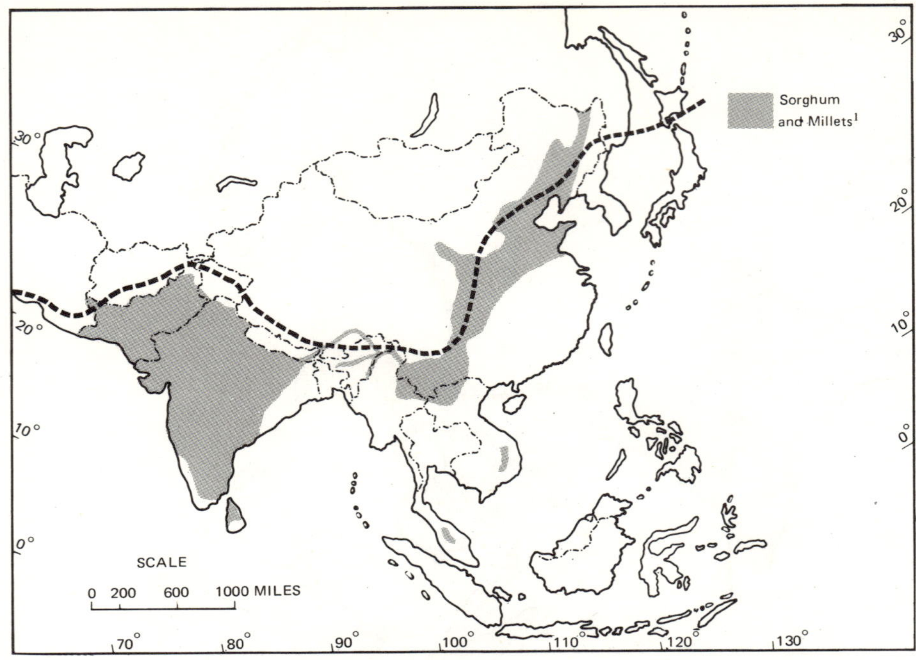

[1] *Eleusine coracana, Panicum miliaceum, Pennisetum typhoides, Setaria italica, Sorghum vulgare, etc.*

FIG. 3/4   The food cereals in agriculture and rural nutrition c. millets d. maize

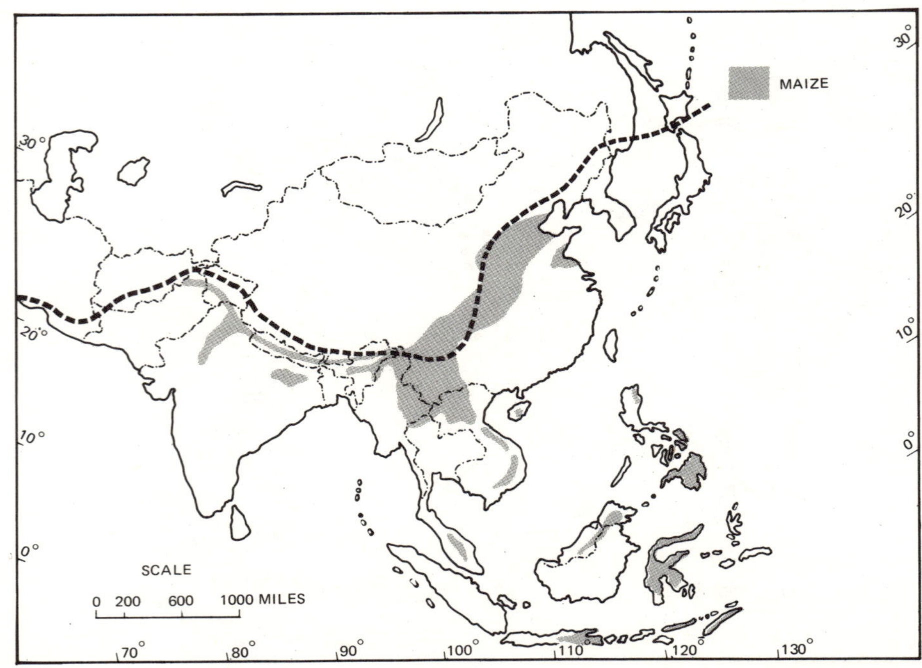

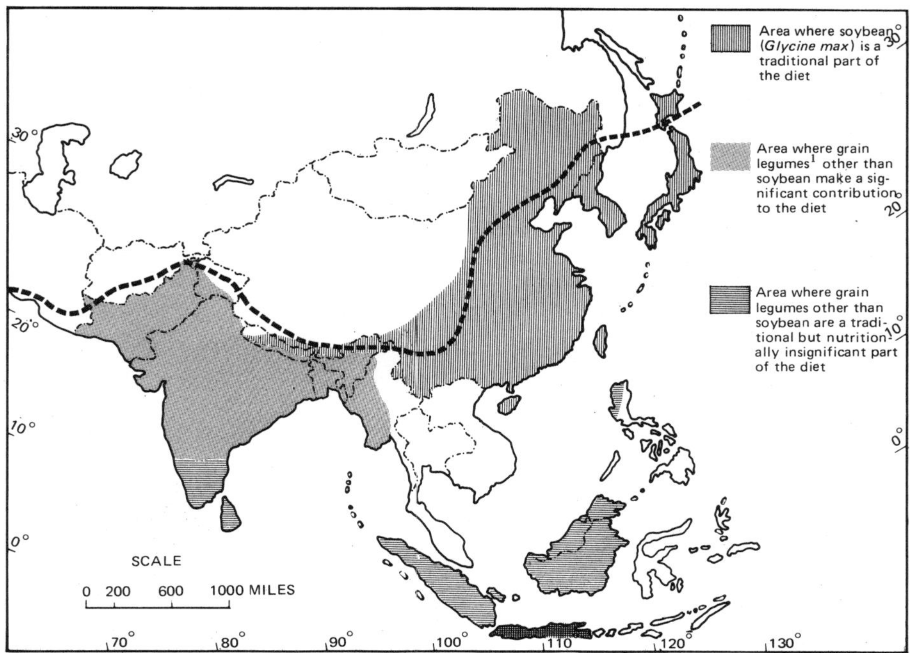

[1] *Arachis hypogea, Cajanus cajan, Cicer arietinum, Dolichos biflorus, Lathyrus sativus, Lens esculenta, Phaseolus* spp., *Pisum* spp., *Vigna sinensis*

FIG. 3/5   The grain legumes in agriculture and rural nutrition

FIG. 3/6   Root crops, tubers and sago in agriculture and rural nutrition

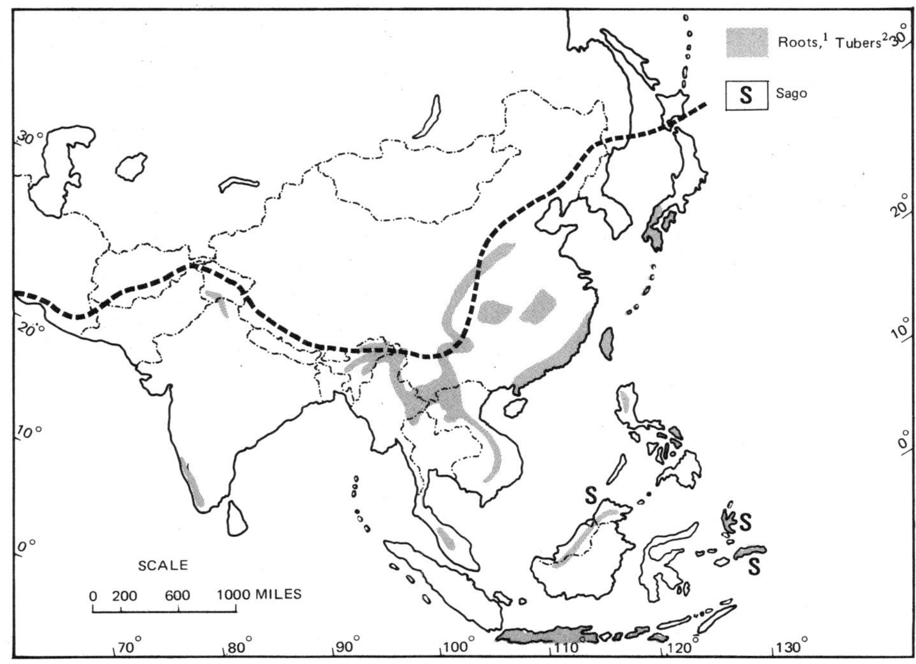

[1] Cassava and taro
[2] Sweet potato and yams

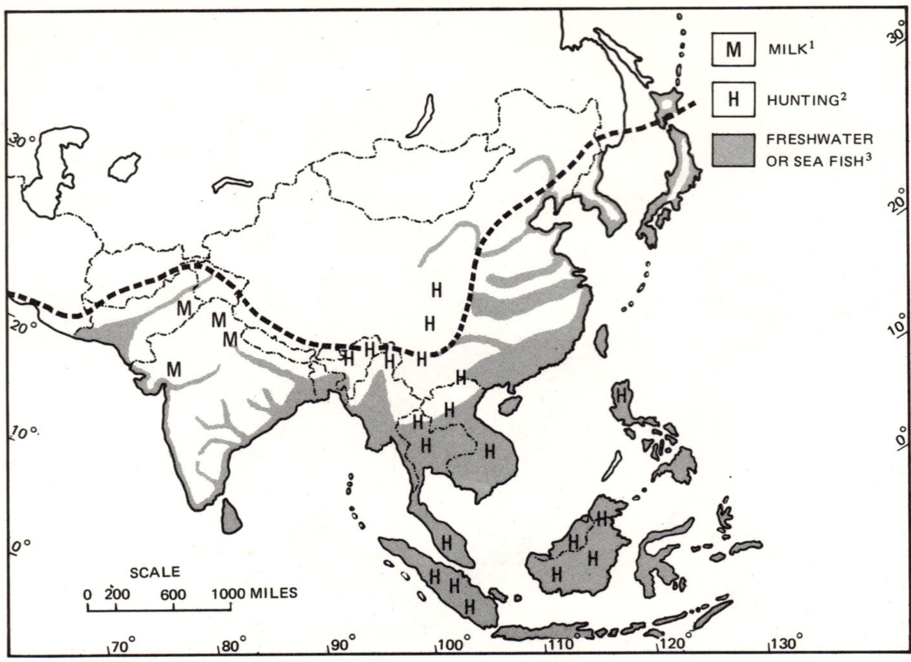

[1] Milk traditionally consumed, but urban marketing policies are reducing consumption.

[2] Hunting in areas of shifting cultivation provides larger animals such as boar or deer, but more frequently smaller game, birds and insects.

[3] Fish part of rural diet, in highly variable and often very small amounts.

Source: Whyte, 1970

FIG. 3/7a   Areas where various forms of animal protein make a significant contribution to the diet

FIG. 3/7b   Livestock potential of Monsoon Asia

Source: Whyte, 1970

Types of livestock which could be developed to provide different sources of animal protein, depending upon ecology of livestock production, ethnic beliefs and preferences, competition of fodder production with food and cash crops, and adequate purchasing power. Milk in India means milk from buffaloes, crossbred zebu x European and zebu cattle; milk in Malaysia, on a very small scale, is from zebu cattle and some crossbreds; milk in Taiwan is from cattle; and milk in Japan is from European Jerseys and Holsteins. Poultry throughout, except where otherwise specified, means eggs and meat from hens and ducks, plus geese in China.

status of rural people who live mostly on a subsistence economy. Others would say that the main factors affecting rural diets are economic, social and ethnic. The economists refer to the poverty of these rural peoples who must purchase part or all of their food or withhold their own marketable produce. They would say that the food problem is not so much one of shortage of food or inability to produce enough food, as the incapacity of vast populations with very low purchasing power to supplement their own production by buying other foods that may be available locally, or could be provided by import from elsewhere.

In a review of the foods that may be produced in a particular environment and the economic capacity of the people to retain them or to buy them, one must also consider the specific dietary practices, preferences and taboos of different ethnic groups. Apart from the dietary habits which have been handed down through generations, different races and the socio-economic groups within those races have different levels of understanding of the importance of good nutrition, and of the correct methods of preparation, cooking and environmental sanitation that must accompany that understanding.

Students may collaborate in cross-cultural studies designed to map the environmental and other factors which govern the present patterns of rural diets. A synthesizing study of this type would bring together data relating to climate, ethnology, land use, natural vegetation and crop and livestock types and methods of husbandry into sub-regions within the overall eco-climates. These would be correlated with the information collected in dietary surveys, such as those presented in the appendix, so that a diet atlas or atlases may be produced. The aspects covered by the Working Party of the Indian Council for Medical Research (Convenor, Dr. C. Gopalan) for the *Diet Atlas of India* (1964) were: population; food production; diet surveys (geographical areas and population groups); patterns of cereal consumption; expenditure on food; monthly consumption of food grains in rural and urban areas; food consumption pattern in different States; calorie intake per person per day; consumption pattern of different foods; monthly consumption of eggs per State; and percentage of vegetarians (Fig. 3/8).

LAND ECOLOGY AND HUMAN NUTRITION

Throughout the world, agriculture has been the main production factor leading to the accumulation of reserves for the different groups within society

(Terra, 1961). Any occupational diversification in which a substantial part of the population is engaged outside agriculture is excluded by the very fact that there is not enough food available for producers outside agriculture. This is due, in the equatorial zone, to:

primitive methods of cultivation, so that much labour is needed per hectare for opening up and preparing the land and tending the crop;

the very rapid weed growth under conditions of high temperature and humidity, and the impossibility of timely weed control when there are long periods of· rainfall;

the small area of land that each family can tend;

poor fertility of the soil, leached by heavy rains, with the exception of recent volcanic and some recent alluvial soils; and

short day length (Terra, op. cit.).

In subtropical areas, the situation may become more favourable, with richer soils, alternations of wet and dry seasons with warmer periods of long days and colder periods of short days, but with long periods of drought making irrigation an essential part of intensification of production and higher yields. A dry-land farmer can cope with a larger unit, but this ratio falls again on an irrigated family-size farm. Approaching the temperate zone, farms again become larger, and surpluses of food become increasingly available for non-agriculturists (Terra, op. cit.).

What are the criteria for recognizing deterioration in the equilibrium between agriculture/food supply/ human population? Imbalance in any rural ecosystem is an expression of hunger, or a deficit in requirements, in one or more members of the ecosystem — deficit of water, soil infertility, sub-optimal temperature range and photoperiod for crop plants, deficit of grazing resources, feeds and fodders with lower quality of intake and excessive seasonal fluctuations in availability for domestic livestock, excessive nutrition density of the human population (persons per unit area of crop land or land under main staple) expressed as deficit of quantity and quality foods, and so as varying degrees of undernutrition and malnutrition. It is recognized that poverty is the major deterrent to improved rural nutrition. But even if it were to become possible to increase purchasing power to a significant extent, it would still be most difficult entirely to eliminate imbalance in the ecosystem and to produce enough food cheaply enough and in the right places to provide a balanced diet for all. Penny (1966) has discussed the characteristics of a deteriorating situation and the evidence of increasing poverty in Indonesia. Reasons for lack of innovation and enterprise have to

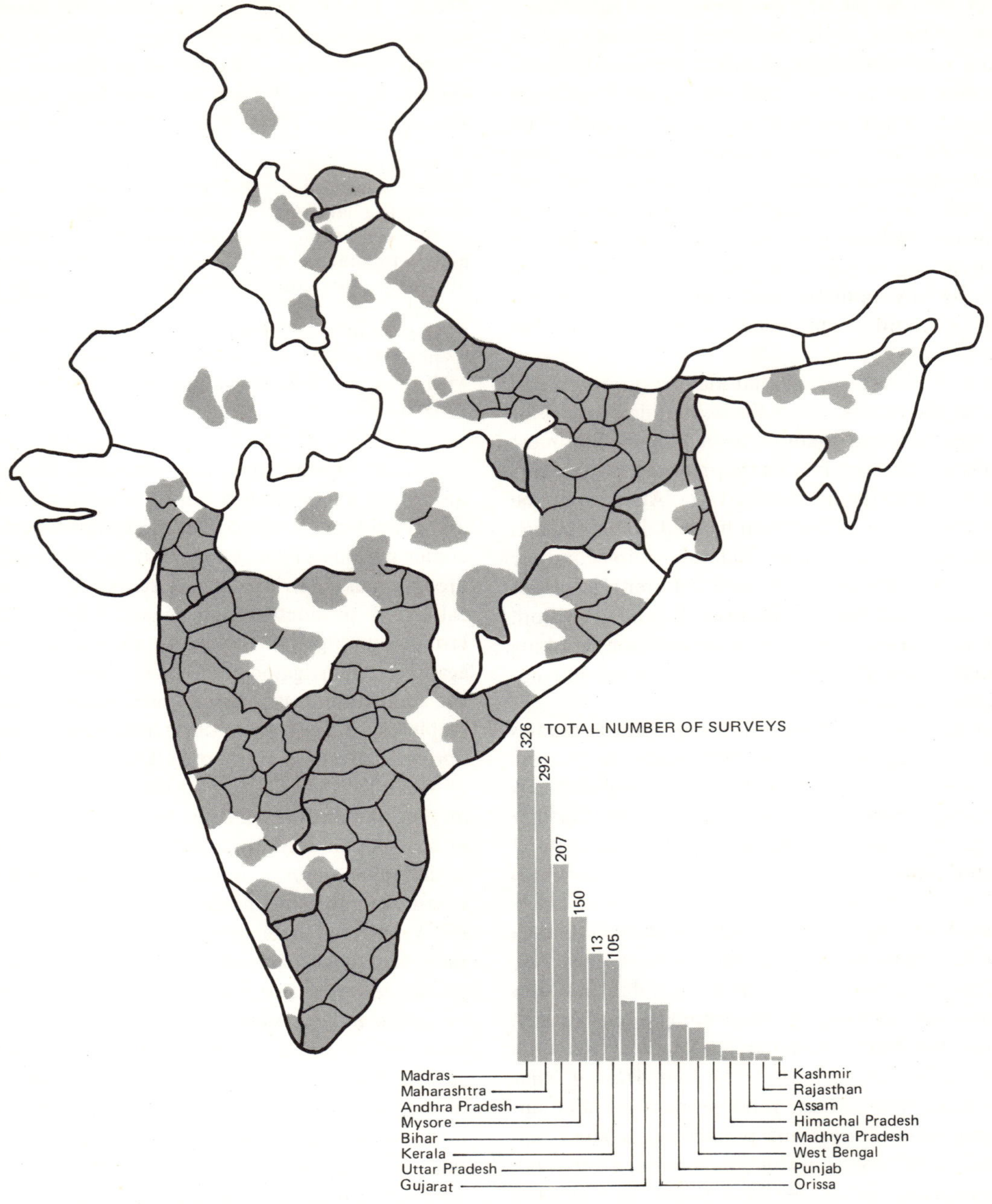

FIG. 3/8   India: Dietary surveys of Indian Council of Medical Research (geographical areas and population groups)

Source: Indian Council of Medical Research, 1964

be considered — labour demands of wet rice cultivation, exhaustion of resources of cultivable land, fall in real income per head, decrease in human body weight, height and girth, and increasing death rate, particularly in marginal areas. Even in resettlement areas where land is still available, for example in north Sumatra, farmers take only enough land for subsistence, not more to grow for profit.

In the terminology of ecological science, equilibrium with the environment is a rare, temporary or transient phenomenon over much of rural Asia. The politicians who put politics first, the introducers of 'development' in the modern sense, and the biased protagonists of one type of crop or animal husbandry to the exclusion of others, all risk creating conditions of ecological regression, or exacerbating the imbalance already created by increasing population pressure. This regression is indicated above all by loss of soil and soil fertility and increasing desiccation of the environment. The tragic introduction and cultivation of maize by lowland farmers on the steep slopes of the mountains of southern China in the eighteenth century led to permanent destruction of vast areas of land. Similar losses have occurred in India with the spread of alkalinity, due to irrigation without adequate drainage.

Regression is also indicated by a progressive change from a higher-fertility-demanding and more nutritious food crop to a poorer one, a decrease in profitability from cash crops, and hence an overall increase in rural poverty and the loss of energy and of enthusiasm for work. However, the change from rice to less valued millets in the mountains of south China or in the Deccan may represent an improvement in the diet; their protein value is higher, though their digestibility may be lower. Penny (1968) states:

Once the man: land ratio rises to a certain point, however, as it has long since done in many parts of Java, farmers begin to grow first maize and later cassava; this is usually associated with a decline in both the quantity and the quality of supplementary food production, the supply of protein foods of animal and vegetable origin declining more rapidly than that of vegetables.

Postmus and Van Veen (1949) and Bailey (1961 and 1962) have described the spread of cassava over former rice lands in Java, the Sundas and Madura. Goethals (1967) has noted how yields from swidden plots in Sumbawa have fallen following increased pressure of population.

The effect of destruction of the environment on nutritional status is not a new phenomenon in Java (but see Pelzer (1968) with reference to Sumatra and other Indonesian islands). On the south coast of central Java at the turn of the century, the staple was still rice. The population was less dense, a great part of the area was covered by woods, and the water supply was good. Then the population increased, the woods disappeared, erosion began and the water supply deteriorated progressively. So did the human diet, changing from rice as the main food to cassava. Heights and weights of the older generation who had subsisted on rice were greater than those of the younger generations who had subsisted mainly on cassava (Postmus and Van Veen, 1949). Food production per head has been declining in Indonesia. The only food crop which continues to show increases in output is cassava (Napitupulu, 1968). When a district produces more than 50 kg. cassava per head per year, it is likely to be the staple of many, who consequently will suffer malnutrition. Thirty-five out of the eighty regencies of Java produce more than 50 kg. cassava per head per year.

Increasing doubts are being expressed whether in Indonesia, with the adoption of better seeds, and the use of fertilizers and pesticides, the projected increases in yields can be achieved without more assured water control. Without the essential rehabilitation of irrigation systems, the rice harvest must continue to be dominated by the climatic fluctuations. The recent increased incidence of hunger oedema in Central and East Java following a long dry season and lower second harvest is a reminder of this critical fact in the Indonesian economy.

The converse, ecological progression, expressed in terms of improved types of land use, of crop and animal husbandry, of human nutrition and general economic improvement and standards of living, must be understood by those involved in development. The overall objective should be greater intensification of husbandry on existing land in preference to the clearance of more virgin or secondary vegetation — intensification defined as the maximum production, in as many cropping seasons of a year as possible, from both crop and livestock products, providing for both economic and nutritional diversity. There have been many examples of extension of the area under cultivation with little or no increase in total production; in the Gangetic Plain in Uttar Pradesh, and in Thailand (deYoung, 1955), there has been a decrease (in Thailand, 60 per cent). Systems of crop monoculture or of all-crop rotations for the production of foods for direct human consumption plus cash crops may be good economics, but are not the correct nutritional objective.

In Table 3/1 are brought together under twelve heads some of the major types of rural economies found throughout the region. Under each head, brief particulars are given of the associated types of land use and the systems of crop and animal husbandry.

The twelve types of rural economies are further classified in relation to the standards of nutrition generally found among the rural people in each individual type. The overall picture which can be seen

TABLE 3/1

Rural economies, land use, systems of crop and animal husbandry, and standards of nutrition

	Rural economies	*Sources of plant foods*	*Sources of animal foods*	*Nutritional status*
1.	Hunters and collectors; low density of population. Few such communities remain.	Wild plants, for roots and tubers, leaves, shoots, seeds, fruits, nuts. Fungi.	Wild fauna, only rarely including larger animals; small animals, rodents, bats, lizards, birds, insects, worms. Some fish trapping. Collection of honey.	Relatively balanced diet, when not crowded and harassed by neighbouring swidden communities. Possible calorie deficiency probably compensated by small physical stature.
2.	Hunters and collectors, in primary and secondary forest, with swidden. Low population density.	As above, but decreasing use of wild roots and tubers. Cultivated cereals and legumes, roots and tubers, and vegetables adapted to local environment.	Wild fauna, plus scavenging domestic fowl and domesticated wild fowl, ducks, goats. Domestic animals mainly for ceremonial use and consumption. Fishing.	Diversified diet, with more carbohydrate from the cultivated crops.
3.	Swidden, with regenerated secondary forest as fallow. Increasing density of population.	Wild plant foods of lower stages in succession, plus the crops as above.	Secondary levels of wild faunal components, following regression of plant cover. Hunting becomes less important. Domestic livestock as above. Cattle and/or buffalo kept by some groups for draught.	Animal protein may be less frequent in diet, depending chiefly on availability of fish.
4.	Fishing communities on sea coasts and inland lakes where fishing as the primary occupation is combined with some agricultural and/or horticultural activities.	Adapted cereal, root, legume and vegetable crops; collection from wild plants and animals of moderate or little significance.	Small amounts of fish eaten regularly, depending on economic status and length of fishing season.	Diet may be adequate or marginal in calories, and consequently inadequate in protein; calcium requirement met where small fish eaten whole. Vitamin and iron deficiencies.
5.	Swidden, with inadequate regeneration of secondary forest; soil fertility tending to fall. Excessive population pressure for this system.	Mainly millets, maize and upland rice, where adapted. Contribution from wild flora less significant. Limited legumes and vegetables on seasonal basis.	Contribution from wild fauna less regular. Scavenging fowl, pigs and goat, dependent upon environment and ethnic traditions. Consumed at festivals. Some fishing.	Diet likely to be inadequate in calories and most nutrients, with very marked seasonal fluctuations.
6.	Settled dryland cropping with swidden on infertile soils. Excessive population pressure per unit of cultivable land.	Adapted cereals and grain legumes. Vegetables few and limited to rainy season in absence of water for small vegetable plot. Up to two-years' store of cereal may be retained.	Scavenging or free-ranging fowl, pigs, goats and cattle, dependent upon environment and ethnic tradition.	Diet dependent on access to markets for sale of produce. Diet marginally adequate in calories, with deficiencies of animal and plant protein, and serious deficiency of vitamin A, other vitamins and minerals. Marked seasonality.
7.	Grazing and browsing communities. Migratory, nomadic or settled, with some cultivated land, dry and/or irrigated, at base village or camp.	Mixed cereals, though not usually eaten at same meal, with some grain legumes. Few vegetables.	Sheep, goats, cattle, buffalo, camel, mostly on free-range grazing, with small livestock around base.	Male diet probably adequate in animal protein, therefore in total protein, most vitamins and minerals. Diet of vulnerable groups adequate only while flocks and herds at base village, calories, plant proteins inadequate; consistent deficiency of minerals and vitamins. Major deficit is water.
8.	Irrigated plus settled dryland plus swidden. River valleys, terraced slopes and hill-sides. Excessive population pressure per unit of cultivable land.	Mixture of several dryland cereals, root crops with wet rice. Few legumes. Highly seasonal vegetable supplies. Some collection of wild green leaves.	Scavenging poultry, pigs, draught buffalo. Eaten only at ceremonies. Small wild-life and insects hunted, fish in paddies and streams.	Calories marginal; protein, vitamin and mineral deficiencies.
9.	Settled dryland agriculture. High to excessive population density.*	As with (6)	As with (6)	As with (6)

* **Greatest cultivated area in Asia**

10.	Paddy monoculture. High to excessive population density.**	Wet rice, with few alternate crops.	Draught buffalo. Ducks. Fish in paddies. Scavenging fowl and pigs near homesteads.	Serious protein deficiencies, especially among vulnerable groups, since animal produce sold and usually only small amounts of fish consumed. Deficiencies of thiamine associated with highly milled rice. Deficiencies of calcium, iron, vitamin A, riboflavine predominant; some other vitamins inadequate.
11.	Irrigated alternate husbandry. High population density.	Major cereals, grain legumes, fodder crops, vegetables, cash crops grown in crop rotations, with irrigation water available in all seasons, integrated with adapted forms of intensive animal husbandry.	Intensive forms of animal husbandry (dairy cattle, chickens, pigs and ducks) fed in stalls or special buildings on feeds and fodders produced from cultivated land.	Farmers tend to sell their cash products of high nutritive value to urban markets until economic status permits some retention for family. Thus most diets deficient in protein, vitamins and minerals.
12.	Plantation agriculture.	Food grains, some legumes and vegetables may be grown or purchased.	Cows for milk kept by Indian plantation workers. All may keep scavenging chickens, pigs, ducks, goats, depending on location and ethnic preferences.	Amount and quality of food intake dependent upon provision by plantation manager to workers and their families. Great variation in number of meals provided per day by management.

** Greatest population density in Asia

from Table 3/1 is of a general deterioration in the diet from the most primitive rural communities down through the swidden dry-land farmers to the wet-rice cultivators, and potentially at least rising again in those areas in which some form of alternate husbandry can be evolved.

The diets of the primitive rural economies can be regarded as relatively balanced, if perhaps quantitatively inadequate, either permanently or following a seasonal pattern, and dependent on pressure from surrounding swidden groups. With increasing population pressure within swidden economies, and among settled dry-land farmers, the diet deteriorates largely because of the reduced availability of animal protein, lower yields from eroded or inadequately fallowed lands or smaller landholdings, and seasonal deficiencies in supply of cereals and vegetables. These swidden and dry-land people, however, may have the advantage of a mixture of grains of superior nutritive value. It is when one comes to the monocultural wet paddy ecosystem that the diet becomes most monotonous, unbalanced and deficient in important nutrients. Here the diet may be improved if farmers have access to upland areas unsuitable for wet rice.

There are only a few areas where both crop and animal husbandry can be and are integrated on irrigated land in various forms of alternate husbandry. Theoretically, these rural people should have a better diet. However, the extraction of animal products such as milk, eggs and meat from the rural areas becomes so efficient that none remains for the use of the cultivator and his family. It might be possible to visualize a future situation in which the economic status of the cultivators is raised to a level at which they would consent to hold back some of their high-value animal produce for the use of their own families.

LAND CLASSIFICATION AND RECLAMATION

The sub-regions and zones in a map of rural nutrition are based on the features of the land, its geomorphology, geology, soils, topography, natural climax and secondary vegetation, present land use systems, and the availability of water for year-round or seasonal irrigation to overcome the limitations on crop and livestock growth and production imposed by annual climatic variations and by fluctuations on the longer term (Williams and Joseph, 1970).

The ultimate objective of any technique for the analysis and classification of the total environment in its widest sense must be to recognize and define Asian land systems, forms, units or types in terms of the present and potential nutritional status of the people living in them. Only if human nutrition at a subsistence, barter or elementary market level is brought into the whole complex of factors to be studied can the blueprint for a long-term development plan be evolved.

The fabled fertility of the equatorial lands is proving to be a myth. The Indonesian Institute of Sciences and the U.S. National Academy of Sciences

Workshop in Food (1968) expressed great concern that most soils in Java are in various critical stages of destruction by erosion. It recommends land classification, with re-zoning maps for planning effective conservation measures. All efforts to increase food production will be seriously affected unless action is taken to conserve and re-forest vulnerable areas in the catchments of the main rivers of Java, which provide the water essential for irrigation. There is a critical deficiency of food in over-populated Java, Madura, Bali and Lombok, and in the other Lesser Sunda Islands. The people in the outer islands are generally better fed, although there are still deficiencies, and in some places the situation is desperate (Indonesian Inst. Sci., op. cit.).

The Workshop also recommended in 1968 that the clearing of forest lands outside Java should be regulated by Government, but by 1970 the situation had deteriorated still further. Indonesia has the largest undeveloped forest resource in South-East Asia, some 122 million hectares, plus the largest man-made tropical forests in the region — the teak forests of Java and Madura. Some 150 extracting companies have been given licences to operate (from the Philippines, United States, Japan, Hong Kong and others), especially in Kalimantan (Manning, 1971). There are no controls, quotas being determined only by the amount of timber they can log — mining a precious natural resource for quick returns, living on a country's capital with no regard for the future of the vegetation, the land, human nutrition and the long-term national economy. These forestry enterprises have drawn some of their labour from the fishing industry, thereby adversely affecting its productivity.

The plant geographers may contribute greatly to background knowledge of patterns of human nutrition, by using their own specialized techniques for surveying and mapping their natural resources. The many types of forest not only provide the usual forest products. They reduce the aridity of the environment, and conserve water resources for the benefit of the cultivated lands and irrigation systems lower in the same catchment. The value of forests for human nutrition was once great, but is now seriously diminished. Cultivators in areas of low-density shifting cultivation and some isolated sedentary and fishing communities still rely on their nearby forest resources to provide food from the native flora and fauna.

Instead of opening up new areas of forest to the shifting cultivators, some consideration should be given to the possibility of reclaiming the vast areas already ruined by this process. Comprehensive studies of ecosystems are required to relate forest succession and the faunal population to the intensity of use by man. It may be necessary in the interests of improved human nutrition to combine natural regeneration of a plant stand with restocking with appropriate members of the original fauna. Reclamation of areas of abandoned shifting cultivation, especially the so-called green deserts of cogon grass (*Imperata cylindrica*) may include:

> regeneration by natural or assisted means of a secondary forest cover, combined with appropriate steps to restore the tuber-bearing and other edible plants, and faunal components of an original ecosystem;
> reclamation to grasslands of improved botanical composition, as a basis for a beef cattle industry; and
> treatment involving ploughing up, manuring and fertilizer application, to provide reasonably good cultivated land for growing local food requirements for the people.

SEASONALITY IN FOOD PRODUCTION AND DIETS

Most parts of the region are subject to marked variations in climate, particularly rainfall, either between one season and another within a year, or in a pattern of cyclic variation over a number of years. Droughts of varying duration are regular annual features of the monsoonal environment; droughts of equal biological effect are frequent in the equatorial environment, but more unpredictable in occurrence and duration. The seasonal swing from sufficiency to deficiency of rainfall in a subsistence dry-land economy is expressed in terms of human nutrition — for example, from a condition of adequacy and diversity of food in the good season to that of scarcity and monotony in another — *lapar biasa,* the usual hunger of Indonesia, and 'the barley pass' of Korea (Rutt, 1964). This is common in areas of shifting cultivation and dry-land farming in the months before the new crop becomes available. There may be a climatic and economic change from a superior cereal to one of lesser value, or from a cereal to a root crop. This may of course, theoretically at least, be overcome by greater trade in superior staple foods, assuming that rural purchasing power is sufficient to buy them. Foodgrains may be conserved for use in the long dry seasons of a monsoonal ecoclimate. Vegetables and other perishable fresh foods are, however, available only during the short growing seasons, without irrigation.

It is essential to recognize the parallel responses in terms of rural diets, which are dependent upon seasonality of production, especially of the perishable foods. Even the specialist, surveying nutrient intakes or clinical and biochemical status, may overlook the fact that, for reasons of convenience, his survey has been conducted at the best time of the year; only rarely is it possible to survey the same area in all seasons. A dietary survey should record food availability, consumption or preservation in all seasons; over most of Asia this is likely to involve at least three surveys. They should be repeated over a five-year period so as to record the effect of annual fluctuations in climate. Ideally, crop and livestock specialists should be members of the team.

An example of a nutritional survey covering different seasons of one year, and confined to pre-school children, comes from Tamil Nadu State, India (Sundararaj, Begum, Jesudian and Pereira, 1969). Significant differences were found in protein intake, which was 2.07 gm. per kg. body weight during the rainy season when groundnuts and freshwater fish were available, but only 1.46 gm. per kg. body weight during the cold season. Fat provided 14 per cent of daily energy intake during the rainy season, but only 4 to 6 per cent in the other seasons. Seasonal differences in intakes of vitamin A, riboflavine and vitamin C were also found. Clinical signs of both vitamin A and riboflavine deficiency appeared during the cold season. A qualitative study of family meals of 111 households in Tamil Nadu was made (Rao, Klontz, Rao, Begum and Dumm, 1961) during four seasons: January to March; April to June; July to September; October to December (Tables 3/2 and 3/3). Cereals provide a high proportion of calories and protein throughout the year. There are widespread deficiencies of protein, riboflavine, vitamin A and possibly vitamin C. Seasonal variation is largely dependent upon time of harvest. Diets are unsatisfactory at all times, but less so in the first season, more so in the third and fourth, and most unsatisfactory in the second season. Intake of calcium is high in the second and third season, due to the consumption of ragi when it is harvested. Vitamin C intake is relatively high during the third and fourth seasons, when more leafy vege-

TABLE 3/2

India: Tamil Nadu: consumption of foodstuffs during the four seasons
(per cent of total food intake of family)

Foodstuffs	Sholavaram:				Pennathur:
	First season (Jan.-Mar.), per cent	*Second season (Apr.-June), per cent*	*Third season (July-Sept.), per cent*	*Fourth season (Oct.-Dec.), per cent*	*All seasons, per cent*
Cereals (total)	65.3	74.7	77.5	73.3	75.2
Cholam and ragi	27.6	45.9	51.2	41.4	38.0
Rice	37.8	28.8	26.3	31.9	37.2
Pulses	6.3	4.1	3.0	5.0	5.3
Leafy vegetables	0.4	1.8	5.8	2.9	2.1
Other vegetables	14.4	8.1	4.2	3.4	8.2
Fats and oils	2.4	0.7	0.7	0.5	1.4
Fish, meat and eggs	0.3	1.2	0.2	1.2	2.0
Milk and milk products	3.6	2.7	2.3	2.0	1.8
Fruits	0.2	0.2	0.4	0.6	0.1
Sugar and jaggery	0.6	0.4	0.2	2.1	0.3
Coconut	0.4	0.2	0.0	0.1	3.7
Ground-nut	0.2	0.2	0.1	3.2	
Condiments	5.9	5.8	5.6	5.5	

Source: Rao, Klontz, Rao, Begum and Dumm, 1961

TABLE 3/3

India: Tamil Nadu: average percentage of nutrient deficiency during the four seasons

Food values*	Percentage of deficiency				Total for all seasons Sholavaram	Penna-thur
	I	II	III	IV		
Protein, gm.	46·4	58·6	55·6	49·9	52·6	42·0
Calcium, mg.	41·4	29·1	36·2	46·0	38·2	44·7
Iron, mg.	41·0	44·5	33·7	42·1	40·3	44·0
Calories	22·6	34·3	28·0	29·1	28·5	28·0
Vitamin A i.u.	86·8	84·0	73·9	78·8	80·9	71·2
Thiamine, mg.	13·0	14·7	13·5	17·0	14·6	18·5
Niacin, mg.	20·9	44·7	48·1	36·5	37·5	23·7
Riboflavine, mg.	70·5	79·0	63·0	56·0	67·1	75·6
Ascorbic acid, mg.	46·5	60·4	26·7	55·9	47·4	48·6

*Carbohydrate, fat and phosphorus are not included in this table, because no recommended allowances have been set

Source: Rao, Klontz, Rao, Begum and Dumm, 1961

tables and cholam (*Sorghum vulgare*) are consumed. The availability of groundnuts during the fourth season contributes to relatively higher intakes of protein, fat and riboflavine. More than 50 per cent of families consumed diets providing less than 50 per cent of recommended amounts of protein, riboflavine and vitamin A during all seasons; less than 50 per cent of recommended amount of vitamin C was consumed in the first, second and fourth season; calcium intake was less than 50 per cent of recommenda-tions in the fourth season, and niacin in the third season.

When this study was repeated in nearby villages ten years later (Sundararaj and Pereira, 1971), no significant differences were found. Calcium intake is less, probably because of preference for rice. Cereals provide at least 75 per cent of the protein. Consumption of milk is negligible. Few use dried or fresh fish, meats or eggs; only during the October-December quarter does animal protein add significantly to total protein

TABLE 3/4

India: West Bengal: seasonal variation in calcium and vitamin intakes from vegetables, due to recession of wet monsoon

	Calcium gm.		Vitamin A i.u.		Vitamin C mg.	
	Total	From Vegetables	Total	From Vegetables	Total	From Vegetables
July (wet monsoon)	0·54	0·37	3220	2780	160	151
November	0·27	0·05	460	250	14	11
January-February	0·50	0·25	970	820	45	32

Source: Roy and Roy, 1962

TABLE 3/5

Indonesia: Gunung Kidul, Java: seasonality of food intake
(gm. per caput per day)

	May to August	*September to December*	*January to April*
Fish and meat	1·4	1·1	1·0
Milk, milk products, eggs	negligible	negligible	negligible
Rice	42	15	26
Maize	2	0	32
Millet	0·7	—	0·4
Cassava (fresh)	75	3	0
Sweet potatoes	4	1	0
Other roots and tubers	11	28	0
Gaplek (dried cassava root)	265	295	269
Sugar	5	4	3
Pulses	22	4	5
Tempe (soybean)	2	2	1·5
Oilseeds and coconuts	17	18	11
Coconut oil	0·1	0·1	0·1
Leafy vegetables and young pulses	38	41	76
Other vegetables	27	54	27
Fruits	3	2	2
Calories	1285	1113	1138
Calories in percentage basal metabolism	132	111	113
Protein	16·5	10·5	13·8
Protein in percentage of requirement	36·3	21·6	27·8
Fat	14·9	9·7	9·5
Vitamin A (i.u.)	2283	2369	2980
Thiamine (mg.)	0·33	0·30	0·30

Source: Postmus and van Veen, 1949

intake. Amounts of energy foods, vitamin A and ribo-flavine are inadequate, and protein sufficient only for the smallest men.

In an agricultural community in West Bengal (Roy and Roy, 1962), differences are revealed in the intake of vitamin A, vitamin C and calcium in three seasons (July, November and January), due principally to the relative availability of vegetables (Table 3/4). In eastern Uttar Pradesh, night blindness is most prevalent during the dry summer season when green leafy vegetables cannot be grown. The villagers, however, associate their night blindness with the heat of the sun at that period, which they think affects the head (Govil, Prasad and Pant, 1958).

A dietary survey (1938-9), followed by a medical survey (1939-41) made in the Gunung Kidul region on the south coast of central Java covered the three seasons, May-August; September-December, and January-April (Postmus and Van Veen, 1949). The rainy season begins in November and ends in April. Five groups of families in four ecological zones were examined. Water for cropping depends on the monsoon except for a small area of irrigated wet rice (Table 3/5).

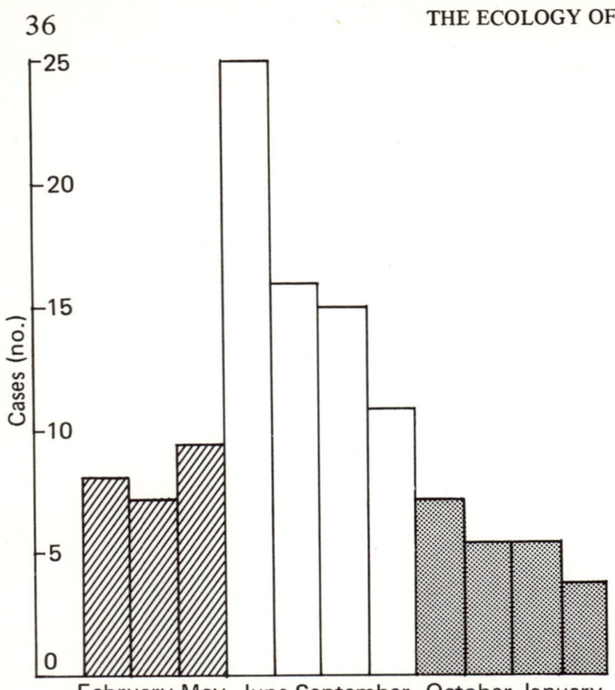

FIG. 3/9 Thailand: seasonal distribution of protein-calorie malnutrition in patients admitted to Chiengmai Hospital, 1 Jan.-31 Dec. 1964

Source: Thanangkul, Whitaker and Fort, 1966

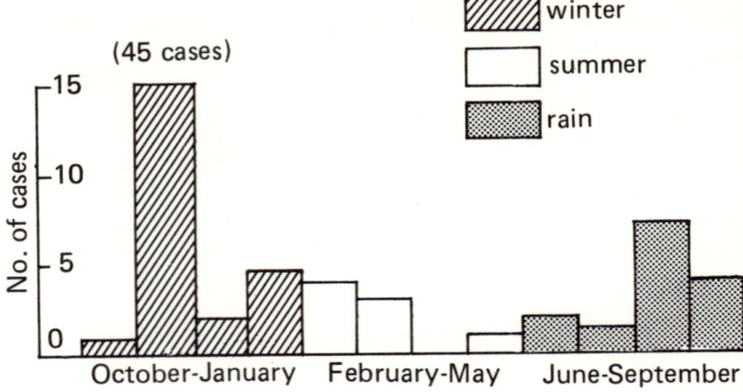

FIG. 3/10 Thailand: seasonal distribution of thiamine deficiency in patients admitted to Chiengmai Hospital, 1 Jan.-31 Dec. 1964

Source: Thanangkul, Whitaker and Fort, 1966

Three seasons are recognized in Thailand: summer (February to May); rainy (June to September); winter (October to January) (Thanangkul, Whitaker and Fort, 1966). A factor involved in the seasonal distribution of protein-calorie malnutrition in the Chiengmai district (Fig. 3/9) may be the diarrhoea which is most frequent during April and May. After this epidemic, 69 per cent of the children with protein-calorie malnutrition were admitted to hospital from May to September. There is also a high incidence of pneumonia during this period. The seasonal pattern of thiamine deficiency in children (Fig. 3/10) may be due to a fall in the thiamine content of rice during prolonged storage, and to the use of highly milled rice during the pre-harvest season when home-processed rice is not available. A contributory cause may be the hard physical labour performed by the mothers during rice planting and harvesting.

In China during the early 1950s, it was noted that there was a higher incidence of beriberi during June, probably due to the length of time that rice had been stored before consumption (Hueck, 1952). Another effect of seasonality is shown in birth weights of full-term infants in west China (Lee, 1948). Despite severe deprivation of essential foods over the preceding eight years, there was little variation in birthweight during that period, but there was a marked seasonal variation. Infants born in January were heaviest, and infants born in September of each year were the lowest in weight. These differences were undoubtedly related to seasonal variations in availability and/or quality of foods.

In Korea there is a variation between seasons in respect of foods purchased and foods grown (Yonsei University, 1967-8). The food intakes also differ as between the four ecological regions, although there is little variation among adults in intake of calories and protein. However, coastal children have better intakes of fat and protein, with low vitamin C intake; diets of children in the plains are rich in carbohydrates, but low in protein, fat, vitamin A, thiamine and riboflavine.

A study has been made in Japan (1949/50) of food intakes of farmers in single- and double-crop districts of Niigata and Aichi Prefectures before the great changes which occurred in the decade 1960-70, following the introduction of power cultivators. A variation in calorie intake is noted between the busy and slack seasons; tables give data for different members of the family (Takagi, Masuda and Kida, 1970).

SEASONALITY IN EMPLOYMENT

ECAFE estimates (1970) that Asian countries must find 1,000 million additional jobs for their populations of working age within the next thirty years. The present working population (age 15 to 64) of 1,150 million will exceed 1,617 million in 1985, and rise to about 2,300 million in the year 2,000. The availability of work associated with the true monsoonal environment is a major factor in the problem of rural unemployment that is causing concern among politicians and planners. This has been the subject of a study in Bangkok by the International Labour Office and the Food and Agriculture Organization of the United Nations.

The green revolution has not generated more work in the rural areas, because farmers have tended to use the proceeds for mechanization. But the major problem is that dry-land farmers in a monsoonal environment are unemployed for up to six months in every year (Fig. 3/11). Swidden farmers are under-employed for part of the year, but they may at this time be hunting, fishing, repairing housing or equipment, or doing other essential tasks. Whether such people would be willing to leave their homes, or be physically able to undertake heavy labour on public works as has been proposed, is another matter.

The introduction of labour-intensive schemes and systems of production, of road construction, house building and crash programmes of rural works are together likely to absorb only a fraction of the populations involved. The employment of rural labour in projects of public works should be limited to the slack season, since permanent withdrawal of labour would reduce agricultural production (Sobhan, 1968). Of course, if wages are good and paid regularly, and the site of the temporary seasonal labour is near a city or large town, the worker may not feel disposed to return to his village and his land.

ENVIRONMENT AND HUMAN DISEASE

The ecology of human disease in rural areas is closely related to the environment, as expressed through clearance of forests, methods of cultivation, introduction of irrigation water, density of population and other factors. In considering maximum production from the land, it must be accepted that disease is a most important factor in rural human ecology, affecting energy, enthusiasm, willingness to undertake more work, optimism and general attitude to life. The rural people have little option but to become adapted to the environment in which they find themselves, because of the dearth of medical attention and supplies.

Intestinal, respiratory and other diseases transmitted by contact with the sick, by unclean water, rodents, snails, mosquitoes, cockroaches, flies, sandflies, larvae, ticks and mites require regular attention by skilled medical practitioners, of which there is a critical shortage throughout Asia. Availability of

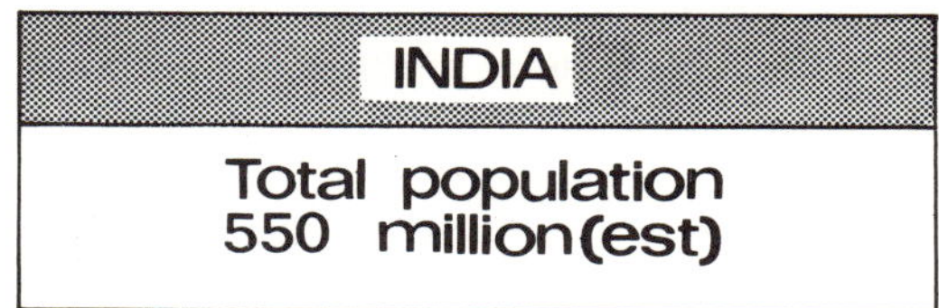

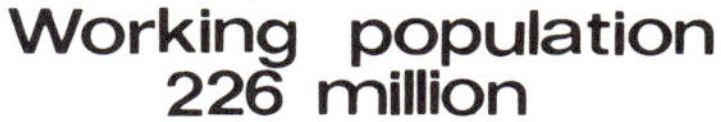

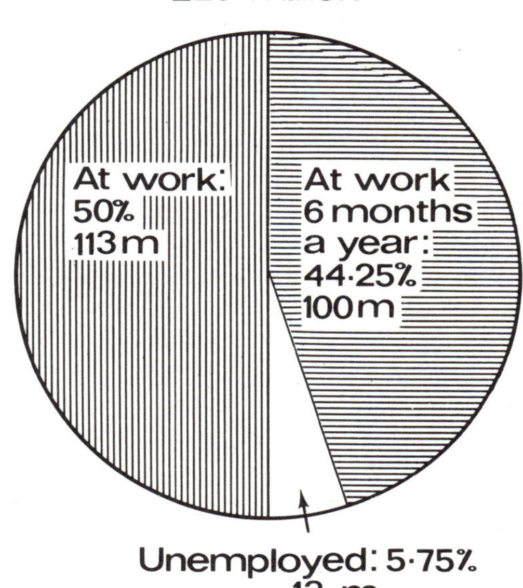

FIG. 3/11   India: seasonal unemployment
Source: Duggal, 1970

medical attention is reflected in differing mortality rates of different groups. In Sarawak, Chinese mothers between 25 and 29 years of age (living within reach of doctors) have lost 3.4 per cent of their children; in the indigenous communities at the same age, the losses range from 17 to 25 per cent (Lee, 1970). The unhygienic practices of traditional midwives and their unsterile and primitive equipment cause many infant deaths from tetanus. This also applies to circumcision in certain Muslim countries. Japanese workers on Lombok, Indonesia, found death from tetanus following circumcision to be an important cause of death of boys from 5 to 10 years (Toda and Mori, 1967).

Some examples of the interrelation between environment and disease may be given. The vegetational disturbances produced by shifting cultivation cause considerable loss of equilibrium in the ecosystems, following clearing of the forest. This is expressed in progressive changes in the numbers of most animal and plant species in and around affected areas, including the human pathogens, vectors and reservoir hosts of pathogens; increases in any of these may lead to an increase in transmission of the corresponding disease (Polunin, 1960). In undisturbed primary forest, many species of vectors or reservoir hosts exist in small numbers. In the range of diversified conditions produced by forest clearance, the total number of species is reduced, but the numbers of individuals in any one species may be greatly increased. The forest edge is a fringe habitat which provides a new range of environments which are neither clearing nor forest.

Methods of cultivation will, however, probably exert more indirect effect on other aspects of the health of shifting cultivators than change of the numbers of pathogens and vectors. A contributory factor is the increasing density of population per unit area of land under shifting cultivation, leading to land degradation, and thus to deterioration of human nutrition. Shifting cultivation based on an ideal 15-year cycle will support a population of around 6 per square kilometre in perpetuity (Lee, 1970), without soil deterioration. When the figure reaches 20 per square kilometre (Freeman, 1955) or 50 per square kilometre (Pelzer, 1945), degradation of land and human nutrition and health occur. Leach (1950) considers that there is no reason to insist upon more intensive forms of land use as long as population density does not increase beyond 20 persons per square kilometre.

Since the low-density swidden communities may not be frequently exposed to disease pathogens, they do not build up resistance, and therefore suffer severely when disease is encountered. As density increases, so does the degree of exposure, but also the degree of resistance. The evolution of the shifting cultivation cycle involving the use of isolated farm huts to watch the ripening grain has proved a considerable obstacle to attempts at malaria control, since mosquitoes which are zoophilic in longhouses become anthropophilic in farm huts. On the other hand, the use of huts prevents a build-up of concentrations of long-surviving infective agents such as the roundworm eggs, hookworm larvae, β-haemolytic streptococci and tubercule bacillus, characteristic of places of continuous habitation.

In 1969, WHO reported that malaria had been eradicated in Taiwan, Japan, the Ryukyus and Singapore, but that it still existed in the Philippines, Brunei, Malaysia, Korea, rural Hong Kong, Cambodia, Laos, South Vietnam, India, Pakistan and Ceylon, with no information available from China, North Korea and North Vietnam.

In 1972, WHO reported a resurgence of malaria in parts of Asia — one million cases, or six times the 1966 figure in India, and 145,000 cases in Sri Lanka, where the disease had been practically eradicated in 1966. Results from Malaysia are more encouraging. Incidence in 1972 had fallen to less than one-fifth, following only two cycles of spraying. The importance of regular control of vectors cannot be over-emphasized.

In Malaysia the immunity gained by the rural people has been achieved at the expense of a high child morbidity and mortality (Sandosham, 1970). It has been said that the rural Malays have a *tidak-apa* or apathetic attitude towards life. This may be due to the continuous destruction of red blood cells by malaria and the consequent anaemia and lethargy. If they could be freed of malaria, the rural people would become more ambitious, work harder, and so improve their lot and their nutrition. The current programmes of land clearance, development and settlement in Malaysia will provide potential grounds for vector breeding. If malaria is introduced from other parts of rural Malaysia (Fig. 3/12), there is every likelihood of a new crisis.

Localized success has been achieved by the regular use of prophylactics under careful medical supervision, in the elimination of filariasis, but these diseases remain endemic in South-East Asia. No biological means of controlling the schistosomiases have yet been discovered.

Water supplies are easily contaminated by faecal material from humans and animals, by seepage during the wet monsoon and by dust during the dry. Myrdal (1968) notes that throughout Asia the incidence of water-borne diseases (cholera, typhoid, dysentery, diarrhoea and intestinal parasites) is extremely high, and protected water supplies rare. Apart from cholera, these diseases are rarely fatal to the adult, but they sap vitality and adversely affect labour inputs and efficiency. The occurrence of these diseases, and of the respiratory diseases characteristic of overcrowded and ill-ventilated housing, especially sleeping arrangements, could be limited if it were possible to provide pure water and adequate housing on the enormous scale required. Their cure calls for adequacy of medicines and of doctors to administer them.

RURAL MEDICINE

Throughout Asia, the number of doctors trained in modern medicine, and who are capable of advising on the prevention and cure of endemic tropical diseases

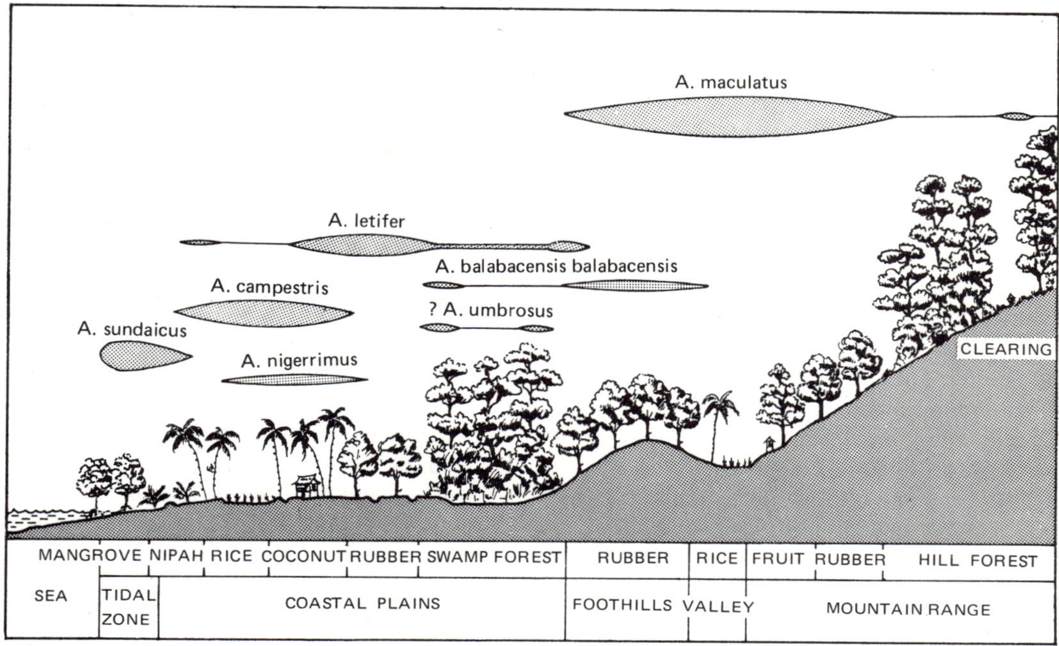

Fig. 3/12 Malaysia: The distribution and abundance of vectors of malaria in different ecological zones

Source: Sandosham, 1970
Note: Size of the ellipses indicates relative importance

and are familiar with the nutritional deficiency diseases, is hopelessly inadequate.

While the religions of Asia have included an obligation of care for the unfortunate, the introduction of a sense of responsibility for those in no way related or bound by traditional ties to one's family has been of truly western origin. This sense of responsibility has been called humanitarianism: ... an active concern for the welfare of all human beings irrespective of caste, economic position, religion, age and sex (Srinivas 1966). One outcome of humanitarianism has been the introduction of modern preventive medicine. In recent decades, with relatively small numbers of mobile technicians and para-medical personnel, it has become possible to eliminate or to mitigate the effects of the major tropical diseases, leading to a great reduction in human mortality. There has not, however, been a proportionate increase in the number of qualified general practitioners, able to deal with recurrent community ailments and accidents, and the detection and cure of malnutrition. Moreover, conditions in rural areas have always been so unattractive to doctors and their families that most are concentrated in urban areas.

In China in 1966, there were 100,000 doctors trained in modern medicine (Orleans, 1969). Mao

Tse-tung said in 1965 that 85 per cent of the farming people had for many years had access neither to doctors nor to medicines. The proposal to move 50 per cent of trained medical personnel to the rural areas, even if wholly successful, can have little impact on a rural population of 640 million. Moreover, since the Cultural Revolution, all education, including that of medical students, has been disastrously disrupted, and is only now beginning again in modified form. The travelling barefoot doctors, who receive brief training in simple first-aid and preventive measures, may have a greater impact if they are available in numbers sufficient to cover the vast areas and populations involved, and if they are provided with the medicines and chemicals in critically short supply. There are not, however, enough fully trained doctors on call in rural areas to advise the barefoot doctors on less elementary matters, usually considered essential for para-medical personnel. The barefoot doctors are also being entrusted with the spread of birth-control measures.

In Thailand, there is one doctor for every 1,100 people in Bangkok and Thonburi, but one for 20,000 people in other provinces; one north-east province has only seven doctors for 600,000 people (Maxwell,

1967). The background to rural medical service has been examined, and proposals made for changes which might encourage young doctors to serve in rural areas. Few students, however, wish to remain general practitioners, and there is 'essentially no interest among students in entering the field of preventive medicine and public health. Less than 1 per cent indicated strong interest in this field.' Five per cent of senior students wish to practise within the Accelerated Rural Development areas — the backward north and north-east region of the country selected for intensive economic and social development. Eighty per cent of students prefer provinces falling outside this area. Few of those interested in general practice are willing to work in the rural provinces, and none in the north-east (Maxwell, op. cit.).

Only 40 per cent of the Indian doctors trained overseas return to India, due to lack of facilities and low salaries in State employment. Within India in 1967, only 36,000 out of the total of 108,000 doctors were practising in the 570,000 villages in which 400 million people lived. Many of the 8,000 maternal and child-care centres in rural areas are without personnel. Half the primary and a third of the secondary rural health centres are without doctors, buildings or a safe water supply. University authorities propose that each college should stipulate that graduates should work for at least three months in the rural areas. A compulsory one-year course in maternal care, child health and family planning should form part of training. The State of Maharashtra is the first to make a two-year internship in a rural health centre compulsory for all medical students before they receive their degree. In Malaysia it has been proposed that all newly-registered doctors should work for Government for two years, during which time they would be available for posting to rural areas. These problems are common to all developing countries.

B.G. Maegraith, Professor of Tropical Medicine at the School of Tropical Health, Liverpool, addressing the 63rd meeting of the Royal Society of Tropical Medicine and Hygiene in London, said that the Diploma of Public Health course in Tropical Medicine should concentrate on training students to tackle the diseases of poverty, rather than the special circumstances arising in urban practice: '90 per cent of the peoples in the rural areas are fighting for their lives against malnutrition and communicable disease. It is no good training (doctors) for work in a small back room in an ivory tower'.

Part II

THE SOCIAL AND ECONOMIC ENVIRONMENT

4 The Study of Rural Life

INTERDISCIPLINARY INVESTIGATION

THE economic and nutritional status of a rural people may be analysed in two ways, by studying statistics in central planning agencies in national and state or provincial capitals, or by conducting primary investigations at the rural or village level. The centralized approach calls for government statistics of food production, trade and consumption in the rural areas. But in most Asian countries these data are not now collected, assembled and presented in a manner which will give a correct picture of rural conditions. Probably, in view of the vast areas and numbers of people in more or less isolated communities, the present facilities, funds and staff are insufficient for the collection of the data that would be required by an objective statistician.

Thus it seems to be desirable to favour the second approach, namely, to collect and consider the reports of field studies made by specialists in practical and scientific disciplines, those studies of the rural people in their *oikos* or home which together comprise human ecology in the broadest sense. Perhaps a statistician may be able to advise how many such studies would represent a random sample, presumably a small number per thousand villages in uniform land systems like the Gangetic Plain or the central plains of Thailand, more per thousand, or perhaps an additional distribution of sample areas in dissected landscapes like Indonesia and the Philippines.

Specialists working on individual aspects adopt different concepts and techniques. There arises the distinction between the specialist and the inter-disciplinary or cross-cultural generalist or synthesizer of data from individual disciplines. What is the full range of subjects to be covered? Do the available funds provide for the appointment of a team to cover all these aspects? If funds are limited, what type of specialist and in which discipline is best qualified to collect and perhaps also to interpret information? If specialists in different disciplines are to make their field studies in sequence rather than concurrently, what would be the best sequence?

Commenting on a project of the Massachusetts Institute of Technology Center for International Studies in Indonesia, which covered economics, political science, history, sociology, anthropology and geography, Benjamin Higgins (Geertz, 1968) states:

> Interdisciplinary research is always a gamble. All too often it results in a series of discrete articles or monographs with no very clear connecting theme. When the interdisciplinary research is applied to a political or geographic area such as Indonesia, the danger is that the spatial limits will be the only common feature of the products of the different disciplines. Accordingly, when the contributions from various disciplines to the study of a particular area produce genuine synthesis, the result is of unusual interest . . . .
>
> The M.I.T. Indonesia project was in any case a loosely defined affair, the precise composition of which changed from year to year . . . . Each of us, using the methods of his own discipline . . . arrived at essentially the same broad analytical framework, and at the same general conception of the task that lies ahead of the Indonesian people if the high hopes of their revolution are to be realized.

SOCIAL DIVERSITY

Dobby (1960) stated that every human type was represented in South-East Asia, from indigenous peoples to immigrants from other cultures; that these different groups had different levels of absorption into the economic, political and social setting; and that frequently each group had a specialized position in society, so that it was rare to find a group that was homogeneous, either horizontally or vertically.

Since Dobby's book was first published in 1951, the effects of economic development and economic independence have led to increased homogeneity

(Phillips, 1963), although great differences still remain. A region characterized by such anthropological and cultural diversity presents problems to administrators concerned with the organization of social and civic life. 'Yet social organization is a vital factor in agricultural output.' The problem is how to create out of plural societies and traditional communities an integrated social and economic structure which can support and profit from the introduction of modern technology in agriculture and human nutrition.

Although the bulk of the Asian population lives in rural areas, the region, numerically speaking, is by far the most urbanized. The population in localities of 20,000 and above amounts to 370 million, or more than the total populations of Africa, or Latin America or North America. Urbanization is biased towards the largest cities; many of these have grown at rates from 5 to more than 10 per cent annually, and much of the increase has been in terms of squatters and slum dwellers. This rapid growth with its accompanying unemployment and family poverty has induced a further precipitous decline in urban living conditions.

The word *peasant* is taboo in U.N. Agencies, but is still used by the anthropologists. Writing in 1955, Lewis stated that, although peasantry constitutes about three-quarters of the world population, and a higher proportion in the developing countries, it had been relatively neglected by social scientists. Anthropologists had specialized in primitive or tribal societies, sociologists in urban societies, and rural sociologists in modern rural societies. A comparative science of peasantry was only then beginning to take shape, to cover the great majority of mankind which formerly had no discipline of its own. Since then, Wolf (1966) has produced a 'primer on peasantry' for economists, political scientists and area specialists, as an essential background to the study of rural life.

DEFINITIONS OF RURAL COMMUNITIES

Government statistics do not always distinguish clearly between the one-fifth of the total populations that may be called urban, and the four-fifths which comprise the food producers in the rural areas and those non-food producers who are dependent upon them, plus the tribal peoples who are usually self-sufficient in food. The United Nations Organizations generally expect the countries themselves to classify their populations into urban and rural, according to their own criteria. Those adopted in India and China are given in Chapters 14 and 15.

FAO also accepts the classification provided by individual countries. UNESCO (1965) recommends that an urban agglomeration should be defined as 'a distinct and indivisible population grouping, irrespective of its size, having a locally recognized name or statute, and functioning as an integrated social entity'.

Rural social unit

No one can claim to study agriculture in Asia without considering the contributions of the social scientist. This is just as applicable to the nutritionist who is urban-oriented and trained, and who is faced with the complexities, obvious or latent, of rural life. There are already many studies of villages and other rural communities, which give not only information on village structure, kinship, caste and related matters, but also refer to the foods, dietary practices and taboos, child-rearing and other aspects that are essential for the nutritionist. A parallel study and review of the village in Asian development is in preparation.

Those who go to work in the rural areas will wish to consider different definitions of the social units in their region, examples of which follow, and will refer to the existing literature in the social sciences, such as the UNESCO publication, *Social Research and Problems of Rural Development in South-East Asia* (1963).

The primary social unit is a small group of families setting themselves off from the large society by some social factor in such a way that (a) they conceive of themselves as *some sort of unit* (i.e. have group identification), (b) they have frequent mutual interaction, and (c) they possess temporal and/or spatial stability (Whiting, Child and Lambert, 1966).

The peasant society is intermediate between the folk (tribal peoples) and civilization (or urbanized society). The peasant society differs from the folk society in that it has developed economic and political relations with urban market centres. In its relations with other villages, the peasant society still retains a good deal of the folk quality of isolation and introversion (Redfield and Singer, 1955).

Further reading on village structure and change 'under foreign or urban influence' on their former 'clear structural definition, high degree of economic self-sufficiency, political solidarity against the outside world, and a sense of ritual integrity' (Marriott, 1955) is given in the bibliography.[1]

[1] General: Burling (1965); Kroeber (1952)
China: Schurmann and Schell (1968)
India: Béteille (1969); Gough (1955); Lewis (1955);
      Marriott (1955); Srinivas (1960); Srinivasan (1956)
Indonesia: Geertz (1967)

SOCIAL AND CULTURAL ANTHROPOLOGY

The present picture of human life and nutrition in rural Asia depends very largely on the anthropologists, sociologists, ethnographers and similar practitioners of field disciplines. Margaret Mead (Burgess and Dean, 1962) has said that there appears to be a good deal of misunderstanding of what anthropology is, and what anthropologists can and cannot do. This leads to difficulties when, for example, public health personnel and anthropologists try to work together. Cultural anthropology is a pure research science – a practitioner or 'applied' aspect hardly exists. A student who from the beginning knows that he wishes to deal with directed social change is a very rare person (Mead, op. cit.).

However, Foster (1969) distinguishes between applied anthropology (which is a role) and pure anthropology (which is an occupation). The applied anthropologist is seen as participating in programmes that have 'as primary goals, changes in human behaviour believed to ameliorate contemporary, social, economic and technological problems, rather than development of social and culture theory', the latter being the realm of the pure anthropologist. Hitchcock has said (1968): 'It is true that most anthropologists have not provided the kind of information needed for health and nutrition surveys; it must seem a conspiracy of silence; but there is a growing interest and the number of useful studies should increase.'

While more attention has been given recently to what are called behavioural sciences, there is not yet an established training school or university course producing recognized 'applied anthropologists'. They would require at least some training in human nutrition, medicine and public health, so that they may collect the right type of information regarding the nutritional status of the rural people they study, and perhaps be able also to recognize the more obvious clinical and other signs of deficiencies. Conversely, it would be desirable if some aspects of social science and anthropology were regularly included in the syllabus of nutrition training.

This is not to say that the reports of field work of most anthropologists are of little value in planning for improved production, distribution and utilization of food and for better nutrition. Those by Geddes (1954), Morris (1953), Leach (1961) and Nash (1965)

Japan: Norbeck (1967)
North Korea: Lee and Kim (1970)
Philippines: Romani (1956)

are of great value to agriculturists and nutritionists. McArthur (1962) and Freedman (1954) are anthropologists who were asked specifically to investigate the socio-economic background to nutritional habits. Bailey (1961 and 1962) is a doctor who studied the social, ecological and agronomic background to nutritional deficiencies and diseases. More recently, a nutritionist with anthropological training has made a long-term study of a village from a specifically nutritional angle (Wilson, 1970 a and b, 1971). Moerman (1968) is an anthropologist who tried to develop data and techniques to enable the work of field ethnographers to be used by development economists concerned with increasing agricultural production of underdeveloped economies.

No attempt can be made to analyse the concepts and techniques adopted by different specialists and by different schools of learning in that broad group of overlapping and complementary disciplines of anthropology, ethnography, rural sociology and human ecology. Some of the problems of South-East Asia for which these are applicable were discussed at the UNESCO/FAO Seminar on Social Research and Problems of Rural Development in South-East Asia, in Saigon in March 1960 (UNESCO, 1963):

Demographic disequilibrium (lack of balance in the distribution of the population by regions, especially as between mountain regions and plains);
Contrast between flooded rice fields and dry lands;
Existence of ethnic minorities;
Existence of traditional civilizations with their laws and customs;
Respect for the family (in the sense of blood relationship);
Intense village community feeling;
Very limited and sometimes unsuitable school instruction;
Unsatisfied aspirations of the peasant masses, together with passivity as regards certain fields of activity;
Spiritual influence of certain beliefs tending to check the desire for material progress;
Tendency towards tolerance, excluding class and religious strife;
Insufficiency of collective equipment, especially sanitary installations and communication lines;
Insufficiency of peasant income, due to under-employment and low farm productivity;
Slowness of technological change, and even greater slowness of social change.

The need for improved education in rural areas is frequently stressed. A specific example of the consequences in Malaysia of such a desirable development is given by Wilson (1967):

A number of children, both boys and girls, attend the secondary school in Kajang and there is a general recognition throughout the village that education is worthwhile. But those who receive this education will, with but a few exceptions, leave the village to work in offices in the larger towns, leaving those with only the minimum education and those with the least abilities to remain in the village as the undeveloped rural masses. Their daily lives and their livelihood will be earned according to the methods and precepts they have learned in the village, mainly in the household, which means that little change is likely. I believe that this process is as basic to any form of development as questions of mechanization, industrialization and so forth. The approach to the solution of this problem lies first in the understanding of the basic tenets and structure of village life, and then in the formulation of a means of effective communication of concepts, methods and values, as well as techniques and the supply of material on which the entire process of change and development rest. I am in effect arguing for a translation of non-village values into a set of concepts comprehensible to villagers. Put in another way, the prerequisite for change is a presentation of the anthropology of the societies from which the changes emanate. Thus the values associated with 'work' in a capitalist or even in a socialist economy are not only different from the values about work in a Malay village, but are integrated in, and help to integrate a total social structure that is different.

The UNESCO/FAO seminar concluded that the problems of rural life may be reduced to a common denominator; the need for modernization, or more exactly, the need to fill the gap between urban and rural life through the introduction of new techniques and ideas in country areas. 'The essential effort still needs to come from the peasants themselves. One must find minds that are open to progress (provided they are willing to remain in the rural areas) and collaborate with them' (see role of innovators in Chapter 8). 'It might, for example, be possible to spread the desire for progress through an improvement in the health situation and by working through women and children, who form the majority of the rural population' (UNESCO, 1963).

THE STUDY OF CHILDREN

For studies in social anthropology in general and in child rearing in particular, a manual has been developed for the field work in the Six Cultures Series supported by a grant from the Behavioural Sciences Division of Ford Foundation (Whiting, Child and Lambert, 1966). The field work was part of a comparative study of child-rearing practices as related to subsequent personality differences and certain other aspects of culture which reflect facets of personality. The manual states the hypotheses to be tested, the data to be collected, and the procedures to be used in obtaining the data. These studies conducted in the Asian region (in Uttar Pradesh, India — Minturn and Hitchcock, 1966; Luzon, Philippines — Nydegger and Nydegger, 1966; and north Okinawa — Maretzki and Maretzki, 1966) contain much incidental information related specifically to rural nutrition. Whiting notes that the field workers in the Philippines (Nydegger and Nydegger, 1966) viewed ecology, economics and social and political organization as largely determining the behaviour of the agents of child-rearing (Fig. 4/1).

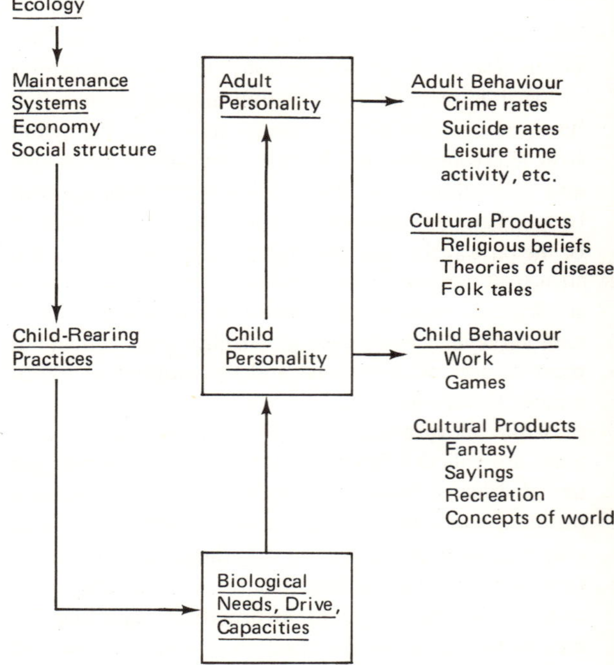

FIG. 4/1   The relation of personality to culture
Source: Whiting, Child and Lambert, 1966

The human ecology of each of the three areas creates differences in the farming communities. In Okinawa and Luzon, men and women work together in the fields (wet rice). In Uttar Pradesh, only men work in the fields (wheat and other food grains). The amount of agricultural work done by women is related to the distance from the dwellings to the gardens and fields, except in Uttar Pradesh, where their enforced seclusion as married women makes field work impossible.

The gardens are closest in Luzon, furthest away in

Khalapur, Uttar Pradesh, which is surrounded by fields that are a fifteen to twenty minutes' walk from the courtyards. In Okinawa, the rice paddies are also on the outskirts of the village, but closer than the fields in Uttar Pradesh. Women do more gardening work when gardens are nearby. Women are better at transplanting the young rice shoots in the paddies, 'a backbreaking and fussy job which requires manual dexterity and patience'. Women do not assist in the season of slash and burn. Men do whatever ploughing is done (buffalo being used in Uttar Pradesh and Tarong). The amount of time and effort women put into agricultural work is one of the several ecological and economic variables which influence the time they can devote to child care and housework.

METHODS FOR FIELD STUDIES OF NUTRITIONAL STATUS

Phillips (1963) has prepared a check-list for use in the introduction of new agricultural methods in areas already cultivated, and for settlement projects in new areas of cultivation. This list covers environmental factors, human and social factors, and the questions to be asked in checking the relative economic and social advantages and viability of a project. Spencer (1966) gives a list of 'seven broad systems' which together may explain why man lives in a particular region, practises a particular type of shifting cultivation, and therefore has the level of nutrition characteristic of that type of farming. The existing check lists do not provide enough detail for the crop agronomist and the animal husbandry specialist to be able to assess the data recorded. It is desirable that such a list be prepared, simple in terminology and limited in scope to meet actual needs.

Other methods relate specifically to the study of rural nutrition, to the determination of the nutritional status of a community or section of a community. It becomes necessary to apply the techniques of clinical, biochemical, anthropometric and biophysical examination to all members of a community, or to a representative sample including persons of all ages and both sexes in the different socio-economic groups comprising the whole. WHO (1963) indicates methods, but states that a medical assessment of nutritional status is of limited practical value without an assessment also of the different conditions of environment, land use and the social and economic structure from which it results (Table 4/1). The health survey in rural Nepal (Worth and Shah, 1969) is an example of this approach.

The village was chosen as the sampling unit. The population was surveyed on the basis of 1:1,500. A large-scale map based on aerial photographs was used, over which was superimposed a small-square numbered grid system. A random sample of twenty-four grid squares was selected; the village nearest the centre of each square was chosen as the sampling site, one to five representing different ecological zones in Nepal. An advance party of four (an engineer and women specialists to conduct household interviews) preceded a medical team of seven, supported by helicopter from the base laboratory in Kathmandu, which had one administrator and two laboratory technicians. A period of two weeks was allotted to each village for the collection of demographic, nutritional and sanitation information, and for examination of prevalence of disease.

The ability to communicate with rural people in their own language is important to gain their confidence and thus to obtain reliable information. In this respect, the anthropologist has two important advantages over other specialists; he usually learns or already speaks the language of the people he is studying, and does not normally expect to complete his work in less than one year. Specialists in home economics, nutrition and medicine, on the other hand, generally work through interpreters, and are rarely able to spend much time with the people they study. Such disadvantages may be overcome by training national specialists to make the investigations, although frequently there is still a wide gulf between these educated urban people and the rural families they are investigating.

The home economist is interested in the social and environmental factors which govern the way of life in the home, and in the best use of whatever meagre facilities may be available. She will study family income and expenditure, particularly on food, and make suggestions regarding more nutritious and possibly cheaper forms of food likely to benefit the family diet, especially that of children. She will investigate local recipes and methods of cooking, and see how these might be improved in ways acceptable and practicable to mothers. In her training course for Malay students, Aleid (1960) emphasizes the need for understanding the common needs and problems of rural families, time and money management, social and ethical aspects of home life, family relationships, food habits in relation to local customs, and facilities for food preparation. Bustrillos (1961) prepared a schedule for young field workers in the Philippines, covering food

TABLE 4/1

Information needed for assessment of nutritional status

Sources of information	Nature of information obtained	Nutritional implications
(1) Agricultural data Food balance sheets	Gross estimates of agricultural production Agricultural methods Soil fertility Predominance of cash crops Overproduction of staples Food imports and exports	Approximate availability of food supplies to a population
(2) Socio-economic data Information on marketing, distribution and storage	Purchasing power Distribution and storage of foodstuffs	Unequal distribution of available foods between the socio-economic groups in the community and within the family
(3) Food consumption patterns Cultural-anthropological data	Lack of knowledge, erroneous beliefs and prejudices, indifference	
(4) Dietary surveys	Food consumption	Low, excessive or unbalanced nutrient intake
(5) Special studies on foods	Biological value of diets Presence of interfering factors (e.g., goitrogens) Effects of food processing	Special problems related to nutrient utilization
(6) Vital and health statistics	Morbidity and mortality data	Extent of risk to community Identification of high-risk groups
(7) Anthropometric studies	Physical development	Effect of nutrition on physical development
(8) Clinical nutritional surveys	Physical signs	Deviation from health due to malnutrition
(9) Biochemical studies	Levels of nutrients, metabolites and other components of body tissues and fluids	Nutrient supplies in the body Impairment of biochemical function
(10) Additional medical information	Prevalent disease patterns, including infections and infestations	Interrelationships of state of nutrition and disease

Source: WHO, 1963

practices, income and expenditure, housing and equipment. Environmental sanitation — the availability of pure drinking water, clean water for washing, and the presence and use of latrines — has an important bearing on community health.

Nutritionists may have more specialized interest, although most study the environmental factors which govern diets or nutritional status. Food consumption surveys are usually organized with an initial pilot survey, to train national staff better able to recognize and evaluate rural foods than can a foreign specialist. If an entire country is to be covered, investigations must be made in representative areas differing in climate, soil, staple food and economic status. FAO has prepared a general formula for estimations in food consumption surveys on a per caput, household or group basis (François, 1970).

The FAO/WHO/UNICEF Protein Advisory Group (February 1970) has drafted guidelines for the design and execution of field studies to evaluate measures for improving the protein status of malnourished people in their urban or village environments. It is essential to define clearly the precise objective of a field study, to begin with a pilot study which will itself be complete and self-contained, and to plan and test all experimental procedures, including the collection of significant data.

The Protein Advisory Group discusses the particular problems involved in a planned field study of anthropometric measurements, weight, height, skinfold thickness, head circumference, etc. of pre-school children. It refers specifically to the work of Greenberg and Bryan (1951) who compared groups of school children on the basis of age-adjusted heights and weights, and again in terms of weights adjusted to age and height; also to Guzman, Scrimshaw, Bruch and Gordon (1968), who used simple linear regression methods to estimate individual rates of gain in weight and height for children of 10 to 60 months of age, measured at monthly intervals[1].

A random sample of families may be chosen from a census or other list of population in each locality. Reh in Brunei (1963) considers that fifteen or twenty

families would give an adequate picture of a rural area. A record of food consumption in each family during one week is obtained and the food weighed. Each investigator is provided with a jeep, a motor boat, rainproof bags for equipment and documents, diet scales to weigh up to 1,000 gm. or up to 5 or 10 kg. scales for weighing people, and steel tapes for measuring height. One worker can cover five families in a week, allowing additional time for selection of the families in each kampong or village, survey work in the field, and subsequent calculations. A thorough investigation must be carried out with the same families in at least two different seasons of the year, to observe variations in the seasonal availability of foods and of income. It is important to evaluate the distribution of different food items within the family. Foodstuffs must be analysed in a laboratory so that standard values may be established as the composition of many rural foods is not known (but see Chapter 12).

Dietary information may emerge from medical investigations on the etiology of disease, for example, Blackwell's work on blackfoot in Taiwan (1961). On a visit to Thailand, Ramalingaswami (1956) studied the causes of goitre and beriberi, covering a wide area and making rapid clinical assessments of samples of the population. Bailey (1961 and 1962) adopted an ecological approach in his study of the nutritional status in different parts of Indonesia.

The FAO/WHO Expert Group on Vitamin Requirements (WHO, 1967) considers that diet surveys are still the best available sources of information about nutrient intake, although they recognize their shortcomings; many have been limited in population coverage, the length of time given, the number of seasons covered, and the attention given to different members of the family. Such disadvantages perhaps apply with greater force to medical experts who have come to assess nutritional status or the etiology of specific diseases. Their visits are apt to be even more brief than those of other foreign visitors; in examining members of a rural community, they may be unaware that those who are too sick to walk have stayed at home. In interviews, there is the danger that the unfamiliar visitor may be told what he seems to want to be told, or that expenditure on food may be minimized or exaggerated according to local standards of behaviour, or the spirit of rivalry between one rural community and another. Natural reserve or shame may colour answers unless the specialist is forewarned by someone familiar with local mores.

---

[1] Methods for the assessment of nutritional status are also discussed in the report of the WHO Expert Committee on the Medical Assessment of Nutritional Status (1963); in the WHO Monograph on Assessment of Nutritional Status of the Community (Jelliffe, 1966); in the Manual on Nutritional Surveys issued by the U.S. Interdepartmental Committee on Nutrition for National Defense (1963a); in Chapter 6 of the WHO Monograph on Interactions of Nutrition and Infections (Scrimshaw, Taylor and Gordon, 1968); and in WHO's The Health Aspects of Food and Nutrition (1969).

5 Evolution of Ethno-Dietary Groups

ORIGIN AND DISPERSAL

FROM within this relatively discrete region have arisen peoples of diverse ethnic origins; from outside the region have come other peoples and influences which have greatly affected the picture. This has led to a wide diversity of agricultural economies, and thus of nutritional standards and practices. There are in Asia today three main ethno-dietary groups, each with variations dependent on latitude, topography, altitude, rainfall or reliability of water for irrigation, exposure to outside influences and access to waterways and forest.

The first group occurs in the Indian subcontinent and Ceylon. Diets are based on the staples, wheat in the north-west and north, rice in the north-east and south, and various millets on the dry-lands; grain legumes of the genera *Cicer* and *Phaseolus* provide the plant protein; milk is valued as a source of animal protein; it is in this area that spice is most important.

The diets of mainland and insular eastern Asia are based on the staples, wheat, sorghum and barley in the north, rice in the south; the predominant grain legume is the soybean; the pig is the major source of animal protein. Along the coasts, major waterways and in the islands, this diet is supplemented by fish.

The third group is the Melanesian of mainland and insular South-East Asia, as defined by Coon (1966). Rice is a relatively new staple, root crops and crops reproduced vegetatively are still important in some places, and fish is the main source of animal protein.

The 'Indian' diets have spread south-eastwards and the 'Chinese' diets southward into South-East Asia, where they have merged with or have replaced earlier indigenous diets. Subsequent trade contacts also brought the characteristics of the Near-Eastern lands, the Muslim diets and taboos, to South-East Asia, to be fitted into the mosaic.

The present types of rural or agrarian structure, with their associated customs and standards of nutrition, may have been acquired by peoples in their migrations from earlier habitats and applied to the new (Fig. 5/1). Or the present techniques of land use and agriculture may represent adaptations of earlier techniques, or may have involved the abandonment of the old in favour of techniques more suited to the new environment in which the peoples now found themselves. On this basis, one can evolve regional patterns on which plans for improvement of food production, distribution and utilization may be based.

The origin and dispersal of peoples are usually discussed from the points of view of ethnology and social history. Primitive man became banded together in communities which increased in size and complexity, and in these a natural human tendency towards social structuring operated. Out of these various types of social structure and of factors such as kinship, caste and religion evolved characteristic types of land use and cropping systems, and therefore also dietary practices and standards.

The opposite view may be taken by an ecologist. The characteristics of the climatic subdivisions, the degrees of aridity and humidity, expectancy of droughts as part of the short-term or long-term climatic changes or fluctuations, and the adaptation to environment of human beings, plants and animals — all these and many other factors of a bioclimatic nature are considered to be predominant. They are regarded as governing the location, shape, size and even the evolving social structure of land-based rural communities, as well as the specific crops and types of domestic livestock which can be maintained in systems of crop and animal husbandry adapted to the environment. The rural Asian has learnt to use that environment, the evolved or economic ecosystem of which he is still a part, correctly and to the full, according to the level of his technological advancement. Above

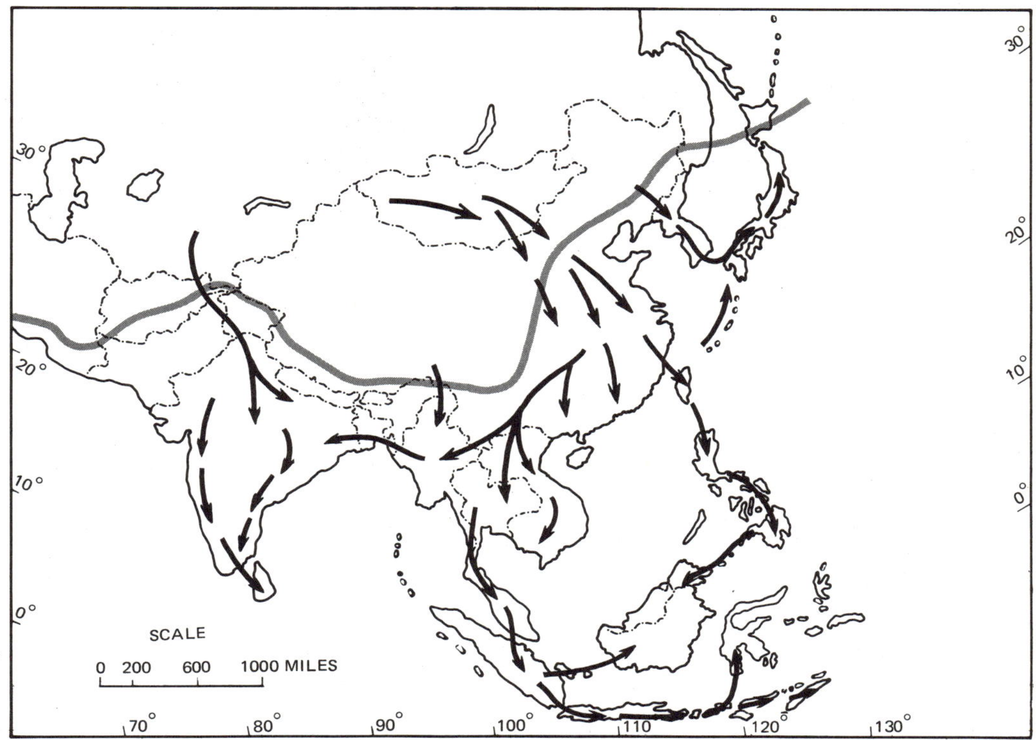

FIG. 5/1   Movements of peoples from early times which have contributed to the evolution of present dietary
patterns

that level, and up to a certain biological limit, he can apply modern knowledge and techniques for improved land use and husbandry. He can change his environment in some particular direction, but may not necessarily also change his dietary habits and nutritional status.

WESTERN MONSOON ASIA

The racial affinities of the earliest inhabitants of the Indian subcontinent are still not known. Primitive hunters and gatherers were driven deep into forests and hilly regions, and can be found today in Sri Lanka, Kerala and Chhota Nagpur. The Munda-speaking peoples of the Chhota Nagpur hills and similar tribes with different languages are descended from migrants who brought the Neolithic swidden technique from South-East Asia into north-east India during the second millennium B.C. (Dani, 1960; Sankalia, 1962).

Coon (1966) expresses the sequence of ethnic history in the subcontinent as follows:

(1)   forest peoples, both Caucasoid and Australoid — food gatherers;

(2)   Neolithic from a South-East Asian Australoid/Mongoloid admixture, tending more towards Australoid in the plains, and towards Mongoloid in the higher elevations;

(3)   Dravidian speakers (now mainly in south India); and

(4)   two Aryan invasions.

The most numerous and latest groups to arrive were the Indo-Iranian-speaking peoples from the northwest. On linguistic evidence, Clark (1966) deduces that there were probably two Aryan invasions:

(1)   peoples accustomed to herding at moderately high altitudes and on broken ground, mainly shepherds from west Asia, crossing Afghanistan into Kashmir and through the western Himalaya into the Nepal valleys and so into Bengal; and

(2)   Sanskrit-speaking peoples related to the Scythians and Sarmatians, cattle-breeders who crossed mountain passes in covered wagons, massive invasions with women and children, continuing their advance to the edges of the hills, for example to the western Ghats and wooded hills of the Deccan, where grazing became poor and wheeled vehicles could not easily proceed. The old class distinctions were brought — earls, churls and thralls, and a fourth priestly class. These became the Indian caste system with its network of genetic isolates.

Why did these peoples move into the north-west of the Indian subcontinent, and whence did they come? In Chapter 2 and again below, under China, we refer to the climatic fluctuations arising in the arid lands to the north, and causing pulsations of climate and population down through the latitudinal zones to the south. Might not the outpourings of peoples from the grazing lands of the heartland of Asia into Iran and the Indian subcontinent have been due also to climatic fluctuations of 100 to 300 years' duration?

The present diets characteristic of the peoples of the Indian subcontinent may be traced back to the early days when primitive groups lived on the resources of the land itself. Others came in from the west and north-west, and from the north-east, bringing with them crops, domestic livestock, systems of husbandry and dietary habits and preferences to create the amalgam of the subcontinent. During its long subsequent history, major developments have contributed to a constantly evolving situation, especially the granting of sanctity to the cow, and more recently the introduction of new plant genotypes from all parts of the world.

The original forest peoples lived on collection from the fruit, tuber-bearing and grain plants found locally in the natural vegetation, climax and/or secondary after burning, and by hunting or collecting the edible fauna. Hunting was more important in the drier tracts, vegetable foods in areas of higher rainfall.

The Allchins (1968) believe that there was a considerable time lag between the appearance of the western Neolithic in the Middle East and Iran, and its spread into north-western parts of the Indian subcontinent. Around the end of the fourth millennium, possibly earlier, new influences or peoples came from the west. Settled agriculture began in the Indus plain, based on a form of wheat, *Triticum compactum* ('one of the three ancient varieties probably native to this site'). During the Harappan period, both *T. compactum* and Indian dwarf wheat, *T. sphaerococcum* together with *Hordeum vulgare*, field peas, lentils and flax, were grown.

Triticum is not a genus of the natural grass covers in the monsoonal ecoclimate; these early wheats must therefore have been brought from beyond the western limits of the region, from Iran, Iraq or Afghanistan. Wheat in the diet may have played an important part in the military history of the Indian subcontinent. The best soldiers traditionally come from the western wheat lands — the Sikhs and Punjabis of Pakistan and India, the men from the North-West Frontier, and the

Rajputs and Mahrattas. Their characteristics may have been partly a response to constant invasion from the west up to Mogul times, but also an outcome of superior nutrition — wheat as a staple, combined with grain legumes and milk.

EASTERN MONSOON ASIA

The ethno-dietary history of China is still largely speculative, being closely related to the sequence of early cultures and the way in which they grew their food crops. It may have been in the river valleys and small basins in the western highlands of north China that Mesolithic hunter and collecting peoples first evolved the Neolithic technique of slash and burn agriculture, slowly developing what came to be known as the Yangshao culture. This subsequently evolved into the Lungshan culture, characterized by settled farming, but still with some hunting and food collecting.

Parallel with this early history, there developed a series of dietary patterns. The first was based upon the flora and fauna of forest and the secondary grasslands and upon fish. With the beginnings of crop cultivation, the first food plants would be grown to supplement the dwindling food resources from the natural vegetation. Thus the staples of the early Yangshao peoples were the three millets, foxtail millet (*Setaria italica*), broomcorn millet (*Panicum miliaceum*) and large millet or kaoliang (*Sorghum vulgare*). They may also have cultivated the soybean, of which the centre of origin is in Manchuria. Their domesticated animals were pigs, cattle, sheep, dogs, chicken and possibly horses.

During the next phase of the Lungshan cultivators, there appeared wheat and rice. It is generally assumed that wheat came in from the Near East. The extension of settled agriculture gave rise to greatly increased population, sending the Lungshanoid further south and south-east. It was only during this period that rice began to appear in the diets of the north Chinese.

Thus in these early stages of the history of China, the distribution of crops and therefore the rural dietary patterns of the present day were evolving. During these millennia, there were climatic fluctuations over periods of 100 to 300 years, as discussed by Eickstedt (1944; Wiens, 1954). Eickstedt introduces his recurring theme of the dynamics of the so-called population chambers of the valleys of the Yellow, Yangtze and Hsi Rivers. It is assumed that pulsations of population pressure arose following long and recurrent periods of excessive drought in the desert lands to the north-west of China (Chappell, 1970), that they would have acted upon the populations of the Yellow River valley, there generating dynamic overflows which in turn had to move southwards into the Yangtze valley. Here the inflows of population are seen as creating pressures which in turn sent forth other dynamic streams southward and south-westward into the lesser pressure chambers of the Hsi River valley and the basin lands of south-west China. From these lands the biodynamic forces spilt over into the Indo-Chinese peninsula. Eickstedt claims that it is possible to trace these movements anthropologically, in the superimposition of racial characters and cultural features by northern groups successively over southern groups. His final conclusion is that this dynamic process represents the history of the sinicization of eastern Asia.

These pulsations and the consequent southward movement of the overflows of population would be due not solely to the occurrence of long periods of excessive drought and the consequent outpourings of nomadic peoples with their livestock from the arid lands to the north into the cultivated areas. There would also be associated occurrence of drought in the Yellow River valley itself, with lesser intensities in the other valleys to the south.

By the middle of the first millennium B.C., there were two major historical movements in China, one from the expanding Chou civilization south, and one from the central Asiatic Steppes — mounted nomads of different ethnic groups (Phillips, 1965). Altogether there have been four great mass migrations of Han Chinese to the south and south-west, caused by droughts, floods, wars, political chaos and lawlessness. The first two took place during the Western Chin and Chao periods, between the third and fifth centuries. The third took place as an aftermath of the Mongol conquest and the Sung retreat into south China. The fourth was the movement during the Sino-Japanese war from 1937 to 1945 (Wiens, 1954). These great migrations had repercussions on non-Chinese peoples to the south. The Chinese came into the Yunnan central highland triangle in response to its climate and agricultural potential, driving out the Lolo, Miao and others. The Miao-Yao and Kam-Tai both originated north of their present limits of distribution, in central or northern China, and have been pushed steadily southward by Chinese expansion.

The significance of these movements of population may again be expressed in terms of diets. They would involve a change for the Han Chinese from the northern diets based on the staples of kaoliang and wheat, to the southern diet of rice, while tribal peoples forced into higher altitudes had to adopt the coarse grains and buckwheat which grew there.

SOUTH-EAST ASIA

The Melanesian family was produced in South-East Asia by a mixture of Australoids — both dwarf negritoes and larger Australoids — with Mongoloids coming from the north in relatively small numbers (Coon, 1966).

Traits common to all these peoples evolved (Coedès, 1964):

Technology
1. cultivation of irrigated rice-fields,
2. domestication of buffalo and ox,
3. rudimentary use of metals — metal culture (bronze and iron), originating in China and Tonkin about 300 B.C.
4. skill in navigation.

Social
1. importance of women and descent by maternal line,
2. organization resulting from irrigated cultivation.

Religion
1. animism,
2. ancestor worship and gods of the soil,
3. location of shrines on high places,
4. burial in jars or on dolmens,
5. cosmological dualism of mountain versus sea, winged beings versus water beings, men of the mountain versus men of the sea coast.

Centuries of migrations, trade and political relationships link the peoples of Burma, Thailand, Laos and Vietnam with the southern provinces of China: Yunnan, Kweichow, Kwangsi and Kwangtung. This entire region of greater South-East Asia forms an integrated whole for the study of racial and linguistic history, ethnic distribution and cultural evolution (Lebar, Hickey and Musgrave, 1964). Persistent pressure of the Chinese caused the Burmese, Tais, Miaos, Yeos and Laos to move southwards and upwards into the higher elevations. The present-day inhabitants of Malaysia and Indonesia came from an area in southwest China, moving down the Malayan peninsula, while other migrants came to the Philippines from the south-east China coast.

A repeating pattern of river valleys or plains and mountain ranges running north and south has been an important factor in deciding the direction of these southward movements — the Ganges/Brahmaputra/Arakan/Irrawaddy/Dawna/Thailand, mountains of Laos and Vietnam, which divide the lowlands of North Vietnam from those of South Vietnam and Cambodia; the Thai lowlands are divided by a low range which turns east to separate east Thailand from Cambodia. Along the ridges, Mongoloid peoples, mostly non-Chinese tribesmen from south China and east Tibet, have been filtering down to the steamy jungles and swamps of the lowlands and deltas, gradually becoming acclimatized through admixture with the resident Melanesians (Coon, 1966).

The so-called march to the tropics of the Han Chinese (Wiens, 1954) was represented by major movements of population for purposes of cultivation and soldiering as far as the present borders of China; beyond that they went mainly as traders. The coming of the Tais into South-East Asia was probably the result of southward and south-west infiltration of a small, Tai-speaking ruling and military élite, and the resulting assimilations and Tai-ization of larger Mon-Khmer-speaking peoples (Lebar, Hickey and Musgrave, 1964; Wiens, 1954). The Tai tendency to social organization (arising from wet rice cultivation) and their assimilating ability were possibly the result of early wet rice cultivation in the middle Yangtze and Chengtu Plain area of Szechuan (Wiens, 1954). There is historical evidence that wars between Buddhist rulers in South-East Asia were aimed at increasing the labour force needed to produce food in these then sparsely-inhabited lands (Moerman, 1968).

Early in the Christian era (Coedès, 1964), Indian culture, brought by Brahman court advisers, spread from the Mauryan and Kushan courts to the coastal communities of South-East Asia which had long been known to Indian traders. Originally they had little influence on the peoples outside these court centres. During the first five centuries A.D., trade centres in South-East Asia became areas of Indian rule and influence, separate from the Indian subcontinent itself. In the third century the Chinese entered into diplomatic relations with the Indianized kingdom of Funan, said to have been founded by a Brahman, Kaundinya, on the coast of Indo-China in the first century A.D. Chinese records refer to another Indianized state in the north Malay peninsula in the early second century A.D., Amaravata, an important centre of Buddhism; images have been found in Siam, Funan, Sumatra, Java and the Celebes. With the overthrow of the Funan dynasty by the Khmers in their pre-Angkor drive southward in the sixth century, a powerful dynasty became established in central Java in the seventh cen-

tury. This was followed in the middle of the ninth by the great Indianized state of Srivijaya, with its capital at Palembang in south Sumatra — the real successor to Funan as the predominant political and commercial power in South-East Asia (Hall, 1968).

Then came Islam. Its founder had been a member of the Trading Company of Mecca, and the expansion of the Islamic faith in Arabia itself was as much an economic drive as a religious and political movement. Their conquest and development of the great commercial centres of Baghdad and Alexandria made possible a great expansion of trade between the Mediterranean, India and South-East Asia. Islam moved east by conquest and trade, reaching the Indus delta in 712 A.D. As South-East Asia had for long accepted Indian influence, it was the Gujarati and Bengali Muslims who brought Islam to that part of the world. The main nutritional consequence was the outlawing of the pig, until then an important animal for sacrifice and feasts.

The arrival of the Portuguese, British, Dutch, French, Spanish and Americans caused a major disruption in the old primitive forms of land use. In the Malay peninsula in particular, the introduction of plantation agriculture, as well as the development of tin mining, caused a new influx of population into the country to provide labour. These peoples were Chinese, Indonesians and south Indians. Chinese plantation labour was also introduced into the Philippines and Indonesia.

In terms of human genetics, Coon (1966) believes that the Indonesians of Java probably absorbed the most Indian genes, especially the upper classes; Malaya the most Arab; the Philippines the most European, and Indo-China the most Chinese. This is reflected in the ethno-dietary history of these countries.

INFLUENCE OF TRADE

From time immemorial a pattern of trade linked the coasts of East Africa, Arabia and all parts of the Indian subcontinent with the mainland and insular countries of South-East Asia. Arabs, Persians, Indians, Malays and Indonesians, and to some extent Chinese sailors and subsequently the merchant adventurers used the prevailing monsoon winds to carry them across the Indian Ocean and the Bay of Bengal, on through the Straits of Malacca to the South China Sea. They carried first gold and tin, later ivory and ebony, but above all spices — pepper from Malabar, nutmeg and mace from the Bandas, cloves from the Moluccas. The expansion of trade and, later, missionary activi-

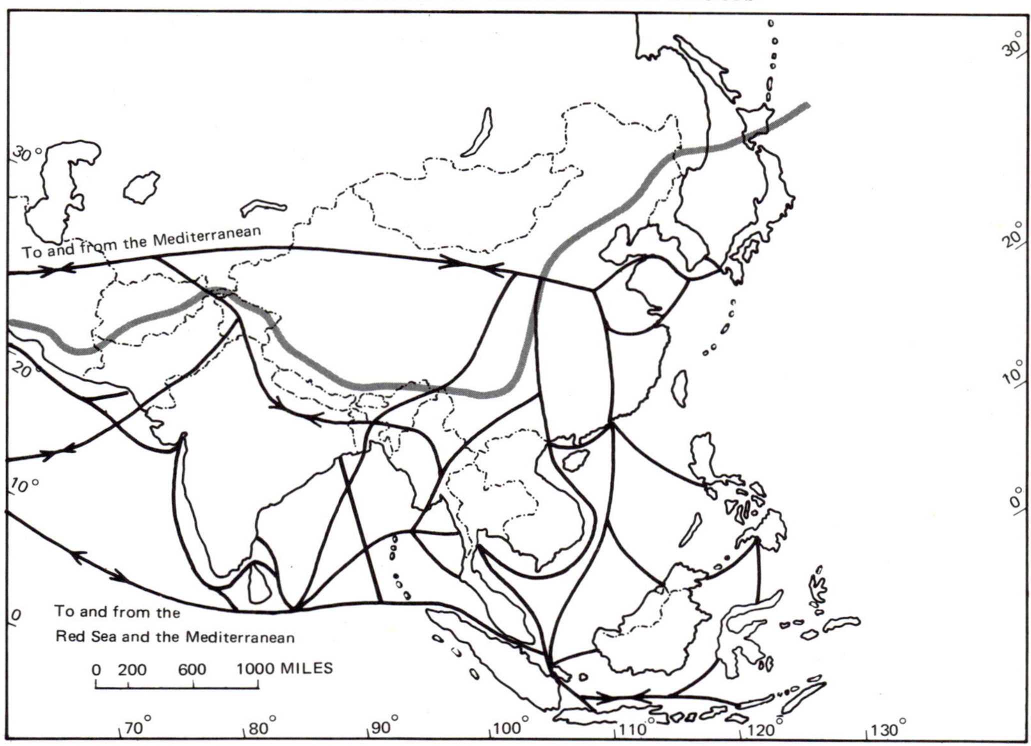

FIG. 5/2   Principal routes of trade, religion, pilgrimage and tribute before the sixteenth century which have affected dietary patterns

ties, with a regular flow of peoples, ideas, caravans and ships, permitted the introduction, either inadvertently or deliberately, of cereal and other vegetable foods and of domestic animals. This took place from the westernmost borders of the Roman Empire to the easternmost ports of call of the traders in the Indianized kingdoms of Sumatra and Java, and on into China. In the fifteenth century the Portuguese, and later the Spanish, brought plants from the New World into Asia. Maize and sweet potato, and to a lesser extent tapioca and peanuts, transformed the diets of large parts of the Philippines, Indonesia, China, Japan and the vast mountainous tract extending from China along the Himalaya to the Hindu Kush.

The anonymous Graeco-Egyptian compiler of the *Periplus of the Erythraean Sea,* the manual of trading and navigation written in A.D. 70 — 71 (Pirenne, 1961) had not travelled further east than the limits of Greek navigation, the Malabar Coast, Cranganore and Broach in Gujarat. But other local ships are mentioned, those that sailed to ports like Kaveripatnam, Pondicherry and Markanum, and the larger ships which traded with the mouths of the Ganges and on to Burma and Sumatra.

Sea traffic from Gujarat and Sindhu and (from the Mauryan period) from Bengal, gave cultural stimulus to the south Indian centres of the Pandiyas, the Cōlas on the Kāvēri delta and the Céras of Kerala and to Ceylon (Maloney, 1970). Traders were attracted by pearls in the Indo-Ceylon straits from at least 300 B.C., while the Chinese came in the second and first centuries B.C. Conch shells and the gems of Ceylon were highly prized in north India. Immigrants, ultimately from the Punjab, settled in Pandiya country in southeast India.

During the first and second centuries B.C., India's main route for the importation of precious metals from Siberia across Bactria may have been cut by Central Asian nomads. In the first century A.D. she sought metals from the Roman Empire; prevented by Vespasian from developing this trade, Indian merchants then probably turned east to the Golden Khersonese (Malay Peninsula).

There is evidence of a northerly land trade route as early as 128 B.C., through Assam, upper Burma and Yunnan. In A.D. 79, envoys from the eastern parts of the Roman Empire visited Yung Ch'ang, a Chinese prefecture with its headquarters on the Salween, founded in A.D. 69 to control and protect the route across the upper Mekong. In the second century A.D., the silk trade followed not only the long trans-continental route to Parthia, but also subsidiary land routes through Siam, Burma and down the Salween and Irrawaddy for shipment to the Mediterranean.

The long sea route from the south China ports to Europe was also used, with the Indianized States of South-East Asia developing as entrepôts (Hall, 1968), and trade routes between India, Burma and South-East Asia were mainly by sea, especially from the coast of Coromandel to the Straits of Malacca. To avoid pirates in the Straits of Malacca and Sunda, short land crossings were used, across the Kra Isthmus by Kedah to Sengma, from Tavoy over the Three Pagodas Pass, by the Kanpuri River to the valley of Menam, and by Moulmein and Raheng Pass to the valley of the Menam.

Sea trade and travel between India and China was further stimulated in the first five centuries A.D. by the spread of Buddhism, with pilgrims from China travelling to India, and scriptures being sent from India to China.

With the coming of Islam, Gujarati Muslims shared the great commercial revival of the twelfth century with the traders from Persia, Arabia and China. They also benefited from the Crusades (1100 to 1300 A.D.), asserting themselves as the principal agents for India's overseas trade with the Far East, Middle East and the Mediterranean. They acted as exporters and intermediaries, selling their valuable textiles or bartering them for spices (Harrison, 1954).

Following the arrival of the Europeans and the great development of seaborne trade in tropical primary products from new plantations, the seaport cities so characteristic of the area expanded to become great commercial centres. These centres of high purchasing power, now being increased still further by the influx of tourists, depend partly for their food on the cropland that is within easy reach, and partly, probably more so, on food imported from outside the region. It is debatable whether the benefits of this modern expansion will reach the remoter settled and swidden cultivators, belonging to the many smaller ethnic groups and sub-groups in South-East Asia.

The diets of the wealthy, particularly those in urban centres, have progressively been changed beyond recognition by the ebb and flow of trading and religious activities throughout the centuries. A fundamental change in the nutrition of the rural Asian was, however, the introduction of new staples, particularly the sweet potato (which gives a higher yield per acre in calories than other Asian crops) and maize, which will grow in dry, unirrigable areas unsuited to rice production.

6 Beliefs: Naturalistic and Supernatural

A complex network of beliefs and traditions, both ancient and modern, determines the foods that people will or will not eat at any given time. Many of these are naturalistic concepts regarding human growth and health, and the properties of foods to disturb or rectify what is considered to be the body's natural balance. The medical systems of ancient India and China, like those of the Greeks and Arabs, were based on the belief that the human body was composed of different elements or humours. According to Ayurvedic medicine, these humours were wind, gall or bile, and mucus or phlegm; some added blood as a fourth element (Basham, 1954). It has not been possible to decide whether India borrowed these beliefs from Greece, or vice-versa (Rawlinson, 1937); the basic Indian textbooks date only from the first to second and fourth centuries A.D., although Indian medicine began to evolve at the time of the Vedas.

In China, early writings have also been lost. Tradition has it that the divine ruler, Shen Nung (Shu, 1963) of 2727 B.C., taught the people the art of agriculture and the use of herbs for the treatment of sickness when the five bodily elements, metal, wood, fire, water and earth were unbalanced. Herbs possessing qualities opposing those of the illness were used; for example, fire (inflammation or infection) was treated with watery, cooling herbs. In fact it appears that the theory of the five bodily elements was brought into China by Tsou Yen (305 − 240 B.C.) (Huard and Wong, 1968). A combination of Babylonian, Indo-European and Chinese conceptions led to the creation of an extensive pharmacoepia of herbal and mineral remedies, a knowledge of poisons, of dietetics, respiratory techniques, physical culture and the study of sex, as well as the quest for the means of obtaining immortality. In the third century B.C., the theory of the Yin and the Yang, oppositeness and complimentarity, was evolved.

From these different sources, the belief in health and sickness being caused by bodily imbalance between the humours, and in the heating and cooling properties of foods and herbs to influence this balance, has penetrated into most of Asia, while a modified version was introduced into Latin America by the Spanish.

The totality of traditional beliefs, both naturalistic and supernatural, influences the selection of food under different circumstances, at different seasons of the year, and in different stages in the human cycle. It is not possible to be sure to what degree traditions are followed in actual practice. Urban influence, improved communications, rural health centres and proximity to a more sophisticated community all tend to break down some beliefs; others are observed simultaneously with 'modern' practices. The more isolated a community, the stronger the hold of traditional beliefs. Even here, however, some may be sceptical; Dentan (1968) notes how some Semai will nibble bits of forbidden foods to see if they cause any harm.

Some practices may be beneficial. Many beliefs are harmless, while some have serious consequences. Those most far-reaching in their effects on health are undoubtedly naturalistic beliefs regarding foods suitable for pregnancy, lactation, infancy and childhood. Rural worship invariably involves some sort of flesh offering, afterwards consumed by the community or family. Such occasions are more frequent among some groups than others, but for many they provide the principal source of animal protein. There may be disproportionate expenditure on prestige items of food deemed to have valuable properties, as with ghee in India. The same amount of money would buy not only vegetable oil for cooking, but other more nutritious items of diet as well.

EARLY BELIEFS

The reaction of these Asian peoples to the precarious nature of their environment is reflected in a multiplicity of supernatural beliefs and practices common to the whole region. The natural world is peopled with innumerable spirits. These are generally divided into at least two categories: those which are benevolent and protective when worshipped according to prescribed ritual and with suitable, usually flesh offerings, and those which are invariably malevolent. The spirit hierarchy is, however, often far more complex than this. Household, village and ancestral gods and many nature spirits come into the first category. Demons and ghosts, especially those of people who have died a violent death, are dangerous and to be avoided at all costs. Among some peoples there is a vague conception of a supreme being or creator, who is generally uninterested in the affairs of men, but whose existence has proved useful to Christian missionaries. Omens, often the call or direction of the call of birds and animals, the condition of the organs of an animal to be sacrificed, or of its bones after roasting, are interpreted and invariably obeyed. Priests, astrologers, shamans and medicine men are important figures; they may be hereditary officers, may have received some special enlightenment or training, or may simply be chosen by their village.

In those areas of mainland South-East Asia where contact with Chinese culture has been continuous, ancestor worship is performed by the head of the household at altars with ancestral tablets. Lunar New Year is an important festival in countries east of Burma, except among the Muslim and Christian communities. In China itself, there have been strenuous efforts to abolish all forms of cult, since they are considered economically wasteful.

Individual festivals of importance occur at birth, naming, attaining of maturity, marriage and death. The new mother may not work, though she may bathe herself and the child frequently. In India, the first ceremonial bath takes place after a few days. Birth seems to have been long associated with a conception of impurity, removed by ritual observances. This idea has persisted into the more modern faiths; by Islamic law, the mother is unclean for 40 days and subject to taboos. The Chinese mother, however, does not take a full bath or wash her hair for one month after giving birth. (Topley, 1973).

Housebuilding is generally an important communal occasion and the subject of ritual and sacrifice, including placating the spirit of the soil to atone for disturbing it.

Many aboriginal hunters and collectors appear to have a strong concept of individual responsibility towards the supernatural and the decisions of life. This does not seem to withstand the transition to shifting cultivation, which imposes collective effort at times of heavy labour such as planting and harvesting. Rituals are also collective.

MAJOR RELIGIONS

All the world's major religions have developed or been introduced in the region in relatively recent historical times. These new faiths have been embroidered onto the tapestry of existing beliefs, becoming an inextricable part of the whole attitude to life. The farther away a community is from an urban centre, the stronger the hold of the supernatural, irrespective of nominal adherence to one of the major faiths. The new faiths have tended to be observed particularly at major events of the human cycle; birth, coming of age, marriage, death, and particularly the after-life. These faiths have, unlike supernatural beliefs, an ethical and moral component. This is not often understood by rural people, who nonetheless devoutly follow prescribed ritual.

Confucianism and Taoism made their mark on non-Han peoples within China's borders and those in South-East Asia who were influenced by Chinese culture. Elements of Brahmanism are found where Hinduized kingdoms existed, or within their former spheres of influence, in Burma, China, north Thailand, Malaya and Indonesia. Buddhism, Islam, Hinduism and to a lesser extent Christianity are major faiths in the region. The eastern religions have an important bearing on the attitude towards the husbandry, slaughter and consumption of domestic animals.

A religion develops a philosophy and rules of behaviour most adapted to the environment in which it originates. Thus Islam and Christianity, which have been transplanted into Asia, have elements most at variance with that world. Islamic dietary restrictions grew up in arid lands where a ban on pork was compensated by the presence of large flocks of sheep and goats. The pig, so well adapted to humid Asia, is unacceptable. Sheep must be imported into Asia, either live, or killed at source by appropriate Muslim ritual. Islamic disapproval of birth control, like that of Catholicism, arose at a time when mortality was high and there was an urgent need to produce as many members of the new faiths as possible. Catholicism can afford such luxurious beliefs in the developed world of falling birth rates, falling death rates, food surpluses and high standards of living. Such views are totally at variance with the demographic, economic and social needs of a country like the Philippines.

Some beliefs and practices may indirectly impoverish the rural diet. The contribution made by many Buddhist people to the food of the monks in the village temple has been calculated in Thailand as representing enough to feed an additional family member per year (deYoung, 1955). Spiro has denied that such practice is 'uneconomic' in Buddhist eyes; the people believe they are acquiring merit which will ensure a more comfortable existence in their next lives (1966). In Cambodia, however, villagers can partake of the remains of temple feasts, and this also bestows merit.

One may not infer that religious and ritual observances will be the same in different communities within the nominal boundaries of the dominant religions. Nor can anything but a general outline be gained from the many studies of ritual behaviour in specific communities. Such behaviour varies from village to village, being influenced by accidents of history and local topography. There are, indeed, different nuances in the practices of different members of the same village, even where these are avowedly all of the same persuasion. It is not uncommon to find differences in the devotions of men and women of the same family.

FUSION WITH OLDER BELIEFS

Just as in the West, Christianity is practised alongside a following of printed horoscopes, trepidation on every Friday the 13th, the throwing of spilt salt over the left shoulder and the annual decoration of the Christmas tree, so in the East, the major religions co-exist with many, far older, traditional beliefs. It cannot be assumed that followers of Mohammed, Buddha or Siva will observe all the injunctions their faiths impose upon the fully enlightened. Thus the effect of new agricultural, nutritional or medical practices may be influenced or offset by admixture with old, possibly conflicting observances. This is more marked in the rural than in the urban areas where, among the educated, there may be greater adherence to the tenets of the major religions. But even here, there may still be private observance of former traditional beliefs; astrology, for instance, remains as important in urban areas as in the villages. In the rural areas, traditional belief systems predominate in guiding everyday decisions, problems and rules of behaviour.

Functionaries of the new faiths, generally unwittingly, perform many rituals of the old. Hinduism has everywhere absorbed older beliefs. A visit from the pre-Hindu goddess of smallpox, though greatly feared, is sacred and will be treated fatalistically; if death occurs, the body is not burned as usual on the ghat, but consigned direct to the river, as it has already been sanctified by the goddess — a swift means of spreading infection. Hindu gods receive vegetarian offerings, while flesh foods provided to older deities reflect their lesser sanctity. In Gopalpur (Beals, 1962), the goddesses of cholera, smallpox and scabies receive both meat and alcohol. Cowdung, which would be of such value in maintaining soil structure, is not only burnt as fuel in a deforested environment, but also used in all forms of village worship, both of Hindu and local, non-Hindu gods. In a Rajput village north of Delhi the usual Hindu devotions are allied with worship of trees (Minturn and Hitchcock, 1966); a Brahman receives milk offerings at certain trees from those whose cows have just calved. A Muslim shrine receives offerings from most villagers and from Rajputs going to collect their brides. The Muslim saint protects the crop from locusts and hailstorms. The women worship local spirits, disease goddesses and family ancestors. Brahmans are the village astrologers. The Magars of Banyan Hill, Nepal, treat gods and godlings alike; the Hindu gods do good, if chicken is offered with appropriate Sanskrit prayers. Godlings cause most harm, but, if appropriately treated, may also cure a sick child, make the buffalo fertile and keep the borers out of the maize (Hitchcock, 1966).

In Indonesia, a priest on the coast may perform exclusively Islamic functions, but his upland counterpart in the interior must be a specialist also in the ritual associated with the agricultural cycle. In the village of Bontoramba in the south Celebes, ancestor worship is the religion of women, Islam that of the men (Chabot, 1967). Thus the reaction of men and women to different agricultural or nutritional changes may be expected to differ. In west Sumbawa (Goethals, 1967), villagers participate in Islamic and pagan agricultural ceremonials; the mosque officials conduct rituals in both. Most Islamic occasions among Malay fishermen in south Thailand have at least some traditional ritual (Fraser, 1966).

In Tarong (north Luzon): 'artefacts of Roman Catholicism are widespread, but their functions have been assimilated to and often fused with those of the indigenous belief system'. The hostile world cannot be placated only by means of prayers to the Christian God — one must trust one's talisman and luck. A crucifix is placed beside the pigsty to ward off disease, but amulets are more effective in human illness (Nydegger and Nydegger, 1966). A farmer must appease the *anitos* (deities) who inhabit fields, forests, lakes and rivers which provide his food. He offers prayers and feasts to San Isidro for a good harvest, and saltless foods and drink to the deities of the field, who will otherwise thwart the good intentions of the Christian saint.

In Laos, the bonze calls the soul of rice to enter the grain at storage after the harvest (Halpern, 1964). Jungle villagers in Ceylon are apt to personify the forces of nature (Leach, 1961) although they are practising Buddhists. In north Burma: 'the system of the nats, predictive, devinatory and medical, together with Buddhism, make a coherent whole, a single set of beliefs and activities to be invoked as instrumentalities, depending on the particular situation' (Nash, 1965).

It will thus be seen that an outsider — doctor, nurse, agronomist or teacher, from outside the region or the national capital — can make no prior assumptions regarding the likely behaviour of the people in a rural community in which he is to work. Behaviour which is regarded as 'rational' or 'moral' or 'ethical' in a government office or on a university campus may merely be thought eccentric in the village.

TRADITION AND MODERN MEDICINE

Under-nourished and malnourished populations are more susceptible to disease than healthy people. Without special supplementary feeding during the course of the illness, and without medical care, recovery will be much slower. Modern medicine is being accepted throughout the region in varying degree, according to the size of the country, its economy and the efficacy and intensity of its rural medical network. But even where familiarity with modern practice, combined with positive experience, is common, many people still resort to traditional medicine either before consulting a health centre, or at the same time. Medical practitioners are frequently called in when all else has failed, too late to be of any help.

Knowledge of rural practice beyond the reach of modern help is still fragmentary, but an example of the effect of traditional cures upon the course of illness comes from India. In Andhra Pradesh, treatment of illness falls into distinctive phases. First, purgatives are given to 'tip the balance back' to health, and dietary restrictions immediately imposed. If this fails, home remedies are tried, including the use of emetics or costly exorcising rituals to remove the poison implanted by enemies of the sick. The third phase of treatment, when a local medicine man is consulted, is

the most harmful. He advises severe dietary restriction, limiting intake to rice, chilli and chutney of garlic and ginger, and carries out painful 'treatments'. Voluntary dietary restriction may continue from nine months to four years. Mercury, camphor and herbal pills are also given. Hospital treatment is sought only as a last resort. The average period of illness is 15.6 months, and during 9.7 months there is total inability to work. Nutritional status of the whole family deteriorates, due to economic hardship, and families may break up (Mahadevan, 1962).

Health is attributed to the naturalistic concept of balance of the bodily elements, based on Indian Ayurvedic theories and on the Chinese theory of the Yin and the Yang. In China, the Taoists concentrated special attention on the inner cause of illness, which they saw as an improper balance between the Yin and Yang. It was believed that a correct regimen in the correct seasons prevented illness. The importance of a complete and balanced diet was fully recognized in the medical classics of the Han period, one of which advises (Needham and Lu, 1962; see also Whyte, 1972a). 'Taking the five cereals as nutriment, the five fruits as assistants, the five meats as chief benefactors, and the five vegetables as supplements, and combining together the *chii* and the tastes in the diet; this blending is what benefits the mind and the body.'

Behaviour in illness may be conditioned by a web of both naturalistic and supernatural beliefs. Hsu (1952) noted that during a cholera epidemic in Yunnan, some of the traditional practices, aimed at placating the gods, such as cleaning the streets and avoiding the use of streams from the mountains (flowing through other villages) were of practical benefit in limiting the spread of disease. Equally helpful were naturalistic beliefs, 'cooling' foods, mostly fruits and vegetables, were to be avoided.

Illness is frequently attributed to supernatural agency. Sickness may be god-given, caused by spirit possession, by soul-loss provoked by demons, or by humans using black magic or the evil eye. Amulets are worn for protection against evil spirits and a host of common ailments. 'Soul loss' is a serious cause of illness throughout the region; the errant soul must be persuaded to return quickly to the body it has left during a vulnerable period — infancy, times of shock, prolonged hardship or even sleep — or the victim will surely die. Black magic practised by witches may involve the entry into the victim's body or his food of a foreign body, such as wool, hair, shrunken buffalo hide, or the *ku* poison of Burma, Thailand and the

Miao, and will cause death unless detected and appropriately treated. A lock of hair or nail parings may also be used to bring illness to their owners. The position in society of a woman suspected of being a witch is not a pleasant one.

Spirits (not-humans) are the chief cause of illness in the Philippines (Nydegger and Nydegger, 1966). The Ifugao of central Luzon (Guthrie,G.M., 1964),believe that sickness may be caused by the displeasure of the ancestors. In Pul Eliya, Ceylon (Leach, 1961), punishment for sin is inflicted by demons in the form of illness or misfortune. Psychological aloneness makes one particularly vulnerable to demon attack. Innumerable demons are placated by a collective ritual, while specific rituals are performed for the blood demon, the great graveyard demon, the sorcery demon and the Sanni demons. In the Sanni ritual, the priest symbolically offers his life to the demons in exchange for that of the threatened sick person (Obeyesekere, 1969). Among the Dusun of Borneo (Williams, 1965), the disease-givers are human in appearance, while the souls of the dead are foul and bent on capture and the destruction of the human soul. The Garo of Assam (Burling, 1965) consider that spirit bite is a frequent cause of illness. Freedman (1954) describes a Minangkabau (Sumatra) belief, shared apparently by qualified doctors, that a baby may be made ill merely by being exposed to the sight of a person who, knowingly or unknowingly, has such power. In south India, children with obvious signs of protein-calorie malnutrition are said to be in the hands of a spirit, and can be cured only by uprooting a certain tree. The local medicine man performs the ceremony, and a small piece of the wood is tied round the child's neck as a talisman (Rao and Balasubramanian, 1966).

The supernatural is frequently invoked in the treatment of common ailments; others may be regarded as inevitable for certain naturalistic reasons; in both cases, medical care is not sought. People have, however, come to realize that certain illnesses are beyond the scope of traditional medicine. In the Philippines modern doctors are consulted for appendicitis, infected wounds and tuberculosis (Polson, 1966). In southern Taiwan, since the turn of the century, prevention and cure of sickness combine traditional and modern methods. In K'un Shen (Diamond, 1969), a measles patient will be given herbal medicines, a modern doctor will be called in, and when the rash begins to disappear, a ceremony asking Buddha to wash away the scars will be performed. For other illness, the supernatural is invoked only if the disease takes an unusual turn. Only in the case of mental illness are solely supernatural methods used. Cantonese women in Hong Kong call traditional practitioners only for diarrhoea, 'fright', and boils (Topley, 1973).

Illnesses may also be attributed to a number of causes which relate neither to naturalistic concepts of balance and imbalance, nor to the supernatural. These are often highly localized in character, and are based on folk beliefs, many of which grow out of hearsay. Thus in Andhra Pradesh, India, pellagra is attributed to contact with inorganic fertilizers or to sexual misdemeanours (Mahadevan, 1962). Anaemia is called 'white jaundice' and white substances should be avoided.

Many practices for curing supernaturally-caused diseases are in no way harmful. They are often an important component of local culture, giving a reassuring framework to a life otherwise full of unaccountable and dangerous phenomena. Unfortunately, the local medicine man/witch doctor does not often — indeed has not the resources to — prescribe physiologically beneficial cures. The sick recover — or not— by a combination of their own reserves and faith in their healers.

BELIEFS REGARDING FOODS OF ANIMAL ORIGIN

There are many cultural factors affecting the success of any attempt to raise the animal protein component of the diet of rural Asians. The first is the widespread belief in the strength-giving, nutritional and mystical qualities of rice in South-East Asia. Burmese say 'I grew up eating rice', meaning that they are not capable of foolish behaviour (Khaing, 1962). People who have had a large meal without rice will say they have not eaten. When asked whether they would eat meat without tapioca or rice, the Semai of Malaysia replied 'Do you think we are cats?' (Dentan, 1968). However, like other swidden peoples, they are accustomed to flesh foods. If they have not eaten meat recently, they may say 'I have not eaten for days'. In India, especially in the north, great faith is placed in the properties of milk, which is also sacred. Elsewhere in Asia animal protein is not considered essential in the diet. Most forms of animal protein, except fish, are prestige foods; meat and eggs are highly valued for sacrifices, and are then consumed by most communities. Important festivals demand sacrifice of cattle, lesser occasions pigs or goats; for more common and frequent offerings, chicken.

East of India, milk is often actively disliked, although scattered rural pockets of milk consumption (goat and carabao) are reported from the Philippines and Indonesia, and sweetened condensed milk has long been popular for use in tea and coffee houses in Malaysia. Otherwise, foods of animal origin are taken as a side-dish to flavour the staple; it is considered ill-bred to take too much. Men nearly always get the largest share, then the boys, girls, and last, the mother. Children are often denied meat, egg or fish dishes, and sometimes pulses, due to widespread beliefs that these are harmful.

Hinduism prohibits the killing of the cow and the consumption of beef; it is rare even for non-Hindu Indians outside the educated classes of urban areas to eat beef. To caste-Indians, animal protein foods are acceptable or unacceptable in varying degrees, according to caste status and the part of India in which they live. While most abhor the domestic pig as unclean, and many apply the same stricture to chicken, some consider fish acceptable, and others eat mutton or goat. All agree that milk is prestige-conferring. It is paradoxical that people who think so highly of milk should follow beliefs which make it impossible to develop an efficient dairy industry to provide that milk in adequate quantity. This belief, like that of certain hill tribes which prohibit the killing of sheep and goats, originally arose in an attempt to prevent excessive slaughter for food and sacrifice of these useful economic animals; factors which were regarded as economic at that time but no longer apply today (Srinivas, 1961).

The Buddhist injunction that animals may neither be killed nor reared for slaughter makes it difficult to create an efficient animal industry in countries following that faith; fortunately fishing is not greatly disapproved of, and plays an important part in the diet of most of these people. Buddhists may occasionally consume the flesh of an animal they have not killed. Leach (1961) reports that no Sinhalese would wittingly eat beef. Some feel that eating eggs does not involve the taking of life (Obeyesekere, 1968). Others buy unfertilized eggs, and still others buy 'Buddhist eggs' — those which are cracked — in transport, or by an astute Muslim shopkeeper. Some ask their servants to break the eggs, transferring the blame; the servants consider the employer will be blamed, according to the Buddhist ethic of intentions. Women appear most reluctant to break eggs (Kalab, 1969). Hindus also consider they may eat unfertilized 'vegetarian' eggs without taking life. In Thailand the young may kill poultry, but not the aged, as they are supposed to be thinking about gaining merit (Hauck *et al.*, 1958). In Cambodia, few below the age of 40 to 50 object to fishing (Kalab, 1969). Burmese keep cocks which decoy and kill wild jungle fowl, providing the owners with a blameless meal (Shway Yoe, 1882).

Muslims are forbidden to eat anything with two or four legs that has died. This, like the ancient Chinese stress on the necessity to eat only cooked food, and to discard anything contaminated by animals or insects (Needham and Lu, 1962), has undoubtedly done much to help limit disease. Nonetheless, the Muslim abhorrence of the pig has prevented the development of a pig industry, depriving Malays, many Indonesians, a large group of southern Chinese and some Thais and Burmese of the meat of the domestic animal most adapted to the humid tropical world.

HUMORAL AND FOLK BELIEFS

The ancient medical theories of India and China regarding the bodily humours and the heating, cooling and other properties of foods and herbs to rectify imbalance have influenced beliefs about food throughout most of Asia. Hart (1969), in his analysis of Bisayan Filipino and Malay humoral beliefs, concludes that the Spanish were the major source of such concepts in the Philippines, whereas the Arabs were responsible for Malay beliefs. He is surprised to find these ideas also among Muslims of the southern Philippines who were converted by the Arabs. Conversion to Islam in the Malay Peninsula and Indonesia was, however, carried out largely by Indians, whose cultural influence in the region predated Islam by many centuries. The food beliefs of the Malays resemble those of rural India rather than the Hippocratic system inherited by the Arabs. In the Philippines, however, where Indian influence was much less important, it does indeed appear that humoral beliefs were brought into the village by the Spanish priest, possibly assisted by vaguely similar folk concepts which may have existed earlier (Hart, 1969).

There does not appear to be a consensus, even within small communities, as to which foods have one or other of these properties. The most dangerous are the 'cooling' foods, an excess of which is to be avoided at all times, and particularly by the new mother and child. Rajput villagers (Minturn and Hitchcock, 1966) generally agree that onion, potato, cane liquor, tea, mangoes, oils, ghee and buffalo milk are heating, while spinach, lemon and curd are cooling, and cow milk neutral. Describing the same village, Dube (1956) states:

> Villagers distinguish between foods that are 'hot', that is, which have a heat-producing effect, and foods that are 'cold', that is which have a cold-producing effect. There are also foods that are intermediate between these two, and thus are neither 'hot' nor 'cold'. Some foods are constipative, some are laxative. Another distinction is that of catarrhal, bilious and flatulent foods. Some foods are supposed to have all three of these properties, some are considered to have two of them, and some are believed to have only one. There are many commonly used foods to which villagers attribute none of these properties . . . . One distinction is that of dry and wet foods. Dryness accentuates the hot quality of a food, while wetness accentuates its cool quality.

In Malaya, it is generally agreed that papaya is cooling and durian heating, but there is great disagreement between kampongs in different parts of the country regarding leafy green vegetables and fruit (McArthur, 1962). Many believe that cucumber, pumpkin, water-melon, some types of bananas and a common fungus are cooling. All forms of meat and poultry are considered to be heating; so also coffee, chillies, black pepper and Lactogen, but not other forms of milk. There are more heating than cooling foods. Heating and cooling foods are not thought to neutralize each other; if eaten together, both effects are produced. In Penang, however, the harmful effects of 'cold' or 'hot' can be offset by balancing; beans are cooked with cold green vegetables, while lard or oil is used to offset the coldness of vegetables (Hart, 1969).

In Telengana, south India (Mahadevan, 1961), milk is believed to offset the heating effect of mango, and *Phyllanthus emblicata* that of fish. Heating foods such as eggs, chicken, fish, duck and duck eggs are preferred during the cold months (winter and the rainy season); also unleavened bread, red gram, bengal gram, maize, *Carica papaya, Colocasia* and their leaves, jowar, sesame and jaggery, bread made of wheat and jowar flour. Cooling foods, such as green leafy vegetables and egg-plant, cucumber, lime, buttermilk, curds, gourds and ragi *(Eleusine coracana)* are avoided. The situation is reversed in summer, although the neutral goat meat and rice are eaten then.

In Indonesia a hot food may also be compensated by a cooling one (Freedman, 1954). Here again, durian is heating and banana and papaya cooling, thus making the last two particularly unsuitable for women and young girls. The definition of 'cooling' given by Zainal Abdin bin Ahman, quoted by McArthur (1962) is: 'cooling to the blood, causing impoverished blood so that you always feel cool, and anaemic'. Meat and fish are both considered heating for young children in Sumatra. Pregnant Chinese women must avoid cooling foods (papaya, vegetables, melon, banana), while heating foods (mango, fried foods, ginger, vinegar, wine) are good (Topley, 1973). Some peoples consider that certain foods are mutually antagonistic. Many Chinese believe that persimmon and crab should not be eaten together, nor peanuts and cucumber, nor onions and honey (Burkhardt, 1953). The Semai hold similar beliefs (Dentan, 1968).

Many of the food beliefs in rural areas in the Philippines relate to digestibility and nutritious qualities, to those foods which cause disease or illness and those which cure them, and to foods which are appropriate to certain times of day. Some beliefs relate the quality (real or imagined) of an animal or a plant to its effect on the human. Thus, crocodile and dog's meat make one courageous (Bustrillos, 1961).

A new set of beliefs appears to be growing up around the high-yielding varieties. Rajput elders feel that the new wheat lacks nutritional value and makes the young men weak and unable to compete with their elders (Hitchcock, 1966). Similar degeneration is believed to follow the consumption of vegetable oil rather than ghee.

BELIEFS AFFECTING THE VULNERABLE GROUPS

Many dietary taboos apply frequently to the vulnerable groups, and relate to pregnancy, lactation, infancy, early childhood and sickness. Restrictions are placed on foods which are believed to cause difficult births, or which may affect the physique of the unborn child. For example, sugar-cane is avoided in Java; also certain plants with horizontal fruits, which might cause the child to be born in that position (Geertz, 1961). Korean mothers fear that eating rabbit or hare will cause hare-lip (also believed by Chinese), that chicken might cause the child to have gooseflesh, or carp, scaly skin, that duck may affect its gait, and many similar concepts (Mo, 1966). Other foods in Asia are claimed to cause a child to be cowardly, courageous, strong or puny, dull or intelligent. A pregnant Filipino woman will avoid octopus, fearing that her child may be born a monster, while egg-plant and banana may cause skin disease (Demetrio, 1969). Indonesian and Indian mothers restrict food intake to prevent the child's becoming too large, and causing a difficult birth. In Indonesia and Malaya, the father should not kill or wound any animal during his wife's pregnancy, or the child may be wounded in the same way. This affects the protein intake of the entire family. Among Melanau, paired fruits are thought to cause twins, and glutinous foods a difficult birth (Morris, 1953).

Some protective foods are avoided because they are thought to cause abortions; in India, papaya, raw eggs, horse gram and jaggery; in China, the banana; in Sri Lanka, the pineapple.

It is generally believed that the special cravings of pregnancy (which are often the expression of a physiological requirement) should be satisfied for the sake of the baby's health. Men may go to extraordinary lengths to obtain unusual or costly foods. Pregnancy cravings are known in India as part of *dola-duka,* the symptoms of pregnancy. It is considered a sin not to satisfy these. They may cause the ears of the foetus to rot. Cravings for certain specific foods are common to most pregnant women. Obeyesekere (1963) has examined the physiological, sociological and psychological aspects of *dola-duka* in a village in central Ceylon. Pregnant women are thought to be 'cold' and weak, and they often reject food because they are expected to be weak. The staples, rice and millet bread, are refused, as are dhal and dried fish, the common components of curry. Sweet foods, sour foods such as tamarind, pickles and citrus fruits, festival foods, costly and unusual foods are all craved. If the mother is reluctant to bear another child, she asks for pineapple and wild boar, thought to cause abortions, and for wild honey, associated with the non-pregnant state.

The full concentration of taboos falls on the post-partum mother and her infant. In a country as large as India, there is great variation in both belief and practice. Mothers in a Telengana village are allowed only spiced rice for 30 days (Rao and Balasubramanian, 1966). In Gujarat, dhals, leaf greens, rice, curds and fruits are avoided; curd, rice and leafy vegetables are considered essential for the nursing mother in Tamil Nadu (Rajalakshmi, 1969).

In South-East Asia, the new mother is usually allowed a little dried fish with her rice, and a limited intake of water. These restrictions last for varying periods, and are observed according to degree of exposure to modern medicine and urban influence. Malay women often return to their native kampongs to give birth; here the traditions of their mothers and grandmothers still hold sway. They may observe the full pantang (denial) of 44 days. In Penang, raw chicken eggs are permitted, but not vegetables (Hart, 1969). The period of restriction in Burma varies from one to three months, though some limit only intake of spices (Brant, 1954). Minangkabau mothers in Sumatra will not eat meat or eggs, but accept anything else; forty years ago, their diet was restricted to rice, dried fish, papaya leaves and herbal potions (Freedman, 1954). Laotian mothers must avoid meat (Olness, 1968).

Severe physical strains are placed on the mother after giving birth. Roasting after delivery to speed recovery is common practice in South-East Asia, although again for varying durations. Mother and child stay in the room where the child was born, near or over a constantly replenished fire. This practice, combined with restriction on liquid intake, causes severe thirst and restricted milk flow. In Kedah, the mother may be propped upright for three days and nights after giving birth, with a heated stone of about 4 kg. wrapped in herbs applied to the abdomen (Chen, 1970). In India, in both Gujarat and Tamil Nadu, drinking water is considered harmful after childbirth (Rajalakshmi, 1969). In Thailand, the new mother is given soupy rice, rather than ordinary rice; while most consider fish, either salted or fresh, as being permissible, some will not take any; eggs, beef, vegetables, pork, poultry, many fruits and glutinous rice are said to be dangerous by some, and vegetables are accepted by others only in fish broth. In Java, the new mother is expected not to lie down for 35 days, even to sleep (Geertz, 1961). Within a few hours of giving birth, she must receive guests, and five exhausting days and nights of entertaining follow. Here too, water and tea intake is restricted. Almost all post-partum restrictions thus permit a totally inadequate intake of protein, minerals and vitamins; the level of water-soluble vitamins in breast milk is certainly affected.

There are exceptions to these damaging taboos. Many Chinese mothers appear always to have firmly believed in the value of animal foods as part of their diets when pregnant, as galactagogues, and also as part of their children's diet. However, actual use is likely to be limited by purchasing power, and animal foods are removed before infants are fed (Jelliffe, 1968a; Field and Baber, 1973; Topley, 1973). These practices are not, however, common to all areas of China (Myrdal, 1966).

Protein-rich seaweed- or meat-soup is favoured by Korean mothers to increase milk though eggs and several kinds of fish and meat are avoided during pregnancy (Yonsei University, 1967-8). In Japan, the new mother is advised to consume a variety of different fish and some vegetables, though sweets are to be avoided (Embree, 1939). Hindu mothers in Nepal consider that rice, meat and dhal are good for pregnancy, while others mention milk, curd, ghee and even fruits, the last rarely eaten normally. In a predominantly Buddhist area, the majority mention only fruits (Brown, Worth and Shah, 1968a and b). On Panay island, western Visayas, Philippines, the mother strictly observes food taboos after giving birth. She must avoid all hot foods (jackfruit, breadfruit, mangoes, pork and fatty foods), but should eat cooling foods (vegetables, white rice, seafood), while chicken and eggs are considered good for lactation (Jocano, 1969). She is also advised to take plenty of water and broth. A high percentage of women in Bataan believe that eating sour foods will curdle their milk (Valdecañas, 1972).

There is widespread faith in herbal decoctions as galactagogues. In Telengana, India, garlic is considered useful, also fish and the intestines, knees and nipples of goat, in the form of soup; vegetarians use spinach and other leafy green vegetables (Mahadevan, 1961). Sour and bitter potions are taken in Java (Geertz, 1961); in the Philippines, *tuba* (fermented sap of coconut palm), coffee, boiled sweet potato tops, cocoa and sugar porridge, meat and fish broth and stewed chicken are used by different groups. Clams and crabs are avoided in Leyte (Nurge, 1965), but not on Panay (Jocano, 1969). In Thailand, hot, sour and fermented foods are considered harmful during lactation (Hauck, Rajatasilpin, Ingrasud, Campbell and Thorangkul, 1958). Astringent fruits, tomatoes and green vegetables are avoided, but a soup of garlic and banana stems is believed to stimulate milk flow. In north China, it was customary to take pork fat and red gram, cuttlefish soup, shrimps' heads in wine and a special wine of glutinous rice together with blow-fly larvae (Jelliffe, 1968a); Cantonese mothers make a soup of fish heads, peanuts and papaya (Topley, 1973).

Because of the Indian belief in the nutritious quality of breast milk, solid supplements are considered unnecessary for the infant, and may not be introduced until well after eighteen months; thus the child has inadequate calories and nutrients from five or six months onwards. In northern India early supplements of cow and buffalo milk are considered useful, solid supplements coming later. Infants in Tamil Nadu, Mysore and Kerala receive a supplement of milk in very small amounts, grossly diluted with water 'to avoid causing indigestion' (Rao, Swaminathan, Swarup and Patwardhan, 1959). The water used for dilution may not have been boiled. In Kerala, only 10 per cent of mothers use supplements other than diluted milk.

In most Asian countries, breast milk is considered bad for a child once the mother becomes pregnant again, thus reducing the physiological strain on the mother. Women from rural areas of Kwangtung wean their infants abruptly, within one day, since they believe that milk not drawn from the breast deteriorates and is bad for the child (Topley, 1973). Rao *et al.* (1959) found that 20 per cent of the mothers studied in south India became pregnant within a year of giving birth; the infant therefore receives a weaning diet very low in protein.

If through sickness of the mother or her death, she cannot feed her child, it is not usually difficult to find a wet nurse. In northern Shensi, however, mothers prefer to use goat milk for an infant they cannot feed. Among the Ifugao in central Luzon, it is considered that a child would transfer its affections to the family of the wet nurse, so this arrangement is never adopted; such a child is inevitably doomed (Guthrie, G.M., 1964).

In most South-East Asian countries, faith in the nutritious qualities of rice is so great that it is introduced very early, often after the first few days of life. In Indonesia, however, many infants refuse it, and are not forced to accept supplements (Geertz, 1961). In Thailand, the feeding of glutinous rice from early days diminishes appetite for breast milk, thus leading to deficiency of protein and to widespread incidence of bladder stones (Valyasevi, Halstead, Pantuwatana and Tankayul, 1967). In south-central Java, maize pudding or mashed banana may be used with rice in the second week. In Leyte, the earliest supplements of mashed banana or congee are introduced at two months (Nurge, 1965). When a child can eat rice, the mothers believe that it has no further need of breast milk.

Many infant diseases in Asia are attributed to meat, milk, fish and eggs. Diarrhoea is, of course, frequently the result of eating contaminated food. In Malaya, however, fish are blamed for worm infestation (Dean, 1961; McArthur, 1962). In the Philippines and Laos, eggs are believed to cause toothache (Nurge, 1965; Demetrio, 1969; Olness, 1968), and mental illness (Demetrio, 1969). Korean mothers do not give their children eggs because it is feared these will make them talk late. In Telengana, India, eggs and meat are believed to cause jaundice and oedema, fruits, curds and buttermilk to be undesirable because they are cooling, and legumes to cause diarrhoea. Fruits, and even more vegetables, are considered bad for children in many parts of the region; not surprisingly such children grow up with a lifelong distaste for them.

There are few studies on the nutrition of adolescents. In Telengana protein foods are restricted for females during puberty; in Indonesia, cooling foods (many green, leafy vegetables and fruits) are considered harmful.

With the onset of sickness almost everywhere, both supernatural and naturalistic beliefs cause the. diet to be restricted to the staple with spices, and even the consumption of the staple may be reduced. Again, China and Japan may be exceptions.

CONCLUSION

It is clearly impossible to provide any firm guidelines regarding nutritional taboos during health and sickness for Asia as a whole, so great are the variations and so complex the multitude of belief systems by which countries and groups explain the phenomena and natural events that surround them in daily life. Certain common factors may tentatively be suggested.

Throughout Monsoon Asia, there is belief in the heating, cooling and other properties of food and their effect on the balance between the basic humours of the body, which dates back to the earliest Asian medical theories. Where rice is the staple, its nutritious qualities are believed to be superior to those of other foods. In the Indian subcontinent while wheat and rice are prestige foodgrains, the supreme food is milk, even though for most it is an insignificant part of the diet. Only where there has been great familiarity and positive experience with modern medical care, is 'western medicine' invariably the first resort in case of illness; more commonly, familiar local practitioners are called in first. Where modern medicines are accepted, traditional methods may also be used as an additional safeguard.

The most burdensome food taboos fall on pregnant and especially nursing mothers in the first weeks after birth. Laboratory analyses of the herbal potions used to stimulate milk flow are lacking. These would appear to increase the mineral and vitamin content of the diet if taken frequently, but only in China and Japan does tradition decree an increase in quality and quantity of protein intake at this time; even here, practice is likely to be affected by purchasing power. In China and Japan also, mothers generally provide small amounts of animal protein and vegetables in the weaning diets of their infants. Elsewhere in South-East Asia, animal protein foods are blamed for a host of childhood ailments. Even in India, only in the Punjab is it customary to provide undiluted milk after weaning.

This chapter can indicate only the broad outlines of a vast subject. The nutritionist, agricultural planner, doctor, home economist or anthropologist who is working in an Asian community for the first time will soon discover for himself an unexpected resistance to questions he may seek to answer, to new crops or food habits he may wish to introduce. Conversely, knowledge of a community's concept of health and correct nutrition will invariably reveal some useful beliefs which can be exploited to improve the status of an entire region.

7 Rural Economy and Poverty

TYPE OF RURAL ECONOMY

STANDARDS of nutrition among rural people can be related to their type of rural economy. Whether the cultivator is operating in a subsistence and/or barter economy or a marketing economy will obviously have a marked effect on the degree to which he may be self-sufficient in home-grown food, with or without the disposal of a surplus by barter or sale through a market.

A redefinition of the term 'subsistence' seems to be called for, at least in relation to nutrition. The term has traditionally excluded the use of money, and usually implies that the unit has no surplus for disposal. There must be very few people living in this type of economy in Asia at the present day. Even the most primitive peoples subsisting on the natural resources — hunting and gathering — operate a form of silent barter with the swidden communities surrounding them. With the spread of cash (monetized) economies and improvement in rural communications, many farm households are able both to meet their own staple requirements and, in some or all years, to dispose of a small surplus. Nonetheless many of these cannot strictly be regarded as regular components of a market economy. The proceeds from the sale of surplus farm produce enable the cultivator to purchase the rest of his needs locally, as well as the items which provide the side-dishes, the supplement to the staple, which he may not grow in sufficient amounts himself.

Wharton (1969b) has reviewed subsistence agriculture within the framework of economic development, bringing to light new theories and empirical evidence on the problem of changing from a subsistence to a commercial economy. Is the self-supporting unit in a subsistence economy the farm or the cultivator's family, or the village which provides essential services and labour at planting and harvesting?

If it is the individual farm household, does the term subsistence, meaning self-dependence, apply to all the family's needs, or only to some of them, particularly the staple? Clark and Haswell (1967) show that a prerequisite for the change from a subsistence to a market economy is the provision of transport, since the cost of rural transportation quickly absorbs profits from the sale of produce. Most rural cultivators sell their produce or barter it in their own village, unless they are within easy reach of a market town.

There have been few studies of the rural social units which operate in various combinations of subsistence/barter and cash economies. Examples are those of rice-growing villages in central Thailand (Table 7/1) and northern Thailand made by Janlekha (1955 and 1968).

Is the economy of Saraphi, in northern Thailand (Janlekha, 1968) more strongly subsistence-oriented? This community is in open forest with interspersed tracts of rice land and upland crops, very cold in winter by Thai standards, very hot in summer, without irrigation and suffering from water deficiency. Nearly three-quarters of the cultivated land is devoted to the production of the staple food — rice. This crop is important not for its exchange value but for its absolute value as food — both for immediate consumption and for security against hunger. In drought years, the farmers clear forest, grow upland crops, sell them profitably and achieve a better standard of living; when rains become more abundant, this land is abandoned and rice is grown again in the old fields, so that the people may be 'assured of their own food supply'. The rich are those who harvest more rice than the family needs, the poor are those who cannot grow enough rice to eat.

Again, many items have to be bought from outside the Saraphi community — dried fish for the preparation of fish sauce, chilli paste, salt, sugar, onion, garlic,

TABLE 7/1

Thailand: subsistence and purchased foods and other items in village

Subsistence Items	Purchased Items	
rice	*food:*	fish, fish sauce, shrimp paste, meat, coconut, onions, garlic, dried chilli, curry essence, limes, tamarind, palm sugar, white sugar, salt and cookies.
fish		
eggs		
fruit	*stimulants and beverages:*	dried areca, betel, lime, tobacco, tobacco binder, liquor and coffee, tea, lemonade, coca-cola, pepsi-cola.
vegetables		
	clothing	
	medicine	
	soap	
	fuel:	kerosene, matches. charcoal and firewood.

Source: Janlekha, 1955

clothing, kerosene, matches, household utensils, tools and equipment, school supplies and cure-all medicines. These are paid for by the export of cash crops from the land. The crop area is allocated as follows, in percentages: rice 73; maize 14; groundnuts 7; kenaf 2; castor 2. The gross income in baht per rai respectively is 187; 198; 370; 630; 362. To the traditional Thai farmer, it is inconceivable that rice growing might be discontinued in favour of a more remunerative crop. Rice is more than a mere commodity; it is food, the source of family security, the very basis for existence.

An average Saraphi family has a total annual cash income (1967) of 2,348 baht (one US$ = 20.8 baht) of which 1,362 baht is derived from farming and from farm wages earned outside the family farm. The family has annual living expenses of 2,630 baht, and to them must be added farm operating expenses, estimated at 570 baht. 'This excess of expenses over receipts appears to be inherent, persistent, and probably cumulative. The net result is debt and/or a low standard of living . . . the less affluent farmers are not only poor, but are actually getting poorer.'

It is hoped that there will be follow-up surveys of Saraphi, say at intervals of five years, and that these may give greater attention to human dietary patterns and standards of nutrition in relation especially to seasonal variations in adequacy and deficit of specific foods. It would be interesting to know whether C.A. Fisher's hopes regarding acceptance of innovation become obvious with the passage of time (Chapter 8).

If these situations are typical for a subsistence food-producing economy, what of the other rural peoples who do not own land, possibly beyond a small garden plot? What is the economic relation between the food producers and those who may be called the village artisans? Perhaps in most cases the artisan, whether resident in the village, nearby or migratory, receives payment in kind after each harvest for the work done throughout the year for the cultivator. This is particularly true in India, where specialization is more characteristic than elsewhere in Asia, and where the ironworker, blacksmith, basket weaver, washerman, barber and musician are still largely paid in grain. The owners of migrant sheep flocks that spend a few days manuring a stubble field of a settled cultivator will receive grain as payment for the sheep manure. Labour may be paid in kind, if it is not intended to repay with a similar period of labour. Within reach of centres of money economy, some of these services are beginning to be paid in cash, which is now of greater interest to the rural peoples. Larger bills, such as Rs.3,000 for a new cowshed for a well-to-do businessman-cum-farmer in a West Bengal village, is paid in cash.

Rural indebtedness to the money-lender is a major factor in some of the rural economies of Asia and has a marked effect on the standard of living and nutrition of the rural people. High figures for indebtedness to the banias of north India and the chettiars of south India and Malaysia are quoted, e.g. 40 per cent of the population of Bihar. The money-lender element in rural Java affects the willingness of subsistence farmers to accept innovation (Penny, 1966). Reviewing the contractual bases for mortgages and short-term leases in Ceylon, Leach (1961) states:

When *ukas* and *ande* contracts are examined individually the terms often seem excessively onerous; how can the cultivator possibly afford to pay such rates of interest? But seen in the larger context of contractual relations between affinal kin we see that the economic burdens of indebtedness tend to cancel out. What Peter owes to Paul, Paul, for some quite different reason, owes to Peter. The residue of the total pattern is not an impossible burden of debt, but an extremely dense mesh of reciprocal indebtedness which binds together not merely the members of a single village, but all the members of a single *variga* living within a few miles of one another.

The bases for the operation of the land contract system in Burma and for the borrowing of money from government or money-lenders are given by Nash (1965). Land reform had been introduced in some districts of Upper Burma before the date of writing; it is not known to what extent it has progressed further under the present régime. Nor whether the statements of Nash regarding the system of money-lending still apply:

Cultivators in Yadaw do not necessarily borrow all of their money from a single lender, but many tend to build up enduring credit relations with the same lender. The money-lenders are often active, and they seek out cultivators who need money for the roundabout rice production cycle. In most transactions the lender runs little risk. He knows the character of the borrower and his land, and the rice is virtually certain to come in. The lender gets his paddy before the cultivator gets his. Default is almost unknown then, and the activity of the lenders keeps interest rates at high, but competitive (given the 10-month period) rates.

EFFECTS OF URBAN MARKETS ON RURAL NUTRITION

Those who advise on economic policy for the rural areas strongly recommend the replacement of the subsistence and barter economies by a market economy. It is generally not a simple matter to effect this complete change in rural economy, and the method and rate at which it is introduced may have a marked effect on the nutritional standards of the rural people. When the urban areas in which the rural produce is to be marketed are surrounded by rural communities with a lower economic and therefore nutritional status, the robbing of rural areas of essential foods for immediate cash return will be evident (McArthur, 1962). In Tokushima Prefecture, Japan, the intakes of milk by dairy farmers, and of vegetables by vegetable farmers are low (Usutani *et al.*, 1971).

This situation is common in India, where large quantities of milk and eggs are siphoned off from rural areas within transportable distance of urban markets. For example, milk consumption per head in grammes per day in Gujarat is: upper class 400 to 500; lower class 60 to 70 (Rajalakshmi and Nanavaty, undated). From the same districts, the Kaira Milk Union collects some 500,000 litres per day for transport to Bombay or for manufacturing into baby foods, butter, cheese and other items for export and sale to the high-income groups in cities throughout India.

In the development of a market economy, it seems that this painful stage of transition and of actual deterioration in rural nutritional standards may be unavoidable and must be accepted. If the ultimate effect is to raise the economic status of the rural food producers, then they may in due course feel justified in holding back a percentage of the foods which they now sell, and their family's nutrition can rise to a higher level than heretofore. This is said to be happening in the Punjab, where the farmers were already relatively prosperous and there is a long tradition of milk drinking. With the introduction of high-yielding varieties of cereals and the consequent higher status of rural economies, marriage dowries have increased, status symbols such as radios, chairs and cosmetics are purchased. The urban milk-collecting centres have some difficulty in obtaining enough milk because it is held back for home consumption on the farms.

Roads and other methods of access from the rural producing community to the urban market are important, but improved access is not an unalloyed benefit. It also improves access from the urban areas to the villages, and exposes the rural peoples to the diverse merchandise, not often of higher nutritive value, and the consumer goods of the urban bazaars or the showcases of the itinerant traders. In the Philippines (Quiogue, 1966a), accessibility to centres of trade does not necessarily improve the quality of the diet. On the contrary, by introducing more foods, usually in a processed or refined form, the diet becomes so expensive that the food budget does not allow for purchase of sufficient amounts of the foods that can significantly improve the quality of the diet.

To what proportion of the population of Asia do Penny's conclusions (Penny and Thalib, 1969) regarding Indonesia apply? The short-term outlook is seen to be gloomy, and the long-term outlook is no better if present trends in production and population continue without change. Although Indonesia is not rich in untapped resources, opportunities for development have not yet been exhausted. But neither policymakers nor farmers nor any other group are sufficiently

TABLE 7/2

India: minimum requirements for an industrial working-class family

(father, mother and two children below the age of 14)

	Protein gm.	Fats gm.	Calcium mg.	Iron mg.		Calories	Vit. A i.u.	Vit. B_1 mg.	Vit. C mg.
Man	60	45	500	25		2816	3000	1·4	35
Woman	50	40	500	25		2150	3000	1·2	35
Children	80	65	1600	50	(0- 5 yr.) 1230		7000	2·2	60
					(6-14 yr.) 2110				

Source: Fonseca, 1968

aware of the severity of the problem. Indonesian farmers will continue to practise inefficient subsistence farming until they gain confidence in markets, and this will happen 'only after there has been a fundamental change in the economic, social and political relationships between farmers and non-farmers'.

The significance to a rural production area of an urban market necessarily depends upon the purchasing power and wage structure of the urban people. This should also be based upon an adequate and balanced diet for industrial workers and their families, who must purchase all their food (Fonseca, 1968). In India, since the ingredients for a formula for a balanced diet put forward by W.B. Aykroyd in 1948 were found in 1957 not to be available, a new set of total minimum requirements (Table 7/2) has now been suggested by the Nutrition Advisory Committee (Aykroyd and Patwardhan, 1960; Aykroyd, Gopalan and Balasubramanian, 1966; Rao, 1969).

The total cost of the cheapest foods which could be used to make up a balanced diet for a family of three adult equivalents is Rs.134.10 monthly (in 1968). If the expenditure on food (Table 7/3) represents 57.1 per cent of the total expenditure (according to Central Labour Bureau, Simla), then the need-based wage of workers in various important centres is (Indian Rupees): Bombay 234.85; Calcutta 240.48; Delhi 191.31; Ahmedabad 224.62 and Madras 180.99.

RELATIVE AND ABSOLUTE POVERTY

Poverty is a relative term which must be related to the national economy in which it occurs. The thresholds of poverty for farm families and other families, and the proportion of poor so defined in the population of the United States of America, are shown in Figs. 7/1(a) and (b). The number of Americans classified as poor decreased from 39.5 million in 1959 to 24.3 million in 1969. The poverty line in 1969 was U.S. $3,743 in annual income for a non-farm family of four. In 1959, 18.1 per cent of white families were classified as poor, in 1969 only 9.5 per cent; the proportions for non-white families fell from 56.2 to 31.0 per cent. Between 1959 and 1969, 5.3 per cent of the black poor moved upward out of poverty, but only 4 per cent of poor whites.

The Canadians define poverty as being not necessarily the same thing as starvation or malnutrition, but as meaning that people do not have access to the

TABLE 7/3

India: the prevailing consumption pattern for industrial workers in the western zone, including Bombay

(in gm.)

Cereals	Animal Food	Milk	Vegetables	Dhals	Sugar and Gur	Oils and Fat
435·44	32·8	83·34	147·42	52·44	43·37	30·6

Source: Fonseca, 1968

FIG. 7/1   Who is poor in the U.S.A., as defined by the Federal Government

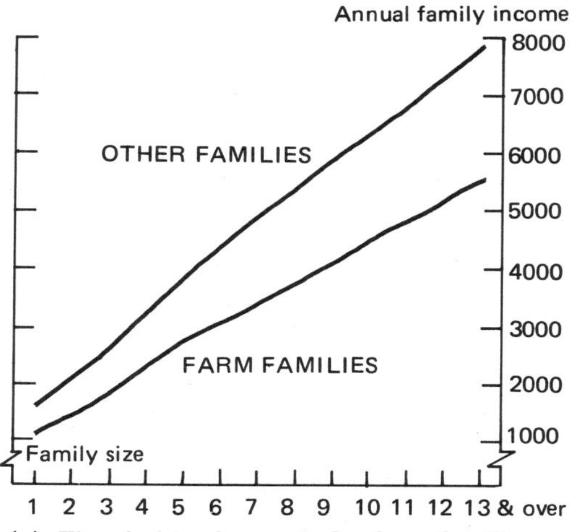

(a)   Thresholds of poverty for farm families and other families

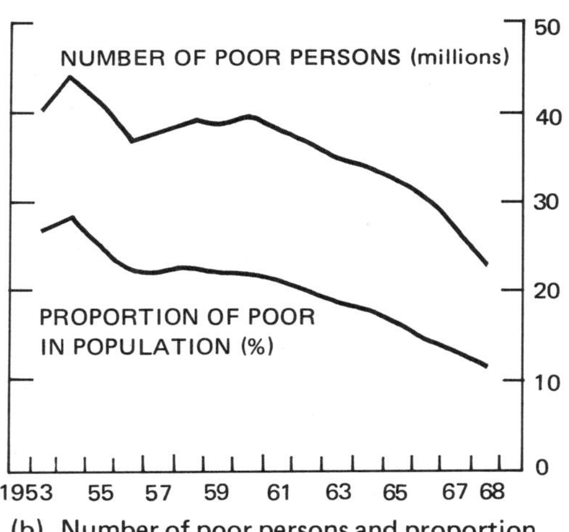

(b)   Number of poor persons and proportion of poor in population

Source: *The Economist*, London, 1 March 1969

kind of life available to everyone else, and which has come to be accepted as a decent minimum. By this definition, a family of five or more needs Canadian $5,000 per year and a single man $2,000 to live a good life. Of the population of 21 million, some 4.75 million do not achieve this standard. A possible short-term solution which has been suggested is a system of 'negative income tax', whereby persons below a certain income level would receive payments from the taxes paid by the upper three-quarters.

Harper (1968) told the Royal Society of Victoria, in Melbourne, Australia, of his survey made in 1967 of 4,000 people living over a wide area of that city. The threshold of poverty was defined as the point where the incomes of individuals or of families were less than Australian $33 per week. One person in fifteen in Melbourne is thus regarded as living in poverty; in families without a breadwinner the incidence is more like 30 per cent. Incidence of poverty rises as size of family increases — 80 per cent among these with four or more children.

The chronic and widespread rural poverty that is so characteristic of Monsoon Asia is completely different in degree and type, as some examples will show.

The rural income in the Philippines is an average of U.S. $15 a year (1964). A nutritional survey in Manila in 1961 showed that few families with an annual income below pesos 2,000 achieved diets which were even 80 per cent satisfactory. Those able to spend between 0.10 and 0.29 pesos per head per day had the lowest average diet rating (49.1 per cent of requirement); and the highest rating was attained at a daily expenditure on food of pesos 1.10 to 1.29 per caput (Philippines, FNRC, 1962). During anthropological work in a village in Pangasinan Province, data were collected on nutrient intakes in relation to socio-economic status (Wilson and Anderson, 1968). Lower-status families consume varieties of indigenous greens of low social status, but which contain substantial amounts of calcium, vitamin A and ascorbic acid, as well as lesser amounts of iron and the B vitamins. Diets of families of higher socio-economic status are deficient in these nutrients.

In a Malay kampong, Wilson (1967) found that household incomes ranged from Malayan $1 to $50 per day, tapping of the rubber trees being affected by the social and religious calendar as well as by rain. The average income for nine sample households in 1965 was M$ 3.45 per day; 24.92 per week and 99.68 per month. Households earning $30 per week generally have enough cash on hand to meet daily expenses. Those with less have often to live on short-term credit and occasionally to borrow. Those with above-average incomes tend not to budget in detail for each day, but to buy what they need when they need it. The poorer households often plan their work for the following day on the basis of what the wife calculates she is going to need in the way of food and other supplies. Apart from these regular daily expenditures, there are the periodic heavy expenditures for dowries and feasts. It is essential to have a large supply of cakes and sweetmeats for visitors, especially during Hari Raya Puasa. The ingredients — essence, eggs, flour, fruit, milk — are costly, and families also like to buy meat at this time. The house has to be thoroughly cleaned and broken furniture replaced. These burdens on the family budget come immediately after Ramadan; efficiency of work and therefore daily income fall markedly as the month of fasting progresses.

Firth (1966) calculated that, in a village of fishermen in the north-east of West Malaysia, a weekly expenditure per head of M$2.50 to 3.50 would maintain a reasonable standard of living. One family spent $3, and another $2. One villager calculated that 'if we only had M$700 a year, we could begin to eat comfortably'. This area of Malaysia has the lowest range of money incomes in the country, around M$600 per year. Half the population had one wage-earner with five dependents. The ratio in 1940 was only one-fifth of the whole having as many dependents.

A correspondent of the *Far Eastern Economic Review* (18 June 1970) states that Malay peasants, Chinese workers and Indian labour cannot earn even M$70 per month. The usual statement that every Malaysian worker is drawing from M$1,000 to 1,500 per annum is not correct.

An example of poverty in Thailand has been given (Saraphi). In the poor lands of north-east Thailand, the Thai Mobile Development Unit Program reports on the economic status of a village. The principal crop and staple is glutinous rice, 75 per cent of which is consumed in the north-east. Water is in short supply, groundwater often brackish, and soils saline. Only 4,000 of 14,000 villages have an adequate water supply. Under-employment is high, but few farmers are in debt. Monthly cash income of an average north-east Thai village family is, in 1966, 249 baht (US$12.45). Average annual income throughout the region is 910 baht (US$45.50), 2,503 baht in towns and 891 baht in villages. These north-eastern village incomes are only 65 per cent of those of villages in other parts of Thailand. Most villages have poor school facilities. Enteric diseases, malaria-induced diseases and vitamin deficiencies are widespread. One sample of 500 school children was entirely infested with intestinal parasites, and 90 per cent had two or more varieties. Babies are born fat and healthy, but gradually succumb to the environment. The villagers do not clean or cook food correctly, nor do they wash themselves adequately. Any change in the pattern of living, such as the raising of chickens, is resisted.

In the eleventh paper in his series on rural nutrition in Indonesia, Bailey (1962e) summarizes the nutritional problems in parts of Java. Because of excessive dependence on cassava as the staple foodstuff, hunger oedema (famine oedema) is endemic and protein intakes are extremely low. As throughout the tropics, so in Gunung Kidul, poverty is a limiting factor in the achievement of adequate nutritional standards. The natural resources of the land around Gunung Kidul are very limited; the poverty of the people, especially such a predominantly peasant population, can be related directly to the poverty of the soil. The limestone hill terrain is unsuitable for any form of agriculture. On the completely deforested and heavily eroded land (in 1850, *Albizia*, teak and other trees were still growing there), there are insuperable difficulties in maintaining water supplies and soil fertility, and in preventing soil erosion. Bailey states that economic development and industrialization would certainly help to prevent hunger oedema, by reducing unemployment and increasing purchasing power. Farmers could then retain more of their cash crops (groundnut and sorghum) and livestock products for home consumption. But the obstacles to industrialization are also enormous.

The Economic Department of the Reserve Bank of India (Ojha, 1970) argues that income inequality is an insufficient measure of levels of poverty in a society. Income inequality represents at best only the relative position of a household in the aggregate income hierarchy; such data cannot measure the absolute levels of poverty — this is a matter of actual facts. Thus a study was made on malnutrition in urban and rural areas, beginning 1960/1, in order to establish an 'Index of Poverty' (Table 7/4).

It has been calculated in India that Reference Man (see p. 73) requires about 2,250 calories per caput per day. In terms of food grain (cereals and grain legumes), this would represent 1,500 calories (66 per cent of total) for urban areas, and 1,800 calories (80 per cent of total) for rural areas, or a daily consumption of 432 gm. per caput for urban areas and 518 gm. for rural areas.

The actual consumption of foodgrains in quantitative terms for different expenditure groups is compared with the estimated norm; the shortfall in relation to the norm measures the level of poverty. The percentage of deficiency to the estimated norm (Table 2 in original paper) represents an index of *absolute* level of poverty. It is accepted that there may be deficiencies in respect of other consumer items as well. It is argued, however, that the deficiencies which exist in respect of items other than foodgrains may be considered 'tolerable' but not so the deficiencies in respect of foodgrains, particularly for the low expenditure groups.

TABLE 7/4

India: index of poverty: 1967/8

(Rural)

Levels of expenditure per caput per month (Rupees)	Foodgrain consumption per caput per day (gm.)	Nutritional norm per caput per day (gm.)	Nutritional deficiency		Population (millions)
			Quantity (gm.) (2-1)	Per cent (3 to 2)	
1. 11·83	252	518	−266	−51·4	20·6 (5)
2. 16·19	287	518	−231	−44·6	20·6 (5)
3. 20·25	337	518	−181	−34·9	41·3 (10)
4. 24·40	330	518	−188	−36·3	41·3 (10)
5. 30·49	379	518	−139	−26·8	82·6 (20)
6. 40·02	414	518	−104	−20·1	82·6 (20)
7. 49·96	471	518	− 47	− 9·1	41·3 (10)
8. 60·72)	481	518	− 37	− 7·1	82·6 (20)
9. 90·63)					
Total no. at poverty (1-6)					289·0 (70)

Note: Figures in brackets in last column are percentages to total rural population
Source: Ojha, 1970

The Reserve Bank finds that, of the total rural population of 355 million in 1960/1 (approximately 450 million in 1970/1) about 52 per cent were to be considered absolutely poor according to this measure. Subsequently the nutritional deficiency in the rural areas widened considerably, until in 1967/8, some 70 per cent of the rural people were at poverty levels, unable to purchase their *minimum* calorie requirements. It is possible, but debatable, that the green revolution may have subsequently halted this trend, temporarily and in certain favoured areas. But again, these conclusions apply to foodgrains and grain legumes, and not also to the special foods needed by the vulnerable groups to provide them with a 'tolerable' level of nutrition.

Subsequently Madalgi (1968) attempted to measure the magnitude of undernutrition in the different States of India, from 1960/1 to 1964/5, and to analyse the factors that contribute to it. There are not sufficient data to break down the analysis further to a district level. Since 90 per cent of the foodgrain consumption is of cereals, Madalgi measures undernutrition with reference to cereals only, and again according to a nutritional norm of 2,250 calories per day, to be obtained from the entire dietary range of cereals, grain legumes, sugar, fruit, meat, eggs, etc. It is estimated that cereal supplies give 1,575 calories per day, or 70 per cent of the norm in rural areas, thus 445 gm. cereal per caput per day.

It is important to know the areas where undernutrition is widespread, so that planning efforts may be directed there. The main causes of undernutrition are low cereal yields, low cereal area per caput, and high percentage of landless labourers to agricultural population. The undernutrition is due partly to lack of purchasing power, and partly to shortage of foodgrains.

Data for the urban and rural areas of East Pakistan (now Bangladesh), for nutrient intake in relation to levels of income, are given in Table 7/5.

Lack of protein in the Indian diet is not always the cause of protein deficiency, but rather that protein is diverted to provide energy in a diet deficient in sources of energy. The total incidence of protein deficiency arising from inadequate intake of energy has been estimated at 40 per cent in Tamil Nadu, and 70 per cent in Bihar (Sukhatme, 1970). The incidence of protein deficiency in India is seen as an indication of inadequate total food intake, the critical factor being energy.

TABLE 7/5

East Pakistan (now Bangla Desh): food consumption surveys—nutrient intakes by income level
(per person per day)

	Calories (No.)	Protein Total (g.)	Animal (%)	Fat (g.)	Carbo-hydrate (g.)	Calcium (mg.)	Iron (mg.)	Vita-min A (i.u.)	Thia-mine (mg.)	Ribo-flavine (mg.)	Niacin (mg.)	Ascor-bic acid (mg.)
RURAL—Rupees/Month/Average	2,251	57·5	7·9	13·7	17·7	—	304	9·7	1,590	1·47	0·53	22·8	39·6
0-99	1,996	49·6	—	—	16·9	411	169	7·5	1,850	1·25	0·38	19·7	34·5
100-199	2,258	57·7	—	—	18·8	465	300	9·7	1,532	1·44	0·48	20·8	40·3
200-299	2,396	64·3	—	—	20·0	490	313	9·8	1,331	1·51	0·50	24·3	37·4
300-399	2,656	69·4	—	—	26·9	534	332	10·7	1,891	1·62	0·62	25·3	45·0
400-499	2,642	70·7	—	—	26·8	530	472	10·7	594	1·64	0·65	26·8	31·2
500 and above	—	72·3	—	—	24·6	637	457	12·0	947	1·85	0·62	28·5	36·1
URBAN—Rupees/Month/Average	1,777	49·7	12·1	24·3	26·1	—	239	8·7	1,875	1·05	0·55	14·6	40·5
0-99	1,549	41·2	—	—	14·8	313	156	7·0	1,337	1·03	0·40	11·6	27·2
100-199	1,751	48·6	—	—	20·2	342	195	7·7	2,026	1·25	0·55	14·0	40·0
200-299	1,722	48·8	—	—	23·5	329	228	9·8	1,745	1·02	0·55	14·0	44·2
300-399	1,812	50·3	—	—	26·2	344	252	8·2	1,744	1·02	0·54	14·6	41·0
400-499	1,805	50·2	—	—	35·0	322	232	8·2	1,441	0·95	0·57	12·8	36·2
500 and above	1,840	54·1	—	—	38·0	320	284	9·8	2,183	1·04	0·67	18·4	41·8

Source: Pakistan, Ministry of Health, 1966

ECONOMIC STATUS AND NUTRITION

The economic status of a population has until recently been expressed as the individual share of the gross domestic or national product per head per unit of time. These figures do not express accurately the relation between purchasing power and rural nutrition, partly because the method of their calculation does not distinguish between urban and rural communities, nor between those working or employed in industrial and agricultural enterprises. In even stronger terms, Galbraith (1970) states that the day of the G.N.P. is over, that a rising G.N.P. does not reliably improve well-being and can be positively damaging, that there will have to be accommodation to a low or zero rate of growth and that the adjustments will include the acceptance of the notion that countries with lower living standards need a higher growth rate than those with higher living standards.

We probably need comparisons like that made by the Ministry of Agriculture and Forestry in Japan, which finds that the standard of living of Japanese farmers is fast approaching that of urban dwellers. The consumption level of farming households in 1967 rose to 156.7 in terms of the overall national consumer index (against the base figure of 100 for 1960). This represents a 9 per cent rise over 1966, compared with a 5.4 per cent rise for city dwellers. In the fiscal year 1967, Japanese farmers and fishermen enjoyed a postwar record increase of 21.5 per cent in their in-

come, although the income was less for those situated far from the major urban centres (see end of Chapter).

The relation between purchasing power and standards of nutrition may be expressed most accurately in surveys of individual communities, showing acreage, monthly income of different socio-economic groups, and family expenditure on food and other items. A few examples are given in the appendix. Another method is followed in India and other countries, where the different socio-economic groups of the whole population, urban and rural, are placed in categories according to average income. The Indian Council of Medical Research (1968) recognizes six income groups, and notes the numerically predominant occupations within each group:

1.   Steady and assured income of over Rs. 1000 (one U.S. $ = Ind. Rs. 7.50) considered adequate to provide for a healthy way of life:

(a) Civil Service — all government officials and employees of local or autonomous bodies with a basic salary of Rs. 1,000 per month or more.

(b) Defence services.

(c) Commercial — industrial magnates, managing directors and directors of large firms and their senior employees, and businessmen with a net profit of over Rs. 1,000 per month.

(d) Artistes — actors, musicians, dancers and allied professions.

(e) All others, including members of former Princely States, zamindars and proprietors with income of similar degree.

2. Income per month of Rs. 500 to Rs. 1000, comprising younger members of the above occupational categories, persons who can with some effort achieve reasonably good nutritional and health standards provided they take full advantage of the knowledge within their reach. This section of the community generally represents the upper middle class of Indian society.

3. Income per month between Rs. 200 and Rs. 500. Families in this group may just be able to maintain a satisfactory standard of living by judicious management of their income. The occupational categories of these lower class families are:

(a) the most junior members in Government services;

(b) junior members of the professions who have just started their careers;

(c) headmasters of high schools, university lecturers and readers;

(d) all other members of non-government services;

(e) members of various trades;

(f) defence personnel of lower ranks.

4. Income per month less than Rs. 200, for persons for whose employment certain basic educational qualifications are imperative. For classes (4) and (5) a distinction is made between families living in urban areas and villages. Families living in villages generally do not have the same facilities with regard to environmental conditions and health services; these are therefore down-graded by one step. In other words, a family from class 4 is taken into 5 it if happens to live in an underdeveloped rural area. Occupations in class 4: clerical staff, inspectors, teachers, tax collectors, mechanics and technicians, cashiers, commercial artists, telephone operators, telegraphists, compounders, nurses, vaccinators, supervisors.

5. Income per month between Rs. 100 and Rs. 200 for persons whose occupation does not necessarily require any educational qualifications; includes all skilled workers and artisans.

Occupations in class 5: tailors, carpenters, painters, modellers, smiths, bakers, drivers, shop assistants, petty traders, constables, non-commissioned defence personnel, linesmen, pointsmen, potters, barbers, dhobies.

6. Income per month less than Rs. 100
All agricultural or other unskilled labourers, fishermen, tappers, gardeners, domestic or other servants. See also table 1 of Madalgi (1968) giving distribution of population — rural and urban — by expenditure for all States in India; his categories of expenditure per caput per month in the rural areas are Rs. 15 or less; between Rs. 15 and 34; and Rs. 34 and above.

A classification by income level, but without breakdown into occupations, has been provided for the Philippines by A.B. Santos. Seven out of every ten Filipino families have an income below US$620 per year, two out of ten (the middle class) have an

TABLE 7/6

Calories provided by nutrients as percentage of total calories, according to
gross domestic product per caput in 1962

	GDP per caput per year	Calories	Separated edible fats	Unsep. vegetable fats	Unsep. animal fats	Sugar	Vegetable proteins	Animal proteins
Japan	521	2230	5·3	5·8	3·6	7·1	9·4	3·0
Malaysia	192	2336	10·0	2·4	4·5	10·6	6·4	2·6
Taiwan	170	2400	4·9	3·3	7·1	7·4	7·4	2·3
Philippines	152	1875	4·6	4·3	5·6	6·7	6·4	3·0
Sri Lanka	138	2049	4·8	12·3	1·7	9·9	7·1	1·7
Thailand	112	2127	1·7	8·3	4·1	1·9	6·8	2·0
India	86	1977	6·3	4·8	1·7	2·9	9·5	1·1
Pakistan	80	1940	5·7	2·5	3·8	1·3	7·7	1·8
South Korea	65	2209	0·6	4·7	1·5	0·9	10·7	1·1

Source: Périssé, Sizaret and François, 1969

income of up to US$1,222 per year, while one family in every ten is in the high income bracket of US$1, 250 and above. Of all families, only 2.5 per cent or 130,000 people have an annual income of over US$2,500, sharing 21 per cent of the total income. The middle income group is said to be increasing, and now represents 28 per cent of the total number of families.

No doubt other countries of the region have made similar analyses, or they may be available. A regional study by competent specialists would be of great value in providing a picture of the important economic bases for greater food production and improved nutrition of rural peoples. An approximation to such a study is FAO's Food Consumption Surveys (1970c), of which vol. 1A deals with household food consumption by economic groups in Sri Lanka, Hong Kong, India, Japan, Pakistan, Philippines, Taiwan, Thailand and South Vietnam. The Surveys included all studies taken on a sufficiently large scale, nation-wide wherever possible, providing information on food consumption of the population classified by income, total expenditure or some other indicator of economic status. Such surveys are acceptable to the extent to which reliance can be placed on national statistics, particularly from the rural areas (Table 7/6).

RESPONSES TO ECONOMIC PROGRESS

While there has been much discussion of the economic effects of malnutrition, little is so far known of the economic impact of the elimination of malnutrition in a population in which this condition was previously endemic. Although there is talk of an economic take-off in Taiwan, South Korea and certain other countries, it will be some time before the effects will be seen in the rural areas. Economic take-off affects the rural areas first, by increasing urban purchasing power for surplus foods from the rural areas, so stimulating increased production, and second, by providing employment in the urban areas for surplus or under-employed rural labour, thus stimulating more efficient and mechanized production of food by a smaller and better-off rural labour force.

It is therefore to Japan that one should look for concrete examples of the effects of improved nutrition on the people and so on the economy as a whole. The structural transformation of the Japanese economy in the 1950s was reflected in the beginning of the absolute decline in the agricultural labour force, in geographic shifts of population, and in the emergence of highly sophisticated industrial complexes. This transformation coincided with radical changes in food consumption patterns. As the level of income grew

TABLE 7/7

Japan: change of nutrient intake per caput per day average

	1961	*1965*	*1971*
Calories	2102	2184	2287
Protein (total) (gm.)	70·0	71·3	78·1
(animal)	25·3	28·5	34·7
(vegetable)	44·7	42·8	43·5
Fat (gm.)	25·8	36·0	48·7
Carbohydrate (gm.)	398	384	378
Calcium (mg.)	404	465	523
Vitamin A (i.u.)	1183	1324	1457
Thiamine (mg.)	1·05	0·97	1·12
Riboflavine (mg.)	0·79	0·83	0·91
Vitamin C (mg.)	73	78	108
Calories from foodgrains (percentage)	70·5	64·7	55·0
Animal protein (percentage of total protein)	36·1	40·0	44·4

Source: Japan, Health and Welfare Ministry, 1972

rapidly, the institutional and technological framework of life also changed. Under these circumstances, a drastic transformation took place in methods of food preparation and patterns of food consumption (Kaneda, 1967).

The Nutrition Section of the Public Health Bureau of the Ministry of Health and Welfare has published (Japan: Health and Welfare Ministry, 1972), a comparison of changes in nutrient intakes over the years 1961 to 1971. These have been considered on a national basis (Table 7/7) and in relation to urban and rural communities and economic status (Table 7/8). (See also Chapter 13 under Japan.)

Improvement in economic status over the decade is revealed by the rising consumption of animal protein and a corresponding decrease in intake of carbohydrate, involving consequential improvement in the intake of all major nutrients.

A comparison of nutrient intakes in rural and urban areas shows the same proportional improvements over the ten-year period 1961-71, with the quality of rural diets still lagging behind those of urban areas. It should be stressed that these are average figures, masking the great differences which exist within both rural and urban areas throughout Japan.

In a study of the increase in average birth weights following the improvement of economy and health in Japan (Gruenwald, Funakawa, Mitani, Nishimura and Takeuchi, 1967), birth weight in relation to gestational age over a 20—year period from the records of three large obstetric services was considered. This covered not only the years of recovery from war-time deprivation, but also the period when there was an increase in birth weights over pre-war levels. The duration of pregnancy is not longer, but foetal growth curves show a striking increase, especially during the latter part of the third trimester of pregnancy. This is attributed to the marked effect of socio-economic factors.

A survey by the Tokyo Metropolitan Government Health Bureau on babies aged from 2 months to children 5 years of age shows that the average heights of boys and girls aged 7 to 8 months are now 69.7 and 67.9 cm. respectively, 1.2 cm. taller than babies of the same age ten years ago. Their average weights are 9.2 and 9.1 kg., respectively, 0.3 and 0.4 kg. more than their counterparts ten years ago. Babies are weaned

TABLE 7/8

Japan: change of nutrient intake of farming and urban communities:
average per caput per day

	Farmer families		Urban families	
	1961	1971	1961	1971
Calories	2194	2285	2042	2290
Protein (total) (gm.)	68·8	75·5	70·8	79·5
(animal)	20·5	30·3	28·6	36·4
(vegetable)	48·3	45·2	42·2	43·1
Fat (gm.)	21·8	41·4	28·6	51·4
Carbohydrate (gm.)	431·2	394·3	375·5	371·6
Calcium (mg.)	401	492	405	535
Vitamin A (i.u.)	1121	1288	1330	1521
Thiamine (mg.)	1·01	0·87	1·08	1·12
Riboflavine (mg.)	0·77	0·83	0·81	0·93
Vitamin C (mg.)	69	96	76	112
Calories from foodgrains (percentage)		59·8		53·2
Animal protein (percentage of total protein)	29·8	40·1	40·4	45·5

Source: Japan, Health and Welfare Ministry, 1972

five months after birth, two months earlier than ten years ago.

These responses to improved economic conditions are not seen among farmers and poor rural communities in remote areas. For example, in Gifu Prefecture (Noguchi and Nonomura, 1970), the diet is inadequate considering the hard work and severe climate — intake is 40 per cent below standard, with little total protein or animal protein. In Aichi Prefecture, farmers, part-time farmers and non-farmers in remote villages (Goto, Takeuchi, Yamaguchi, Sasaki, Oszawa, Toda, Masuda and Niwa, 1969) have little egg, milk or meat, soya products, green or yellow vegetables, fruit, oil or fat; their diets are therefore deficient in protein of animal origin, calcium, vitamin A, thiamine, riboflavine and vitamin C.

In India, the National Institute of Nutrition has made anthropometric measurements of schoolchildren in high and low income groups, by age and sex (Table 7/9). Among both boys and girls, there were differences in height and weight in the two groups at the age of 6. Among girls, these became most marked at the ages of 11 and 12, and tended to diminish by the age of 17. Among boys, the greatest differences were found at the ages of 13 and 14, decreasing only slightly thereafter. (See also Boyne, Aitken and Leitch (1957) for comparable studies in Great Britain.) Some 6,500 Indian children from families with incomes over Rs. 1,000 per month had heights and weights similar to those of American children between 5 —14 years (boys) and 5 — 12 years (girls).

The impact of an Applied Nutrition Program on the nutritional status of selected expectant mothers and their infants (Devadas, Shenbagavalli and Vijayalakshmi, 1970) may be taken as an indication of a probable response to improved economic conditions. The effect was expressed most markedly in increased birthweights, head circumference and chest and abdomen measurements of the infants. After four years, an Applied Nutrition Project in Bayambang, Philippines, had raised the nutrient intake of the entire community, but had not brought about the intended amelioration specifically in the diets of the vulnerable groups (Bulato-Jayme, Villegas and Miranda, 1970).

The severe calorie deficiency noted in Nepal is not characteristic of an entire village, but only of a small number within villages (Worth and Shah, 1969). It is especially prominent in villages where a significant proportion of the families are wage earners rather than subsistence farmers. 'One may conclude that in times of normal harvest, calorie deficiency is related to socio-economic status, is more likely found among those who are wage-earners, and is seldom seen among subsistence farmers except for those of lowest caste, and even there it is an infrequent phenomenon.'

The nutritional status of children of resettlement villagers growing kenaf is superior to that of children of traditional rice cultivators in Thailand (Thurnam, Migasena, Vudhivai and Supawan, 1971). The former must buy all foods and are prepared to spend a little on meat and to grow vegetables. The latter do not purchase rice, and find vegetable-growing a burden.

Agrarian development may introduce new problems of health, for example in the endemicity of disease following the construction of dams in northeast Thailand (Harinasuta, Jetanasen, Impand and Maegraith, 1970).

NUTRIMETRICS

A new discipline within nutritional research, nutrimetrics, proposed by the Nutrition Division of FAO, is based on the possibilities opened up for mathematical statistical analysis, once data of food consumption have been collected on a sufficiently large scale to find statistical regularities or models (François, 1969a). Nutrimetrics is defined as the statistical and mathematical measure of the food intake and nutritional levels of large numerical sets, whether integrated in a socio-economic context or otherwise. Lörstad (1971) has evolved a basic model from which it is possible to predict the proportion of deficiency in any nutrient if the distribution of individual consumption and requirement are known. Further collaboration between statisticians and nutritionists may lead to a more sophisticated model capable of taking other factors into account.

To what degree do the rural peoples of Asia live in a money economy? For people who do, and for those for whom money has already made a break in the traditional economy, the income factor can account for many changes in the structure of the diet. In a study covering 85 countries in Europe, the Americas, Africa, Asia and Oceania, with a total of 1,880 million inhabitants in 1962, an attempt has been made to determine the general trends of consumption patterns as a function of income (Périssé, Sizaret and Francois, 1969). The conclusion is: (see also Table 7/6).

the gradual restructuring of the diet as a function of income appears to be a general phenomenon. However, each country moves in this direction from features basic to it, and which reflect its dietary heritage.

TABLE 7/9

India: anthropometric measurements of school children in different socio-economic groups

A. *High income group (showing mean and standard deviation)*

Males					Females		
Height *cm.*	*Weight* *kg.*	*No.*	*Age*	*No.*	*Height* *cm.*	*Weight* *kg.*
96·86 ± 4·46	14·21 ± 1·54	45	3	130	94·75 ± 4·72	13·50 ± 1·84
103·82 ± 6·46	16·21 ± 2·62	35	4	181	101·71 ± 5·83	15·08 ± 2·09
112·13 ± 4·85	18·34 ± 2·26	39	5	231	107·72 ± 5·87	16·48 ± 2·10
116·14 ± 5·14	20·45 ± 3·02	48	6	251	113·16 ± 5·88	18·04 ± 2·61
123·13 ± 5·03	22·65 ± 3·78	66	7	232	118·92 ± 6·19	19·98 ± 2·78
126·71 ± 12·36	24·26 ± 3·86	96	8	240	124·23 ± 6·36	22·03 ± 3·05
132·16 ± 6·17	27·19 ± 4·10	94	9	252	129·59 ± 7·05	24·51 ± 3·83
136·81 ± 5·97	28·57 ± 3·51	93	10	194	135·19 ± 6·83	27·53 ± 4·95
143·50 ± 7·05	32·89 ± 5·92	97	11	271	141·23 ± 7·63	31·34 ± 5·95
147·34 ± 7·32	35·14 ± 6·19	101	12	287	146·92 ± 7·09	35·25 ± 6·63
154·04 ± 7·84	40·25 ± 7·19	82	13	245	150·38 ± 6·31	37·97 ± 6·36
158·32 ± 7·97	44·89 ± 7·73	80	14	183	152·82 ± 5·56	41·36 ± 6·63
164·06 ± 7·39	49·54 ± 6·67	66	15	116	153·80 ± 5·71	42·50 ± 6·12
167·70 ± 7·67	53·63 ± 10·54	36	16	103	155·13 ± 5·42	42·94 ± 5·57
173·90 ± 6·97	56·89 ± 7·59	7	17	58	154·29 ± 5·08	43·72 ± 6·20

B. *Low income group (showing mean and standard error)*

Males					Females		
Height *cm.*	*Weight* *kg.*	*No.*	*Age*	*No.*	*Height* *cm.*	*Weight* *kg.*
105·40 ± 0·6069	15·16 ± 0·1923	102	6	46	102·33 ± 0·6091	14·22 ± 0·2401
112·18 ± 0·5467	16·95 ± 0·1944	111	7	72	109·17 ± 0·6180	16·19 ± 0·2194
116·51 ± 0·5059	18·38 ± 0·1856	123	8	56	116·31 ± 0·8368	18·14 ± 0·2791
121·77 ± 0·5530	20·28 ± 0·2397	118	9	55	121·49 ± 0·7878	20·30 ± 0·3662
126·98 ± 0·5646	22·34 ± 0·2605	102	10	91	128·35 ± 0·6949	23·29 ± 0·3671
129·99 ± 0·5766	23·76 ± 0·3175	107	11	87	131·44 ± 0·8006	24·72 ± 0·4650
135·15 ± 0·6072	25·98 ± 0·3445	127	12	108	136·95 ± 1·0969	28·44 ± 0·4765
139·66 ± 0·7824	28·68 ± 0·4502	81	13	86	142·95 ± 0·7455	31·85 ± 0·5276
144·00 ± 0·9795	30·61 ± 0·5920	63	14	83	146·82 ± 0·5892	35·98 ± 0·4374
153·04 ± 1·1745	37·32 ± 0·8302	47	15	69	148·01 ± 0·6345	37·10 ± 0·6378
156·35 ± 1·0374	40·01 ± 0·8439	47	16	53	149·10 ± 0·6564	38·87 ± 0·6249
158·53 ± 1·5761	43·75 ± 1·5471	12	17	14	154·69 ± 1·6480	40·89 ± 0·9990

Source: India, National Institute of Nutrition, 1969

The speed of the evolutionary process will depend, on the national level, on the rate at which per caput income rises, but the prime movers in this evolution will be those classes which, particularly as a result of urbanization, will enter a market economy and acquire wider freedom of choice of foods.

This contribution to the methodology of the FAO Indicative World Plan has been extended to a study of the effects of income projection on the protein structure of the diet (Francois, 1969b) as applied to a theoretical low-income rice and livestock-producing country, more especially as an examination of protein consumption among the rural people as a function of income. This highly complex statistical study shows that the most immediate solution should involve a combination of dietary safeguards through education, development of new foods capable of integration within the traditional subsistence farming patterns, and action to promote the greater use of high-yielding varieties of high nutritive value.

CONCLUSION

In money terms the middle, and even the upper middle class incomes of rural Asia do not reach the threshold between poverty and sufficiency recognized in the developed countries. A rural community far from markets is poor if it cannot provide a reasonable living and a minimal effective diet to all members of its families, according to their needs and to the locally accepted standards of housing, clothing and general amenities. The objective of the members of a rapidly increasing population living on a static or declining land resource is to try to achieve and maintain the standards of their forbears. The more the rural people come under the influence of marketing centres and urban demands, the more the money factor enters into the rural economies, both for selling produce to the markets, and for buying the merchandise to be found in the markets. The main problem of rural economies in Asia is, however, how to increase the purchasing power of that 80 to 85 per cent representing the rural part of a total population around 2,000 million. If people with an increased purchasing power can be educated to appreciate the meaning of good nutrition, then their mental and physical capacity and energy will be increased. Greater production and purchase of better foods would become possible, again within the limits which the environment permits.

But in the meantime, there is widespread poverty of land, and of man himself as an economic resource, due to poor nutrition and loss of health, provoking that indolence and apathy for which the Asian is so incomprehendingly blamed. Myrdal's conclusion to *Asian Drama* (1968) is that, in the underdeveloped countries of Asia, levels of living are so low as seriously to impair health, vigour and attitude towards work. Any significant increases in most types of consumption represent at the same time 'investment, as they have an immediate and direct effect on productivity'. The indicators of standards of living adopted by Myrdal are: food and nutrition, clothing, housing, including sanitation, health facilities, information media, energy consumption and transportation. But in all these respects, only general and tentative conclusions can be drawn because of the total absence or unreliability of statistics.

Autret and Paul-Pont (1971) describe how planning, 'that new deity of the developing countries', is to be introduced into family life through an educational programme which aims at providing opportunities for families to plan for a balance between their present and future needs and their available and potential resources, on the following lines of progress: improved diet ⋯ improved nutrition ⋯ lower infant and pre-school mortality ⋯ lightening of family burdens ⋯ parental motivation to seek a better future for surviving children ⋯ family planning ⋯ quality of life. This Planning for Better Family Living Programme was introduced to the First Asian Congress of Nutrition, Hyderabad, India, January 1971 (Boerma, 1971):

If the quality of life means anything, it means that human beings everywhere have the food they need to keep them in good health. This, to be sure, is in large part an economic question. But it is also much more than that. People have to be educated in the kinds of food that they and their children need. They can be educated too, in ways of producing more of this food at minimal expense. Since the population explosion was triggered by a fall in death rates, it may seem curious to suggest that improved nutrition — which would save even more lives, especially among young children — could help in solving the problem. But there is definite evidence that it could. For the continued thrust of the population explosion is far less due than is often supposed to ignorance or lack of contraceptive methods. The fact is that a large number of people, especially in primitive societies largely bereft of social security systems, *want* to have more children than either they or society can afford in order to be sure that at least one or two survive. Quite clearly, then, if measures were taken to greatly increase the assurance of survival of, say, the first two children as a result of better nutrition, the parents would feel much less necessity to have further children, and would accordingly be far more psychologically receptive to the ideas and methods of family planning.

8 Tradition and Acceptance of Change

RESPONSE TO CHANGE

PERHAPS nothing is more daunting to the advisory officer, full of good will and helpful ideas, than a sluggish response or downright hostility, for no reason he can discern, to the benefits he promises. It is beginning to be realized that change cannot be introduced by outsiders who are urban-oriented and have little conception of rural ecology, psychology or poverty. Change is best introduced by someone whose shrewdness the rural people admire. This is almost always someone from their own community, as discussed under 'Innovators' below. These leaders of opinion closely resemble other villagers, but for different reasons they are able or prepared to take just a little more risk than the others. A new idea or technique must be seen by the rural people to be good, reasonable and to their advantage. Their targets are family targets; national targets of planning authorities are without meaning for them. The urban-trained adviser and the rural cultivator have completely different values in terms of time, attachment to the land and prestige, and set quite different values on movable possessions. Thus the advisory officer first needs to identify local leaders of opinion and convince them of the value of his innovations.

There is a conviction that rural people are apathetic to change involving the introduction of new techniques, new crops and new foods. Yet the cultivators have for centuries adapted their methods to the changing environment, absorbed different techniques from newcomers, and changed their foods when necessary. The dry-land and swidden cultivator has constantly to adapt his crops and field methods to a deteriorating environment. When soil fertility falls progressively, he has to change to different, less demanding crops in order to keep his family fed. The success of the high-yielding varieties on 10 to 15 per cent of the cultivated area of Asia has been possible because of their acceptance by relatively advanced cultivators on the best land, who had already invested their limited capital in irrigation pumps, field machinery, seeds of new varieties, fertilizers and plant protection material. These cultivators see the high-yielding varieties as being merely a further stage in the economic development of their enterprises.

Experience from the Comilla project in former East Pakistan led to the conclusion that if the farmer believed that the new agricultural technology would work, if he could market the increased crop, if credit were assured, he would invest the necessary effort. If, however, he distrusted local government, he would resist change, because he believed it would bring no advantage to him and his family (Blair, 1971).

It is sometimes believed that technological change in the rural areas is an unmitigated benefit to the rural people. This is not always so. When new access roads change cropping patterns or provide new markets to rural communities, only rarely does their nutrition improve; quite frequently it deteriorates. A green revolution may increase yields of wheat or rice per hectare, but is too often accompanied by increased rural unemployment due to more mechanization. Schemes for dairy, pig or poultry development may greatly increase the production of animal protein, but little remains in the rural areas which have learned and adopted the new techniques involved. Factors of human ecology and the welfare of rural people must always be considered in economic plans designed to improve urban living standards.

There is a growing literature on experience in introducing change (Nash, 1966; Moerman, 1968; Wharton 1969b). The few examples which follow relate to response to change in agricultural methods and diet.

In July/August 1969, a joint United Nations Development Program/FAO mission reviewed the agricultural work of the Mekong Committee in Thailand,

Laos, Cambodia and Vietnam, with special reference to the programmes of research, demonstration and training (FAO, 1969c). An inspection was made at the Eakhat Agricultural Experiment Station, Banmethuot, Vietnam. The agronomist on the mission, G. Perrin de Brichambaut, decided that an irrigation system is not justified in this area:

The 'montagnards', shifting cultivators, are not psychologically prepared to accept such a sophisticated system of agriculture which is the opposite of their actual way of life and cultivation. They will not show any interest in the proposal because they are able to realize that the new systems will be expensive for crops which they can now grow with God's water. They are far from being interested in continuous cropping and they certainly want to keep the opportunity to go hunting or fishing in the dry season. A preliminary survey would probably demonstrate that, if such a project is started, a large part of the population will move a bit further into the forest.

The agronomist recommends that a study should be made of the montagnard group, to try to understand their way of life and the reasons for their methods of cultivation. Then it might be possible to decide whether to start with social or economic development in the improvement of their lot.

Indigenous people still constitute the majority of the population of the Moluccas. They live in 'primitive affluence', having plenty of land and sufficient food from the sago palm. In terms of rupiah, their income is low, but they seldom suffer shortage and need little effort to satisfy their needs. Few are therefore willing to change their traditional way of life, to produce beyond their requirements for subsistence, or to seek employment at a wage (Burhamzah, 1970).

Transmigrants from Java have been shipped to the wholly different environment of South Kalimantan, to farm poor-quality soil in the traditional Javanese way. Inevitably many fail and drift away. Out of five areas designated as transmigration areas since 1959, only one is now officially regarded as developed, and four as 'retarded'. The reasons given officially are lack of pioneering spirit, incapacity to adjust to the new environment, and lack of perseverance. In the wilderness of South Kalimantan, the opening up of land to obtain a better living is a challenging venture indeed. Merciless mosquitoes, poisonous snakes, the blazing sun, frightening torrents of rain and other scourges of nature are severe tests for all but the most rugged individuals (Partadiredja, 1970).

However, in reviewing the Saraphi project in Thailand (Chapter 7), Fisher (1969) sees the emergence of a readiness among the villagers to make significant changes in established agricultural and other practices, when it has been demonstrated that such changes are both practicable and economically beneficial. In parts of the developing world, the vicious spiral of poor land, poor health and poor farming has gone on for so long as to induce a degree of apathy, which constitutes a built-in resistance to innovation. This is not seen to be so in Saraphi: 'It is because there are so many other areas which resemble it in this respect that this study is of vital importance far beyond the bounds of north-eastern Thailand'.

ENVIRONMENT AND INNOVATION

The priorities assigned to research in south-east Asia by the U.S. Agricultural Development Council are relevant (Wharton, 1965). Attention is to be focused upon the 'motivational and attitudinal variables in so far as they affect the processes of production and development, farmers' goals of production, decision-making processes, and the influence and patterns of diffusion of change on the adoption of new practices and enterprises'.

It is perhaps not always recognized that many, if not most Asian cultivators are professionals within their own indigenous limits. They are accustomed to making those environmental and agronomic decisions which may mean the difference between sufficiency and starvation, even between life and death, for their families. In the main, they succeed, under conditions of climate, soil, standard of living and nutrition that would baffle their British and American counterparts. But can they see any good reason for greater effort of their tired and under-nourished bodies, any more than a New Zealand dairy farmer can see any good reason for increasing his total production of milk to full potential when most of the proceeds will go to the Government in taxation? This is one of the facts of life that are not always fully recognized by the urban planners, utterly dependent as they are upon rural enthusiasam to produce more for their special benefit.

But this Asian land on which so many human beings have to find subsistence and profit is not a fixed and stable resource. In a world where all men are equal, there is nothing more unequal than the environment with which man is endowed and his capacity to utilize that environment correctly. Thus in estimating the success of any new crop, new form of cropping or new type of animal husbandry, one has to assume that in every community, perhaps one-third will make 100 per cent utilization of the environment, including new seeds and advice from government; one-third will make 50 per cent utilization, and the remainder will be intermediate between these two. This distinction does not relate only to the people in an individual community. It must also be applied to categorize those communities which lie at greater or lesser distance from the stimulus of urban communities, markets, government services.

A related aspect is the transfer of farming populations from their former homes and place of cultivation to an entirely new location, as with Javanese farmers to Sumatra (Utomo, 1967), or the internal migration, state-assisted or otherwise, in the Philippines (Krinks, 1970). Since 1905, wet rice farmers from over-populated Java have been transferred and resettled in south Sumatra. They readily adopted the techniques of dry-land shifting cultivation of local farmers. However, the excessive clearance of the forest resource by excessive numbers of new immigrants has by now upset the delicate balance between the indigenous communities of shifting cultivators and the land.

Since the beginning of the present century, Filipino farmers have been encouraged and sometimes assisted to migrate to sparsely populated areas such as the central and southern provinces of Mindanao. Migration to Mawab in Davao Province began in 1919 and continues to this day. Krinks (op. cit.) did his field work there in 1967. The conclusion is that, if a short-term increase in the population-carrying capacity is the measure of desirability, then Mawab, or Mindanao, can continue to absorb settlers. In terms of long-range benefits, neglect of conservation of resources will reproduce the condition of the degraded environments of the migrant source areas. This type of colonization will merely perpetuate the land problems of the Philippines rather than solve them.

It is probably inevitable that rural change in the broad sense, and particularly in respect of intensification of agriculture and animal husbandry, has operated and will continue to operate under the radial influence of centres of population. This applies particularly where urban development in the form of industrialization has also taken place and created a greater urban purchasing power for the produce of the land. Thus, at the more advanced lower end of our ecological scale in Table 3/1, one would expect success from high-yielding varieties, given ample fertilizers on irrigated land, within reasonable access of these centres of population. The factors which would operate would

be proximity to markets, good road, river or rail connections, rural electrification for irrigation pumps, and the emulation by the rural people of the economic and nutritional standards and habits of the urban peoples. But until they progress a certain distance from the poverty levels to which they have long been accustomed, the rural people will sell everything they can to the towns, especially those types of animal protein which would mean so much in the nutrition of their own families.

It becomes possible also to introduce improvements in the less intensive forms of land use, by recognizing their position in the whole radial structure with markets at the centre, and by planning accordingly, up to the limits imposed by the environment, the communications and the technological experience of the producers at the different levels.

DISSEMINATION OF NEW IDEAS

In the introduction of measures for improved nutrition and health in the Philippines (Tiglao, 1964), the minimizing of social distance between health worker and people is important; programmes need to be planned with and through local health staff and accepted community leaders. Here, however, there is close correlation between opinion leaders and direction in the adoption of health innovations.

There are numerous incidental ways in which new ideas may reach a village. For example, new opportunities for modernization and income growth are created by impersonal forces that link a formerly remote village to its region and the nation; these may be all-weather roads, regular bus routes, electricity, radio, newspapers, facilities for postal savings, etc. A village may produce educated people who go to work in cities and send money home, which villagers then spend in towns. Thus growth in purchasing power and better access to cities are agents of modernization (S.R. Simon, in Mellor, Weaver, Lele and Simon, 1968). In addition, migrant labour, either travelling daily into urban centres or moving for long periods from areas of chronic over-population, will always bring back new ideas. Examples are the plantation workers of Malaysia, who return from time to time to their villages in Kerala and Tamil Nadu; the Nepali soldiers, who are scattered in Gurkha regiments in India and throughout South-East Asia; the overseas Chinese, who visit their relatives on the mainland; and young people everywhere who seek a better life in the towns, returning periodically to their homes. To a lesser extent, newer ideas may be brought in by brides, where it is customary to seek brides from areas sufficiently far away. Initially innovation by a bride is difficult, since she is closely observed by her mother-in-law and others of the husband's family, to see whether she measures up to local standards of behaviour.

In strongly traditional societies, where the aged are honoured and respected, change is not likely to be swift. Nair (1961) finds that refugees have brought innovations into various areas of India, which the local people have not been inclined to accept. In Rajasthan, Sikhs from the Punjab have successfully adapted practices brought from their more fertile homeland, greatly increasing productivity; but the local people have no faith in methods not traditional to them, and will not emulate the newcomers. Muslims from East Pakistan (Bangladesh) have successfully pursued market gardening in Assam, which local people disdain for reasons of dignity. Where a village is surrounded by hostile country — because of endemic diseases such as malaria, or because of aggressive neighbours or political antagonisms — what comes from the outside world is regarded with deep suspicion. Nationalism and regional religious revivalism can also produce strong resistance to anything 'foreign'. Where villages are already self-supporting, the people may at best be indifferent to, or apathetic about any improvements. Change is most likely to be adopted fairly rapidly where an impoverished environment, due to pressure of population and unemployment, has caused an initial breach in social customs. Where households become nuclear rather than extended, it is easier for the young mother to adopt practices explained to her by a trained nutritionist or nurse.

INNOVATION IN FOOD PRODUCTION

Since better rural nutrition is based primarily upon the improvement of food production, it is almost impossible to consider the introduction of change in nutritional habits and standards without at the same time considering the introduction of change in agricultural methods. How may one introduce progressive changes in food production or provide incentives to cultivators to change their agricultural practices so that their own and their neighbours' standards of nutrition may at the same time be improved?

The usual approach is to plan demonstrations and to establish extension services and farms, allowing one extension officer for a certain number of cultivators within access of his centre. This would mean the provision to individual cultivators through land reform of holdings of optimal size, the *lot viable,* on which a family would be able to subsist and also make a reasonable living through the sale of surplus produce. The main incentives would be the ownership granted to the farmer and accessibility to profitable markets.

Over the vast areas of rural Asia, however, such an approach is impracticable as a short-term measure. Depending on the ideology of the planners, one would either rely upon the direction given by the political commissar (not necessarily with agricultural and nutritional knowledge) in the more remote communes, or alternatively, upon the guidance and example by the one-third or less of farmers in each community who, because of their above-average natural capacities, are able to make 100 per cent utilization of their land. In a totalitarian regime, there is pressure from above on selected individuals to take up the tasks of village leadership; these tasks are generally of a political nature, but when villagers are given land up to their needs, they tend to abandon politics (Bernstein, 1968).

Anthropologists refer to these natural leaders within the community as entrepreneurs. Geertz (1968) has put forward hypotheses to explain the process of economic change in Indonesia, starting with an innovative economic leadership or entrepreneurship which occurs in a fairly well-defined and homogeneous group. This group is said to have crystallized out of a larger traditional group which has a very long history of extra-village status and inter-local orientation. 'Ideologically the innovative group conceives of itself as the main vehicle of religious and moral excellence within a generally wayward, unenlightened or heedless community.'

Nash (1965) defines the difference in rural Burma between the subsistence farmer and the entrepreneur who will try growing new crops for cash, as the possession of at least 10 hectares of land and access to a market with its concomitant facilities for money lending and commodity speculation — the catalyst from the 'get along' to the 'get going' farmer. There is not in this Buddhist community the same emphasis on religious or moral superiority associated with economic success. Again, Nash finds that:

the household head who with good rain and decent yields can meet his customary standard of living, is not an innovator. His domestic economy is tightly balanced, and he cannot take even the enticing speculative risks. This is the element that has brought and held a kind of stasis, or slow change, to agricultural life. The moderates have worked out the close fit between land, crops and labour; they have adjusted to a level of living to fit the returns, and they are content to move within these limits. They are without debt, free of economic bondage, their own masters, and hardworking, practical farmers. Such men only shift their modes of production when an outside agency — human or natural catastrophe — forces them to do so.

The caste hierarchy in the Indian village is still largely correlated with the economic stratification of rural society based on ownership of land (Fukutake, 1967). The members of the dominant castes (not necessarily the highest) still own more land than members of other castes. They would, due to their social contacts with the officers of local research or improvement stations, regard themselves as the introducers of new ideas, crop varieties and better bulls to the village; first for their own benefit, and ultimately, for the village as a whole. This has been one of the factors keeping the Untouchables in subjection. They do not own land; even if occasionally they are able to obtain some, they do not have sufficient capital to be able to farm it. Nor are they assisted towards economic independence by the caste farmers who rely on their labour.

Redfield and Singer (1955), in their foreword to a series of articles on Indian villages, state:

Widespread also are general processes of change: the disintegration of social systems based on group or corporate relations of status; the decline of occupational specialities; increasing use of money; growth of factionalism; changes in the interdependence of castes and a tendency for the depressed to find common cause in economic or political interests; the double process of Sanskritization and Westernization (Srinivas, 1966).

In Thailand, the Lue Village Headman is regarded as the synaptic leader, who must protect the villagers and their interests from the dissemination of government ideas by district officers whose standards and aspirations are foreign to rural life. 'What the government suggests is the government's way, the way of "men who eat a monthly salary", and who are not familiar with or sympathetic to village productive considerations' (Moerman, 1968). However, when the son of a wealthy headman who had trained in the National University of Agriculture has fertilizers spread on his fields and the villagers can see results, then an impression is made.

Conflict between the official view and the village view was discussed in a study of Gopalpur, Mysore State, India by Beals (1962).

Government officials tend to lay the blame for lack of progress upon the people of such villages as Gopalpur, who in turn tend to lay the blame upon the government officials. Both groups feel helpless and apathetic. The new wind blows in an unchanneled and undisciplined way, stirring up new problems for every one solved. The source of the difficulty seems to lie in the government officials' failure to perceive the inter-relationships among the things they are trying to change. The culture of Gopalpur is an organic whole; its religion and its social organization are adapted to the economic tasks traditionally carried out in the village. The reform programmes stimulated by the new wind are not organic wholes. The new wind offers some hopeful and some frightening prospects, but it does not offer a new way of life.

In Rajasthan, most farmers come to know of an innovation or are influenced to try or to adopt it from progressive farmers within their own caste or lineage (Bose and Saxena, 1965). The experienced persons from other caste groups usually act as innovators when there are none within the caste group. *Gram Sevak* and extension officials figure less prominently in influencing the trial or adoption of innovations. There is centralization of leadership in farm matters at the village level, but even among opinion leaders, very little information-seeking from one another. All opinion leaders are not innovators, but the rate of adoption of new ideas is higher among them than among others. Opinion leaders have a larger irrigated holding, own more livestock, practice commercial farming to a greater extent, have tried and adopted more innovations, have higher literacy rates, greater social participation, and come from castes having agriculture as their caste occupation. There is, however, hardly any difference in the diversification of the source of their livelihood or in their ages. There is little overlapping between leadership in farm matters and leadership in non-agricultural spheres of life (Bose and Saxena, 1966).

INNOVATION IN NUTRITION AND HEALTH

The qualities which distinguish agricultural innovators are also those which characterize innovators in health and nutrition. Those rural families around a Rural Health Demonstration and Training Center in Luzon, Philippines (Tiglao, 1964) who are most ready to adopt improvements are those of higher socioeconomic level and higher occupational and educational status. They also have more children in school, come from larger families, and have more married children. They live near the centre of innovation, are conscious of community problems and aware of the identity of opinion leaders. Thus they are those with the most diversified contacts with the world beyond the home, and most interested in and informed about topics of general concern. Tiglao found that improvement in socio-economic status might trigger off a chain of other changes; more education leads to more income; this in turn leads to better housing, a change of values and greater receptivity: 'There seems to be a direct relationship between buying power and the adoption and use of up-to-date ways of life.'

As with agriculture, so those entrusted with the task of introducing nutritional and health changes among rural peoples are frequently faced with a marked degree of social resistance. The reasons for this are rarely simple and attributable to one cause only. Rather are they usually due to a complexity of factors relating to ethnic origin, social conditions, politics, religion, illiteracy and perhaps above all to the overriding economic factors such as the absence of purchasing power needed to obtain the more essential but generally more expensive foods. Jaspan (1967) considers that impediments to change are greatest where there is lack of understanding of the reasons for plans and change. Similar findings come from a ten-year Community Development Project in Orissa (Fraser, 1968a), and from a group of Chinese farmers in Malaysia (Clarkson, 1968). Thus it is clear that change can be introduced only gradually by the agency of respected local leaders, whose trust has been gained by the outsider responsible for such change.

Opinion differs regarding the amenability of women to change. Srinivas (1966) notes that women are slower than men in India in discarding traditional standards in the processes he has called westernization and secularization. However, elsewhere women are frequently more amenable to change than men, and particularly more willing to adopt new foods for their children and to drop taboos relating to their nutrition

The desire for improved social status is a strong catalyst for change. In India the desire for enhanced caste status has induced many lower castes or outcasts to adopt the style of life proper to higher castes — a process given the term Sanskritization by Srinivas (op. cit.). This always involves a change in diet, and in particular the avoidance of flesh foods and eggs, and the adoption of vegetarianism. Among the educated, particularly in the cities, there is the opposite trend, of westernization, which includes the adoption of the concepts of nutritious foods and hygienic practices, rather than ritually pure foods and bodily purification. This involves, even for Brahmans,

the consumption of eggs, and for others, some flesh foods.

A native of north Thailand, accustomed to glutinous rice as his staple, upon being given a government position in the same area, changes to ordinary rice, the indication of officialdom and of central Thai origins (Moerman, 1968). In Taiwan, rural innovation has been facilitated by the absence of the guardians of traditional values, the gentry/literati class, who disdained manual labour and sought leisure (Diamond, 1969). (This class, of course, no longer has any impact on the mainland). In Taiwan, long hours of hard work are not seen as something to be avoided: 'The new word, "science" has taken on a very positive connotation and fatalistic attitudes are dying out . . . . In the economic sphere, strict adherence to traditionalism in and of itself is rejected. It is perceived as dysfunctional'. Here, innovation is accepted because it is seen as increasing economic status, which in turn enhances social status.

SOCIAL ATTITUDES TO FOOD

Change must be considered in both directions — regression and progression from an existing level. People living in a deteriorating environment are obliged to accept the foods which can be produced in that environment; while this sometimes means the coarser foodgrains of greater nutritional value, it often involves inferior root crops. Bailey (1962e) traced the regression in Java from rice to maize to cassava. Such deterioration is due to population pressure — more mouths to be fed from the same amount of now less productive land.

A large proportion of Asians live in an environment which fluctuates widely within each year, and are accustomed to an annual seasonal change from a food crop they value to one or more which they do not. For swidden cultivators and settled dry-land farmers, there is invariably a period of considerable nutritional deprivation before harvest at a time when energy is at a premium. In Hsin Hsing, Taiwan, the period before the harvest is marked by a greatly increased consumption of low-prestige sweet potatoes, and little if any rice (Gallin, 1966). The proportion of nutritionally superior barley in the diet of Korean farmers increases greatly until there is no rice left in the period before harvest. If the harvest should fail, such crop substitution may continue until the next harvest. Seasonal changes in Indian diets are marked in certain areas, and are regular, accepted facts of life.

Where income remains static and family members increase, there is an inevitable reduction in the availability per head of the side dishes which are the protective foods, both animal and vegetable (Kaneda, 1967). Eventually the situation deteriorates to a point where only the staple is used, with decreasing amounts per person, and some flavouring is added to make it palatable, such as soysauce, chilli or minute quantities of fish sauce. Such change is invariably for the worse.

Asian peoples are ready to purchase more of the foods which their society values; these foods are frequently and fortunately more nutritious ones. First, with increasing income, they will buy more of the staple, sometimes a better food grain, with their ancillary spices, relishes or lubricants until satiety is reached. Then increasing amounts of animal protein and to a lesser extent vegetable protein, including the grain legumes. Hunger is first satisfied with the preferred staple, which automatically involves more of the spices and more side dishes to make the increased quantity palatable. There is also increasing purchase of foods of low nutritional value, such as highly-milled carbohydrate snacks and carbonated drinks; this has led to a great increase of dental caries. Diet is improved only up to a certain level of expenditure: after this the prestige objects valued by urban societies are also purchased.

Plant breeders have come to realize that they must submit their new 'miracle' varieties to the test of acceptability at village level. There have been difficulties with new high-yielding varieties of wheat in India, because they were the wrong colour for chapatis, and new varieties of acceptable colour had to be bred. Dube (1958) reports that the flour of new varieties is less suitable for making chapatis than the indigenous varieties; once made, they become tough and unpalatable unless consumed immediately. New rice varieties are disliked by Asian peoples on account of taste, texture and cooking performance. It is claimed that these difficulties have been overcome with the newest varieties. Thus change cannot be imposed against popular will, without knowledge of daily preferences and practices.

PHYSIOLOGICAL AND PSYCHOLOGICAL INTOLERANCE

Intolerance exists throughout the region with regard to certain items of diet which would otherwise have the merit of increasing the proportion of animal protein in the diet. For example, the Muslim anathema of pork, that of the Hindu and other Indians

for beef, even as soup or stock, and the dislike of dried fish throughout the Indian subcontinent. The Japanese dislike of mutton is giving way only very slowly.

More recently there has been noted the purely physiological intolerance of milk by Asians, Negroes and some Caucasoids (Bayless and Rosensweig, 1966 and 1967; Davis and Bolin, 1967; Bolin and Davis, 1969; Huang and Bayless, 1967, 1968; Flatz, Saengudom and Sanguanbhokhai, 1969; McGillivray, 1968; Flatz and Saengudom, 1969; Korn, 1971). Lactose intolerance occurs in several peoples of Asia, who do not as adults produce the enzyme lactase, which breaks down the lactose molecule into its digestible components, glucose and galactose. However, infants of all races possess the lactase enzyme for the digestion of their mother's milk. The capacity to produce lactase is lost on weaning when milk no longer forms part of the diet (between the age of 1 to 4 years in trials in Chiengmai University). Naturally this does not occur with young Europeans and North Americans. If Asians are given milk, diarrhoea follows if the maximum safe dose of lactose is exceeded; this is about 14 gm. per day, the quantity contained in half a pint of whole milk or in about 35 gm. of powdered skim milk. Naturally the margin of safety varies with individuals.

Some distinction should obviously be made between Asians of different ethnic origins. Pakistanis and Indians, especially those from the north and north-west of the subcontinent, like Caucasoid peoples elsewhere, find milk highly acceptable and regard it as an important item of diet, particularly for the young. Some lactose intolerance has been found among south Indians, who do not get milk in their diet. Also in Africa, Nilotic pastoralists are accustomed to milk, and therefore have low levels of intolerance; agricultural peoples, for whom milk is not a regular part of the diet, have high levels of intolerance (Hunter, 1971).

The consumption of milk has been accepted only relatively recently by the Japanese, largely as a result of successful habituation in school-milk programmes. Sweetened condensed milk has for long been consumed in Malaysia. It has often been stated that the Chinese are allergic to milk. It was, however, customary in the past to give human milk to the aged and the sick. S.C. Hsu of the Joint Commission for Rural Reconstruction, Taipei, finds that skim milk is tolerated even by elderly Chinese people when it is highly diluted. Young people from Hong Kong who go to study in Australia drink milk regularly there. Young

Singaporeans have taken enthusiastically to milk flavoured with Ovaltine and Milo.

In view of the potential importance of milk protein, whether produced within Asia itself or imported, in the nutritional programmes designed to combat dietary deficiency in respect of animal protein and vitamin A in particular, the problems of lactose intolerance require clarification. Findings to date may be interpreted (Korn, 1971) as signs that the ability to produce the milk-sugar splitting enzyme, lactase, is genetically determined to dwindle in the later years of life. The speed of that process is presumably slowed down by continued use of milk after weaning. Studies are necessary to determine whether the ability to produce lactase can be regenerated once it is lost, and whether intolerance of milk in aid programmes increases with the higher age groups of schoolchildren. For older people, the technique of training to eliminate the acquired intolerance also requires investigation.

The U.N. Protein Advisory Group has recommended that a study group be formed to examine milk intolerance, its prevalence and nutritional implications.

NUTRITION EDUCATION

International and national bodies concerned with food and nutrition have done much to provide a basis for designing programmes of nutrition education. FAO has published a Nutrition Study, *Learning Better Nutrition* (Ritchie, 1967). The background of the problems of nutrition education is discussed, for example: (a) cultural and psychological influence on food patterns; (b) social organization in relation to changing food habits; (c) methods of changing food habits; and (d) incentives for better health and economic progress. The planning, development and evaluation of Applied Nutrition Programs, the concepts and content of education of the public or school children, and the choice of methods, techniques and aids are also covered. *Visual Aids in Nutrition Education* (Holmes, 1968), and *Communicating Home Economics Information* (Fewster, 1970), an analysis of the best method of using radio for the training of women, are also valuable guides based on practical experience in nutrition education.

However, again one is faced with that dilution of effort, effect and result between the well-appointed planning rooms through all the intermediate stages to the faraway rural communities of Asia. One may ask, will it be possible to bring enough educational pressure to bear on the housekeepers and women of reproductive age in a population of 1,600 million, rapidly enough to influence the traditional nutritional habits of the hundreds of millions in rural China, India, Pakistan and Bangladesh, or to reach the forgotten outer islands of Indonesia and the Philippines? Who is going to provide the education in the rural areas? Certainly, there will never be enough nutritionists and nutrition educationists trained and willing to go far from the relative comforts of urban areas.

Even if all the rural workers, village level workers, technical officers of the commune, nutrition midwives or barefoot doctors were to be given a basic knowledge of the principles of nutrition for all groups of society, they still could not cover more than a minute proportion of the vast area and populations involved. And are enough rural specialists being trained at a rate sufficient to meet the new demands created by an increase of more than 50 million per year in the human population of rural Asia? Already the number of even partially qualified rural specialists per 100,000 people is lamentably low in most Asian countries, and the proportion is not improving.

Perhaps here again, reliance must increasingly be placed upon those innovators, entrepreneurs and leaders of rural communities mentioned above. The problem of nutrition education is to find some way of educating these people, in the hope that they will pass on what they have learned about better food and feeding and preparation to the other members of the same community who look to them for guidance and example. It has, for example, been suggested that the *Lembaga Sosial Desa*, or Organization of Village Social Development, which has offices in more than half of Indonesia's 60,000 villages, could serve as centres for preventive medicine, first aid and education, in preference to Maternal and Child Health Centres, since the village organizations are maintained by the villagers themselves (Sutedjo, 1970). Rural improvement by members of the community has been the foundation of the Community Development Programme of India.

One of the United Nations' programmes designed to make full use of the power of rural innovators to disseminate improvement is the FAO/WHO/UNICEF Applied Nutrition Program. This provides material aid to rural communities, such as equipment for establishing and operating poultry units, fish ponds, fruit and vegetable gardens, legume fields and dairy units, and for training selected members of these communities in correct agricultural practices to sustain this production. The Applied Nutrition Program also encourages local consumption of useful foods by widespread nutrition education, directed to key members of the community, through schools, health centres, agricultural centres, youth and women's clubs. Free distribution of foods to vulnerable groups is arranged from local production as a practical demonstration of their benefits. These projects start by identifying problems of agriculture and nutrition within a country; a pilot project is then set up, from which trained personnel may establish comparable projects in other areas. In India, the Applied Nutrition Program covers about five per cent of the population; it is spreading throughout all regions of the Philippines; and there are projects in most Asian countries.

FAO has published a manual (Latham, 1972) designed to guide national governments in setting up and evaluating applied nutrition programs, conducted with or without the assistance of U.N. Agencies.

UNESCO sees nutrition education as an essential element in a comprehensive adult education programme, such as the World Literacy Programme (Bowers, 1966, UNESCO, 1959, 1961, 1964, 1966a, b). The Rural Teacher Training Project at Ubol, north Thailand, trained teachers both as rural educators and community leaders, to help improve living standards by giving guidance in health and sanitation, agriculture, crafts, home-making and adult education (Fresnoza, 1969).

One must be realistic in attempting the introduction of desirable standards of human nutrition in rural Asia. Great progress could nevertheless be made even by improving the standards of production and utilization of the foods which are already available locally. This applies more particularly to vegetables (the Applied Nutrition Program lays special stress on school gardens and vegetable consumption). It may be hoped that, in due course, rural housekeepers may be persuaded of the value of retaining some of the plant and animal proteins for their own families.

Great benefit can be derived from the correct preparation of the foods which are a regular part of the diet, particularly in the preparation of rice. When highly milled and cooked in excess water, rice loses 80 per cent or more of its vitamins and 50 per cent of its protein. One cannot recommend a return to the time-consuming and exhausting labour of home-pounding, by which more of the vitamin content of rice is retained. Parboiling retains a large proportion of the vitamins in the kernel. This method has been adopted in some areas, but elsewhere both the colour and smell of parboiled rice have made it unacceptable.

Some Asians cook their rice only in sufficient water to permit cooking; this is clearly preferable to the more common method of cooking and discarding excess water. The best ways of cooking vegetables to retain their nutritive value are being demonstrated in some countries.

Most Asian countries have recommended diets for their own people, with advice on the best methods of preparation (see chapter 9). The WHO monograph for the Western Pacific Region, *Nutrition in Maternal and Child Health* (1968b), has recipes based on familiar and acceptable Asian foods for different age groups.

Long-term improvements in nutritional practices are best introduced by the younger members of the community. School children are quick to adopt new foods they find palatable, and will introduce these to other members of the family. A Japanese grandfather is puzzled when he sees eggs on the breakfast table (Norbeck, 1967). All children like to drink milk, even in small quantities at home, but not grandfather. The Japanese child may eat boiled oatmeal with milk and sugar, or a piece of toasted bread and marmalade like the one eaten on a school excursion to Kyoto, but not grandfather. The young will experiment with foods advertised in magazines and television. Fruit has only recently become part of the daily menu. Fish is now served four or five times a week — grandfather remembers when it was food for the sick or for special occasions.

Practical demonstration is the most effective means of convincing rural people of the value of new practices. Maternal and Child Care Centres can play an important part in demonstration, but their impact on the whole population is limited, as only a few mothers attend them regularly. A new approach has been adopted in Central Java, whereby nutritionists of the Health Department visit villages with a mobile kitchen unit. The nutritionist talks to the women and demonstrates how beans, peanuts, eggs or fish will make the traditional congee more nourishing and make the child grow better; green leaves will prevent the night blindness with which they are so familiar. Modifications may be made, depending on the village source of protein (Tie, Lian, Ong and Rose, 1967).

Ten years after the Rural Health Demonstration and Training Center in Luzon had been set up, there was general improvement in health practices and nutrition status. Intestinal parasitism, however, had hardly decreased, despite an increase of toilet facilities from 7.9 per cent in 1950 to 71.11 per cent in 1960 (Tiglao, 1964). This is ascribed partly to the fact that these facilities are not used by small children, and partly to inadequate hand washing before meals. This demonstrates that only 100 per cent construction and utilization of latrines, together with improved personal hygiene, improvement of food and market sanitation, correct handling and storage of food in homes and public eating places, and safe sources of water supply, could remedy endemic parasitism. Again, far more than merely health education is involved.

Part III

NUTRITION AND MALNUTRITION

9 Balanced Nutrition

RECOMMENDED INTAKES

IN order to ensure growth, the replacement of body tissues and the maintenance of optimal health and energy in the human organism, it is essential to provide an intake of minimal quantities of all the basic components of the diet — the minimal effective diet.

All attempts to deal with nutrient requirements have met with the difficulty of arriving at clear-cut concepts of the amounts of nutrients needed by the body. Thus, a number of terms such as *minimum requirements, optimum requirement, recommended allowance* and others have appeared in the literature. Often the terms are ill-defined and may have different meanings for different people. Recognizing this difficulty, the Group found it convenient to adopt the following term: *recommended intakes*: the amount of a food or food component considered sufficient for the maintenance of health in nearly all people (WHO, 1967).

The optimal or minimal levels of intake of nutrients vary according to age, sex, environment and occupation, and between individuals. The basal components are carbohydrate, protein, fats, vitamins and minerals. All recommended allowances apply to large groups and are not necessarily applicable to individuals, who show great variation between one and another. The widespread adaptation to a low level of intake of nutrients among Asians does not imply a lower actual requirement; studies in India showed no difference in protein requirement between groups living at higher and lower socio-economic levels. Standards are, however, useful as a yardstick against which diets of different socio-economic groups can be measured. National standards are therefore an essential part of any practical national food policy, and for the planning of agricultural policy, but require revision at appropriate intervals (Davidson and Passmore, 1966).

The American National Research Council, the British Medical Association, WHO, FAO and many national medical associations have recommended stand-

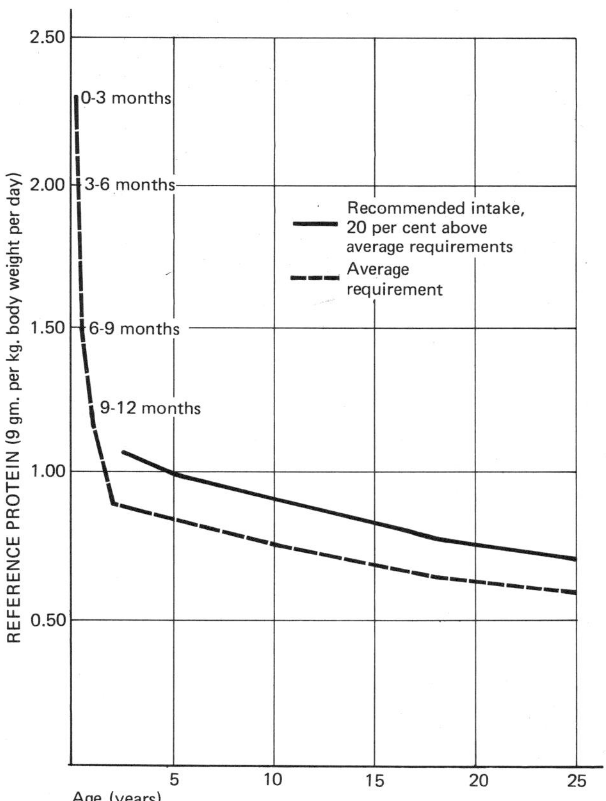

FIG. 9/1   Requirements for reference protein

Source: Protein Advisory Group (1970a)

ards of human nutrition in terms of safe intake of nutrients and calories. FAO/WHO recommend protein intake at 20 per cent above and 20 per cent below average requirement (Fig. 9/1). The upper level covers all but a very small proportion of the population; the lower level is the limit below which all but a few would suffer from protein deficiency. The protein requirement is made up of two components: (a) a basal

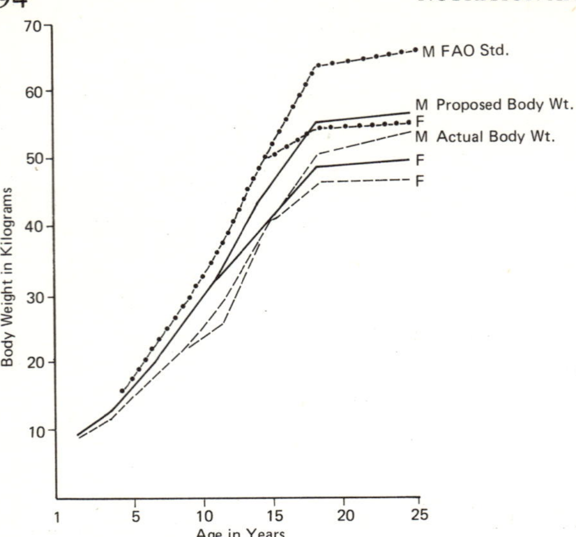

FIG. 9/2   FAO reference man and reference woman,
together with proposed standards for Filipino men and women, and their actual body
weights.

Source: Intengan and FNRC, 1970

amount, below which it is believed that normal health
and growth cannot be achieved, and (b) an additional
amount to provide for the stresses, including minor
infections, to which everyone is exposed. European
and American evidence has shown that protein requirements may vary from 21 to 65 – 70 gm. per day,
with an average of 44 gm. (Davidson and Passmore,
1966). A revision of *Recommended Dietary Allowances* by the U.S. National Academy of Sciences
(1968) estimates that 65 gm. protein daily is required
for an adult, or about 0.9 gm. per kg. of body weight.
This is based on an average basal requirement of 1,750
kcal., of 20 mg. ideal protein per basal kcal.,[1] an allowance of 30 per cent for individual variability, and
a utilization value of about 70 per cent for food proteins.

Dietary recommendations made by Asian nutritionists correspond more closely to locally available
foodstuffs, dietary habits and physical characteristics
than can those made outside Asia. Even here, however,
recommendations are often beyond the realms of at-
tainment for socio-economic reasons. Workers in Gujarat (Rajalakshmi and Ramakrishnan, 1969) have
drawn up dietary recommendations which they consider more realistic than those of the Indian Council
of Medical Research. In particular, they have reduced
the recommended intake of protein from 90 to 55 gm.

per head per day. Conversely, some Japanese workers
have recommended an intake double the FAO figure
(Yoshimura, Yoshioka and Fukushige, 1969).

In the early 1920s, an attempt was made, on the
basis of existing knowledge, by G. Dòuglas Gray of
the British Legation, Peking, and Bernard E. Read, of
Peking Union Medical College, to evolve a minimal
diet for a poor Chinese farming family in north China,
using locally available ingredients (Mallory, 1926).
This, for a family of five, called for a daily amount in
grammes of: kaoliang 125; wheat 90; millet 70; vegetables 40; oil 30; and in winter, 45 gm. cabbage. Money available was, however, insufficient to provide
even this simple diet. Allowing for a period of inaction
during the winter when the people were able to reduce
their food intake, the allowance was 'sufficient to
maintain life'. A common diet for north China at that
time consisted of two meals daily of corn bread and
salt turnips with, in times of crisis, other unpalatable
commodities to keep alive. This is one of the more
extreme examples of an attempt to recommend a minimal, rather than a safe diet.

Recommended intakes are designed for a well-de-
veloped, healthy human being, usually called Reference Man (Fig. 9/2). Such recommendations may not
apply to the average rural Asian, who often carries a
heavy load of intestinal parasites and infections due
to poor environmental sanitation and the need to perform heavy labour under extremes of climate. During
periods of nutritional stress, these parasites and infections increasingly undermine health and energy.
Man can adapt himself to suboptimal intakes of nutrients without obvious signs of deficiency, until he
becomes subject to stress caused by disease, or a high
expenditure of energy, or during pregnancy and lactation in women, or associated with a sudden spurt of
growth in children. The diseased and sick have much
higher nutritional requirements than healthy individuals.

The specific calorie requirements of Asian peoples
have been defined on the basis of average body
weights, which are not necessarily characteristic of an
individual of the same race who has been correctly
nourished throughout his life. This has given rise to
anomalies, such as the differential levels of calorie intakes recommended for Indians and Pakistanis.

Studies of basal metabolism and energy expenditure of Koreans were made to determine calorie requirements (Kim, 1968). A normal young adult requires an average of one calorie per kg. bodyweight
per hour (Rajalakshmi, 1969) with a lower require-

---

[1]kcal = kilocalorie = 1,000 calories.

ment for adolescent girls and adult women; children have a higher requirement per kg. bodyweight, but a lower total requirement due to stature. There are higher requirements for pregnancy and lactation, sickness or emotional tension. Numerous calculations have been made in different countries for the calorie requirements of people carrying out different activities (See also Chapter 10).

NATIONAL RECOMMENDATIONS

Dietary recommendations have been made by authorities in most Asian countries. Some of these are given in Tables 9/5 to 9/12. It will be seen that several tables relate to nutrient intakes; some countries have recommended dietary sources of these nutrients; India has made recommendations for different socio-economic groups, and Malaysia has devised a low-cost diet for pregnant women. The special needs of the vulnerable groups are, however, given in more detail in Tables 10/9 and 10/10.

CARBOHYDRATES

Carbohydrates provide most of the energy in almost all human diets, up to 90 per cent in the tropics, and less than 50 per cent in the U.S.A. Neither extreme is desirable, and probably 55 to 65 per cent is a suitable figure (Davidson and Passmore, 1966). Aykroyd has said (Aykroyd, Gopalan and Balasubramanian, 1966): 'In working out diet schedules, the requirements of protein, fat, vitamins and minerals should be first attended to; subsequently carbohydrate-rich foods can be included in sufficient amounts to meet the energy requirements.' While in the advanced countries much of the carbohydrate in the diet comes from sugars, in Asia cereals are the principal source. This is fortunate, since cereals contain protein, vitamins and minerals, which are absent from refined sugar; 70 to 90 per cent of the Asian diet is derived from cereals (see Chapter 12 and Appendix). It is, however, difficult to provide increased calories from cereals or root staples for children, since total bulk becomes unacceptable (see under *Fat* below).

PROTEIN

The three main forms of food — carbohydrates, fat and protein — provide energy, but it is only protein that can supply the nitrogen and amino acids necessary for growth and replacement. A Joint Expert Committee of WHO and FAO states (FAO, 1965): 'perhaps the most important nutritional problem that is still not fully solved is that of meeting the protein requirements of man ... protein nutrition for young children is the main nutritional problem of the world, and protein malnutrition, if both its direct and indirect effects are considered, is a major source of ill health'.

Protein may be used in two ways:

(a) to provide energy in a diet low in carbohydrates; an inadequate intake of energy food will by itself cause a loss of protein from the body and thus aggravate protein deficiency in the diet (FAO, 1965); and

(b) to act as protein *qua* protein in a correctly balanced diet.

Proteins of the required composition may actually be consumed, but frequently in amounts quite inadequate to ensure a balanced diet, because of large grain in vegetable protein, inadequate absorption due to the fibrous nature of the food, or incorrect cooking.

The pattern of amino acids in egg or milk (Table 9/1) is now adopted as being the most desirable. The protein of milk or egg is therefore taken as reference or ideal protein (Fig. 9/1). The FAO/WHO *Ad Hoc* Committee of Experts on Energy and Proteins; Requirements and Recommended Intakes, is revising the recommendations made in 1965. These have been found inadequate for Indian children aged 1 to 3 years, and excessive for adults (Swaminathan, 1970).

The 1965 Expert Committee stated:

Protein needs, whether expressed as requirements for amino acids or for nitrogen, involve two components: the essential amino acids that must be obtained from the diet because they cannot be synthesized within the body, and the nitrogen of 'non-essential' amino acids, that is also necessary for the synthesis of protein and other nitrogen-containing compounds.

Because of the interest that has rightly been concentrated on the body's need for essential amino acids, it has not always been realized that, under certain conditions, it may be the amount of non-essential nitrogen in the diet that is limiting. For example, in the case of both cow's milk and egg, the minimal quantity that will maintain nitrogen balance in the adult provides more than double the estimated requirement of each essential amino acid. Therefore, after the required pattern of the essential amino acids has been specified, the proportion of the total nitrogen intake which these amino acids form must also be indicated. This proportion, the E/T ratio, may be expressed as mg. of essential amino acids per gm. of total nitrogen or per gm. of conventional protein (N x 6.25).

Some essential amino acids, if not present in the diet, can be synthesized but only from essential amino acids, thus increasing the requirement for the latter.

TABLE 9/1

Essential amino-acid patterns of egg and human milk
(proportion to total essential amino acids mg. per gm.)

Amino acid	Human milk	Hen's egg
Isoleucine	132	129
Leucine	184	172
Lysine	128	125
Total aromatic amino acids	226	195
(Phenylalanine	(114)	(114)
Tyrosine)	(112)	(81)
Total sulphur-containing amino acids	87	107
(Cystine	(43)	(46)
Methionine)	(44)	(61)
Threonine	99	99
Tryptophan	34	31
Valine	147	141

Note: Either of these patterns may be regarded as the desirable pattern for reference purposes.

Nitrogenous equilibrium can be maintained with a mixture of eight pure amino acids: isoleucine, leucine, lysine, methionine, phenylalanine, threonine, tryptophan and valine. To maintain growth in infants, histidine and perhaps also arginine are needed.

Cystine can be synthesized from methionine, and tyrosine from phenylalanine.

Source: FAO, 1965

BIOLOGICAL VALUE OF PROTEIN

In human nutrition, the term 'animal protein' has tended to become synonymous with protein of high biological value, which it certainly is, and to be differentiated from 'vegetable protein', which has tended to be synonymous with protein of low biological value. This broad differentiation is now somewhat archaic, since the importance of amino-acid patterns came to be understood. This is because the nutritive value of many vegetable proteins can be made similar to that of animal protein by combination with other vegetable proteins. Thus one is left with a general division into proteins of high biological value, including those that can be up-graded by combination or supplementation, and proteins of low biological value; it is only a matter of time and priorities before protein products of uniform and high biological value can be made from the judicious blending of natural products of plant and animal origin with the appropriate supplementation of amino-acid products, as a separate enterprise. Whether and how they may be introduced into the Asian rural diet is another matter.

In the meantime, however, one has to consider the ordinary sources of foods of plant and animal origin in Asia in terms of their biological value, i.e. the proportion of absorbed nitrogen that is retained in the body for maintenance and growth (Table 9/2). The protein of hen and duck eggs heads the list, closely followed by the protein of milk. Attempts to make a protein score for different foods have been only partially successful, because digestion of proteins is rarely complete. Some plant proteins may be held so firmly

TABLE 9/2

Percentage of absorbed nitrogen
when foodstuff is sole source

Animal sources		Plant sources	
Whole egg	94	Various millets	80–90
Milk	85	Rice	80
Beef liver	77	Potatoes	78
Pork ham	74	Whole wheat	66 to 67
Beef muscle	69	Oats	65
		Maize	60
		Various pulses	40–60

Source: FAO, 1965

in the cellulose structure of the plant that they are not completely absorbed in human digestion (Patwardhan, 1960). The nutritive value of such foods is clearly less than chemical analysis of their amino acids would indicate. In 1938, the Commission on Nutrition of the Chinese Medical Association recommended a daily protein intake of 1.5 gm. per kg. of body weight (twice the allocation for western man) due to the lower coefficient of digestibility and lower biological value of Chinese diets (Shen, 1957). A Dietary Committee in Taiwan recommends that one-third of total protein should come from animal protein; during adolescence, net protein should be 8 per cent of total calories; for a nursing mother, 9 per cent. Experiments in Taiwan showed that if wheat is the staple, 8 gm. of pork and 4 to 5 gm. fish per head per day are adequate to provide a balanced diet; if rice is the staple, 24 gm. pork and 20 gm. fish are required.

The efficiency of nitrogen utilization declines as the concentration of protein in the diet is increased; even utilization of the most limiting amino acid declines, although full protein requirements may not be met (Donoso, Miller and Payne, 1964). Conversely, following a period of protein-calorie malnutrition in children, there is increased efficiency of food utilization and rapid growth until normal heights and weights for age are reached (Ashworth, 1969).

It is thus impossible to state the amino-acid requirements for a given purpose in terms of grammes per day; essential amino acids may be katabolized in proportion to their concentration in the diet.

Some animal proteins have been found to be more nutritious than expected, a fact that has led some to think that animal proteins may contain a factor ('the animal protein factor') which adds to their value over and above the value of the essential amino acids they contain. This may be at least partly due to vitamin B_{12} which is found only in foods of animal origin; however the existence of a specific factor in animal protein has not been proved. Protein utilization depends upon the efficiency of the enzyme systems concerned with digestion, synthesis and interconversion of amino acids. These enzymes in turn depend upon the state of nutrition of the body, including its supply of pyridoxine.

PROTEINS OF VEGETABLE AND ANIMAL ORIGIN

There are two schools of thought with regard to the provision of protein from plant, animal and manufactured sources in Asian diets.

One group considers that the difficulties of producing animal protein within the region, and the economic and logistic problems of importing sufficient supplies from outside the region, are too enormous to be contemplated. This group would concentrate on vegetable sources of protein and the fortification of food grains with manufactured amino acids. They do not recognize the dangers of one-sided fortification of cereal-based diets deficient in most nutrients, nor do they state how one is to treat the predominant food grain, rice, on the farms and in the villages in a subsistence economy, nor again, how the serious deficiencies in vitamins, fats and minerals are also to be corrected. The addition of synthetic amino acids will improve only the quality of the protein without increasing the concentration of protein in the food or the diet; the need to increase the latter is often the more important problem.

A second group argues that everything possible should be done to produce animal protein from intensive, commercial or scavenger forms of animal husbandry, and from forest wildlife, to supplement that available from fish, since the protein taken in this form is superior *qua* protein to that from vegetable sources. As most forms of animal protein have a higher content of and better balance between the essential amino acids, even quite small quantities will meet the minimal daily requirements for protein and other vital components of the diet. It is because of the chronic deficiency of animal protein in Asian diets and because it is consumed only sporadically that the parallel deficiencies of vitamins, minerals and frequently fats become critical.

Nitrogenous equilibrium in the human diet may be achieved when a legume is the source of protein, provided this forms 10 per cent of the dry weight of the total intake (Aykroyd and Doughty, 1964). With an adult diet of 2,200 calories per day, 30 gm. of legume per day are adequate as a source of protein when the staple is rice, millet, wheat or maize; 90 gm. of soybean with wheat is adequate for a pregnant mother; 45 gm. soybean in a child's diet of 1,100 calories is adequate with all cereals; 30 gm. soybean is adequate if wheat is the cereal; only with wheat are 45 gm. legume grains other than soybean adequate, but with groundnut, even this amount is not sufficient. Cassava and a cassava/maize mixture cannot be made adequate for young children, even if the daily diet contains 45 gm. soybean and 15 gm. skim milk or fish flour (the latter being the most valuable addition).

TABLE 9/3

Amounts of foodstuffs required for a balanced diet for children*
A. Food mixtures each supplying 360 calories
and a protein value of NDpCal 8 per cent

	Wheat	Rice	Maize	Sweet potato	Taro	Cassava flour	
Egg	93 / 22	92 / 23	89 / 28	270 / 33	279 / 28	90 / 50	Egg
Fish	100 / 10	98 / 20	97 / 24	270 / 33	300 / 30	104 / 47	Fish
Chicken	100 / 9	94 / 28	91 / 27	267 / 37	281 / 31	93 / 50	Chicken
W.M.P.	93 / 8	75 / 19	69 / 23	190 / 29	203 / 26	59 / 35	W.M.P.
S.M.P.	98 / 5	91 / 11	88 / 13	259 / 18	269 / 16	88 / 24	S.M.P.
Soybean	90 / 7	86 / 32	80 / 20	231 / 25	245 / 22	75 / 33	Soybean
	Wheat	Rice	Maize	Sweet potato	Taro	Cassava flour	

* Children 1-2 years old need about five small meals daily; aged 2-3 years, four meals, and thereafter, three meals. For purposes of calculation a child can be considered to need about three main meals daily of 300-400 calories each. The table therefore relates to a single meal. In addition to the main components of the diet, small quantities of vegetables and fruits should also be given.

Notes:
1. All figures in the top left corner of each square indicate the amount of staple food (in grammes)
2. All figures in the bottom right hand corner of each square indicate minimum amount of protein food necessary (in grammes)
3. All weights are in grammes of edible portions
4. Fish = fresh sea fillet
5. W.M.P. = whole milk powder (grammes x 8 = mls. liquid cow's milk)
6. S.M.P. = skimmed milk powder
7. In practice all weights should be converted to quantitative measure in local cups, tins, spoons, etc.
8. If fresh cassava is used the quantities given for flour should be trebled
9. Other dried beans would be required in about double the quantity specified for soybean, because of inferior quality

Source: WHO, 1969

WHO has suggested various combinations of Asian foods which will provide balanced diets for small children (Table 9/3).

VITAMINS

In 1965, FAO and WHO convened an expert group to review the available knowledge on vitamins, and to make recommendations on requirements (WHO, 1967). Because of the number of vitamins significant in human nutrition, it was decided to consider them in groups. The choice of the first group, namely, vitamin A, thiamine, riboflavine and niacin, was determined by two considerations: (a) one had to take note of the magnitude of the problem of protein deficiencies, and (b) sufficient knowledge had accumulated about the metabolism and function of these particular vitamins.

Nutrition surveys conducted in different parts of the world during the last three decades, and the available hospital records and morbidity and mortality statistics, clearly show that nutritional disorders attributable to deficiencies of vitamin A, thiamine, riboflavine and niacin occur widely in many developing countries. Their incidence and degree of severity vary from country to country, depending upon many factors, some of which are known and some as yet unexplained. These deficiency diseases occur largely among the population groups of low socio-economic status, usually with defective diets and living in poor sanitary environments which increase the hazards of infection. Poor dietary intake, however, appears to be the principal factor. It should be noted that reliable figures for the prevalence of these deficiencies are lacking. They are usually multiple and those which predominate determine the character of the clinical manifestations (WHO, 1967).

A number of factors governs the distribution and availability of these vitamins in common foods of the region. It was proposed that further research be carried out on the degree to which an alteration of the relative proportions of carbohydrates, protein and fat in the diet can affect the requirement for vitamins; the availability and utilization of the total amount of a vitamin in food, particularly those of niacin and the carotenes; and the effects of different methods of food preparation.

Again, it is not possible to state requirements of vitamins, because these vary from one individual to another. A general guide is given by Davidson and Passmore (1966):

Vitamin A. Clinical effects of deficiency are usually seen only where the diet has long been deficient in dairy produce and fresh vegetables, especially in hot, dry climates. Dried fruits and foods exposed to sunlight lose much of their vitamin A potency. About one-half of the carotene in leafy vegetables, and one-quarter that of root vegetables is converted into vitamin A. Recommended intake, 2,500 international units of vitamin A, or 7,500 international units of carotene (Davidson and Passmore, 1966).

An Indian worker has estimated that 50 to 60 gm. leafy green vegetables per day would meet the requirement for vitamin A (Rajalakshmi, 1969).

Vitamin C. This has a more limited distribution than other water-soluble vitamins, the best sources being citrus fruits, currants, berries and fully grown green vegetables. Dried pulses and cereals form the vitamin on germination, and sprouting pulses are a valuable antiscorbutic. As this vitamin is easily destroyed, foods containing it are best eaten raw.

A controversy exists regarding the desirability of total saturation with vitamin C. The British Medical Association does not consider this necessary, and recommends 20 mg. per day for adults, 30 mg. for adolescents, and 50 mg. for nursing mothers. The U.S. Food and Nutrition Board, however, recommends 60 mg. for men, 55 mg. for women (U.S. National Academy of Sciences, 1968). In the Philippines (Cam-cam, 1968), it is suggested that even 70 mg. daily may be inadequate; in India, where average diets contain only 10 to 15 mg. daily, this amount is considered sufficient, although increased amounts would be helpful for iron synthesis (Rajalakshmi, 1969).

A Joint FAO/WHO Expert Group concerned with requirements of ascorbic acid (FAO, 1970b) notes that the total body pool of ascorbic acid is greater than 1500 mg., while the metabolically active pool is much smaller, katabolizing at a constant rate of 2.6 per cent. When the active pool has been depleted to somewhat less than 300 mg., the onset of clinical scurvy occurs. The Group has decided that a daily intake in the neighbourhood of 10 mg. ascorbic acid prevents scurvy in most individuals, but recommends a daily intake of 30 mg. for normal adults, to allow for variation between individuals. The amounts of ascorbic acid needed during infancy and early childhood are not known precisely. During breast-feeding, most infant needs are met, at least during the first six months, when the maternal diet is adequate. The Group recommends that all infants and children up to 12 years should have a daily intake of 20 mg. ascorbic acid, and from 13 to 19 years, 30 mg. Women during the second and third trimesters of pregnancy and during lactation should receive an additional 20 mg. daily.

Vitamin D. This fat-soluble vitamin requires bile, and possibly fatty acids, for absorption. It promotes absorption of calcium and phosphate from the gut. A deficiency alters the processes involved in the growth of bones. There is, however, no evidence that adults require dietary supply, although it is usually recommended during pregnancy. This vitamin is obtained by the action of ultra-violet light on the skin.

A Joint FAO/WHO Expert group which has studied vitamin D requirements (FAO, 1970b) observes that minimum requirements are not known, chiefly because of the lack of information on the amount of vitamin D resulting from exposure to sunlight. In full-term infants, a daily intake of 2.5 μg. (micromilligrammes) vitamin D prevents rickets and ensures adequate calcium absorption and growth rate, and normal mineralization of bone; since there may be inadequate exposure to sunlight, a higher intake is advised. The Group recommends a daily intake of 10 μg. from birth to 6 years, 2.5 μg. from 7 years and over, and 10 μg. daily during the second and third trimesters of pregnancy and lactation; however, part or all of these requirements may be supplied through sunlight.

Thiamine. The only rich source of this water-soluble vitamin in the biological world is in the seeds of plants; the germ of cereals, nuts, peas, beans and other pulses, and in yeast. It is also present in significant amounts in all green vegetables, roots, fruits, flesh foods and dairy produce except butter. Pork is a richer source than either beef or mutton. Much is lost in cooking when excess water is discarded; in mixed cooking, the loss is 25 per cent. There is a clear relation in animals between the utilization of thiamine and the amount of carbohydrate in the diet, but this has not yet been proved in man. However, intake is usually related to the amount of carbohydrate and protein, or total calories consumed. The British Medical Association recommends 0.6 mg. per 1,000 non-fat calories for all but nursing mothers; for these, with a diet of 3,000 calories per day, 1.4 mg. of thiamine per day are recommended. Such recommendations are sufficient for healthy people on British diets. The Indian Council of Medical Research recommends 0.3 mg., and FAO 0.4 mg. per 1,000 calories.

Beriberi is not a disease of famines, but of poorly balanced diets. The concept of a thiamine/calorie ratio is considered more useful by Davidson and Passmore than a thiamine/carbohydrate ratio. Whole wheat, containing 1.2 mg. thiamine per 1,000 calories, gives protection against beriberi. Raw polished rice, containing only 0.15 mg. per 1,000 calories, produces beriberi.

Most fruits, vegetables and flesh foods have a ratio just above the critical level of about 0.25 mg.

Nicotinic acid (niacin). This water-soluble vitamin is widely distributed in small amounts in plant and animal foods, with more in meat, especially organs, and in fish, wholemeal cereals and pulses. In foods such as potatoes and maize, much of the vitamin may not be absorbed, unless treated with an alkali. It is not possible to state the recommended intake, as in the absence or deficiency of niacin, tryptophan may be converted into this vitamin: 60 mg. tryptophan are required to produce 1 mg. niacin; 15 to 20 mg. daily are probably required by adults.

Riboflavine. Liver, milk, eggs and green vegetables are good sources, but this vitamin is relatively lacking in cereal grains. Exposure to sunlight results in heavy loss. Recommended intake has not been determined, but 1 to 2 mg. daily may be satisfactory.

Vitamin B_{12}. This vitamin is not found in any plants; it is not known how strict vegetarians taking no milk get their supply. Many Asian peoples do not obtain B_{12} regularly in their diets; they may have become adapted to this, or the deficiency may be partly compensated by synthesis of folic acid. This vitamin participates in some essential enzyme system or systems. Attempts to link vitamin B_{12} directly with protein synthesis have not been successful. Absorption may be affected by a variety of intestinal diseases.

The Joint FAO/WHO Expert Group (1970b) considers requirements on the basis of three different types of study designed:

1. to determine the amounts needed to prevent or cure megaloblastic anaemia resulting from vitamin B_{12} deficiency;

2. to study the relationship between the levels of vitamin B_{12} in serum and the levels in liver in deficient and healthy subjects, and

3. to determine body stores and turnover rates of this vitamin.

In order to maintain 200 pg.[1] per ml. serum concentration and to allow some B_{12} to accumulate as body stores (recommended by WHO Scientific Group on Nutritional Anaemias, 1968a), the Group recommends a daily intake of 2 μg. for a normal adult. Deficiency in breastfed infants occurs only when mothers are deficient in this vitamin. The Group considers 0.3 μg. vitamin B_{12} daily to be sufficient up to 12 months. Little is known about the requirements of children; the Group therefore calculates desirable in-

---

[1] 1 pg. (one picogram) = 10^{-12} gm.

takes in relation to calorie intakes, recommending 0.9 µg. from 1 to 3 years, 1.5 µg. from 4 to 9 years, and 2 µg. from 10 years and above. Additional intakes of 1.0 µg. during pregnancy, and 0.5 µg. during lactation are recommended.

Folic acid (folate). Fresh green vegetables and liver are the best sources. Beef, wheat flour, ham and eggs all contain a little of this vitamin, while milk, fruit, mutton and poultry are poor.

The amount of folate excreted or lost by the body each day is uncertain. Total body stores in a healthy, well-fed man are usually assumed to be between 5.0 and 12 mg., and the minimum daily requirement between 50 and 100 µg. To allow for differences between individuals, the Joint FAO/WHO Expert Group (FAO, 1970b) recommends an intake of 200 µg. per day. Daily requirements increase during periods of rapid growth; the minimum for infants has been assessed at 5 µg. The Group recommends a daily intake of 40 µg. per day (approximately equivalent to daily intake in breast milk) for infants from 0 to 6 months, 60 µg. for infants from 7 to 12 months, 10 µg. for children between 1 to 12 years, and 200 µg. daily thereafter. Requirements during pregnancy may be up to four times the normal (daily intake of 400 µg. throughout pregnancy, 300 µg. during lactation).

FATS

Fat provides a readily available source of energy, and is essential for very active workers, especially in cold latitudes (Davidson and Passmore, 1966). Any community wishing to feed well must receive at least 20 per cent of its calories from fat. There is, however, no good clinical evidence that man ever lacks a sufficient dietary source of essential fatty acids. While these are likely to be necessary for the nutrition of the individual cell, it is probable that only 1 gm. per day is required, which the poorest of diets supply. The PAG *Ad Hoc* Working Group on Feeding the Preschool Child has recommended that an infant's diet should provide 35 to 50 per cent of calories from fat sources, with essential fatty acids present at 1 per cent of calorie intake (P.A.G., 1970c). It is often simpler to raise the calorie content of the diets of children by means of fat, rather than carbohydrates, since bulk is not thereby greatly increased.

In most prosperous countries, fat usually contributes 35 to 40 per cent of total calories, and in some poor countries, the figure is 15 per cent or less. Diets of lower socio-economic groups in India provide from 10 to 15 gm., while those of higher socio-economic groups provide 40 to 60 gm. (Rajalakshmi, 1969). In the present state of knowledge, Davidson and Passmore consider it is not possible to state a minimum fat requirement for man. Human diets low in fats are almost always low in protein and other nutrients necessary for health, making it difficult to ascribe disease specifically to deficiency of fat. Mitra's study (1941) of the Hos, an aboriginal tribe in Bihar, revealed a fat intake of from 2.4 gm. to 3.8 gm. per head per day, providing at most 2 per cent of the calories in the diet. Their health was no worse than that of their neighbours who used vegetable oil.

MINERALS

Calcium. This mineral is particularly important for skeletal and teeth formation in childhood. Even in the adult, about 700 mg. of calcium enter and leave the bones daily, as well as playing an important role in extracellular fluids (Davidson and Passmore, 1966). Between 20 to 30 per cent of the calcium present in food is normally digested, aided by the presence of vitamin D. Proteins also facilitate calcium absorption. A higher proportion of calcium is absorbed during bone formation. When dietary intake is low, faecal loss is reduced, and balance maintained. Studies in India (Begum and Pereira, 1969) on children with low calcium intake show that there is 50 per cent absorption of calcium in the diet, increasing when additional calcium is provided. Positive calcium balance can be maintained provided the protein intake is adequate. Seasonal differences in retention of calcium by adults were noted in China (Chen, 1948); retention is greater in autumn (14 per cent) and summer (9 per cent) than in winter and spring (3 per cent). People living in the tropics appear to be able to utilize compounds of calcium which are not readily available to others (Jelliffe, 1968a).

Recommendations for intake tend to be based on experiments with people accustomed to a diet rich in calcium; children in Asia and Africa often develop healthy bones with less than half the recommended intake (Table 9/4). The presence of sunlight and the consequent synthesis of vitamin D help absorption of calcium (FAO, 1962 and 1969a). Milk (caseinogen) is the richest source of calcium, but pulses, other vegetables and particularly cereal grains often contribute the bulk of the supply because of the large amounts consumed. Phytic acid, of which there is a considerable proportion in cereals, has been thought to inhibit calcium absorption, but subsequent studies show that this is not so for those accustomed to whole cereal products from childhood. Perhaps this is because the enzyme, phytase, can break down phytates, making calcium available (Rajalakshmi, 1969). However, the presence of oxalates in vegetables does inhibit the utilization of their calcium. During pregnancy and lactation, 1,000 to 1,200 mg. calcium a day are recommended (WHO, 1965a). It is generally agreed that every child after weaning should have 500 ml. cow's milk daily, which not only provides 600 mg. calcium, but also other useful nutrients, including the amino acids that facilitate calcium absorption.

Phosphorus. A deficiency of this mineral is not known to occur in man.

TABLE 9/4

Recommended intakes of minerals for different age groups

A. *Calcium*

Age	mg. per day
months	
0–12 (not breastfed)	500–600
years	
1–9	400–500
10–15	600–700
16–19	500–600

Source: WHO, 1965a

B. *Iron*

Recommended intakes according to type of diet

	Absorbed iron required (mg.)	Animal foods below 10 per cent of calories (mg.)	Animal foods 10-25 per cent of calories (mg.)	Animal foods over 25 per cent of calories (mg.)
Infants 0–4 months	0·5	[1]	[1]	[1]
5–12 months	1·0	10	7	5
Children 1–12 years	1·0	10	7	5
Boys 13–16 years	1·8	18	12	9
Girls 13–16 years	2·4	24	18	12
Menstruating women[2]	2·8	28	19	14
Men	0·9	9	6	5
Pregnancy } Lactation }		See text page 105		

[1] Breast-feeding is assumed to be adequate
[2] For non-menstruating women the recommended intakes are the same as for men

Source: FAO, 1970b

TABLE 9/5

India (Gujarat): diets suggested for age groups in lower and upper classes

Age (yrs)	Economic level (a)	Amount (gm.) per day								
		Cereals	Pulses (b)	Milk	Leafy vegetables	Root vegetables	Other vegetables	Fruits	Fats and oils (b)	Sugar
1	I	100—150	50	200	5—10	25	25	25	10	25
	II	50— 75	25	500—600	5—10	25	25	25	10	25—40
2—4	I	150—175	50—60	150—200	35	25—40	25—40	25—40	15	25—40
	II	75—100	25—40	400—500	25	25—40	25—40	25—40	25	25—40
5—6	I	175—200	50—60	100—200	50	25—50	50	50	25	25
	II	100—150	25—40	400—500	50	25—50	50	50	25—30	25—40
7—10	I	250—300	60—70	100—200	50	50	50	50	25	25
	II	150—200	50	400—500	50	50	50	50	25—40	25—40
11—12	I	275—375	60—75	100—200	50—75	50—75	50—75	50	25	25
	II	225—275	50	400—500	50	53—75	50—75	50	25—40	25—40
13—15	I	300—450	75	100—200	50—75	75	75	50	25—30	25
	II	300—325	60—75	400—500	50	75	75	50	25—50	25—50
16—19	I	375—475	75	100—200	50—75	75	75	50	25—30	25
	II	325—375	60—75	400—500	50	75	75	50	30—50	25—50
20—40	I	375—550	75	100—200	50—75	75	75	50	25—30	25
	II	350—375	60—75	400—500	50	75	75	50	30—50	25—50

(a) I—low income; II—middle and high income
(b) Groundnut and nuts can replace part of the pulses and fat suggested
Source: Rajalakshmi, 1969

TABLE 9/6

Malaysia: recommended daily dietary allowances

	Age Years	Weight kg.	Calories	Protein gm. N.P.U.[1] = 70	Calcium mg.	Iron mg.	Vitamin A		Thiamine mg.	Ribo-flavine mg.	Niacin equi-valent mg.	Ascorbic acid mg.
							80% β-carotene[2] i.u.	µg.				
Men	18—35	55	2,500	55	450	10	7,500	750	1·0	1·4	16·5	30
	36—55		2,300	55	450	10	7,500	750	0·9	1·3	15·2	30
	56+		1,900	55	450	10	7,500	750	0·8	1·0	12·5	30
Women	18—35	50	1,700	50	450	12	7,500	750	0·7	0·9	11·2	30
	36—55		1,600	50	450	12	7,500	750	0·6	0·9	10·6	30
	56+		1,300	50	450	12	7,500	750	0·5	0·7	8·6	30
Pregnancy (2nd half)			2,000	60	1,200	15	7,500	750	0·8	1·1	13·2.	60
Lactation			2,700	71	1,200	15	12,000	1,200	1·1	1·5	17·8	60
Infants	0—1		110 per kg.	2·3—1·2 per kg.	550	7	1,000	300	0·4	0·6	6·6	30
Children	1—3		1,180	20	450	8	2,500	250	0·5	0·6	7·8	30
	4—6		1,550	25	450	10	3,000	300	0·6	0·9	10·2	30
	7—9		1,910	35	450	12	4,000	400	0·8	1·1	12·6	30
Boys	10—12		2,280	44	650	15	5,500	575	0·9	1·3	15·0	30
	13—15		2,820	59	650	15	7,000	725	1·1	1·6	18·6	30
	16—17		3,280	61	550	15	7,500	750	1·3	1·8	21·6	30
Girls	10—12		2,280	44	650	15	5,500	575	0·9	1·3	15·0	30
	13—15		2,370	55	650	15	7,000	725	1·0	1·3	15·6	30
	16—17		2,180	55	550	15	7,500	750	0·9	1·2	14·4	30

[1] N.P.U. = Net protein utilization, a term used to describe the biological value and the digestibility of a protein
[2] It is assumed here that 80 per cent of the vitamin A in the Malaysian diet is derived from plant sources in the form of the biologically-active carotenoids of which β-carotene preponderates
Source: Chong, 1969

TABLE 9/7

Malaysia: suggested low-cost menu for pregnant woman for one week

Day	Breakfast	Lunch	Tea	Dinner	Supper
Monday	Coffee with milk, bread with margarine	Rice, fried Chye Sim, Ikan Tinggeri in Curry, Papaya	Green gram porridge	Rice, Beef fried with ginger, Taw foo steamed, Overlay with fried onions, ikan bilis steamed with sauce.	Milk drink
Tuesday	Coffee with milk, bread with margarine, half boiled egg	Rice, Pork fried with Tow Chew, Bayam Soup, Tow Gay fried, Fruit 'Nanka'	Sweet Potato with coconut	Rice, Fish tow chew steamed, Long beans fried with pork	Milk drink
Wednesday	Coffee with milk, Bombay toast bread, Margarine	Rice, Ikan bilis fried with groundnut, Kankong sambal, Dhal curry with tomato, brinjal	Biscuit, Coffee drink	Rice, Prawns fried with onions, french beans fried, Dessert —pineapple	Soybean drink
Thursday	Tea with Powdered milk, Bread with margarine	Rice, Liver fried with sauce, Tow Gay fried, Banana	Coffee drink, Maize	Rice, Cuttle fish with asam chilli, Bayam fried	Milk drink
Friday	Coffee with milk, Chapatti with dhall curry	Rice, Fish with tomato sauce, Karang fried with Kuchai, Watermelon	Steamed yam with coconut	Rice, Steamed egg with spring onions, Cucumber fried with dried prawn, Bayam Soup	Milk drink
Saturday	Milk drink, 'Chee Chong Fun' with soya sauce	Rice, Yong Tow Foo and brinjal, Cekur Manis fried with coconut, Banana	Tea drink, Sweet potato fried	Rice, Liver fried with ginger, Chye Sim in sauce	Green grams porridge
Sunday	Coffee with milk, bread with margarine	Fried Mee with Karang, Tow Gay and Chye Sim, Papaya	Maize broth with coconut milk	Rice, 'Fu Chok' cooked in sauce with Pork average, Kankong fried	Milk drink

Note: This diet is adequate in all nutrients except riboflavine (for which supplements are required) and niacin (which may be offset by conversion of tryptophan)

Source: Chan, Lee and Tan, 1967

Magnesium. Deficiency arises due to excessive loss, for example, from chronic diarrhoea, rather than to a dietary lack. In kwashiorkor, diarrhoea may cause a depletion of magnesium in the cells, possibly contributing to the apathy and weakness characteristic of this condition.

Iron. A good diet should provide at least 12 mg. per day; absorption is, however, more important than dietary intake, as only a small proportion is absorbed. This is regulated by two factors: the amount of iron in the body, and the state of activity of the bone marrow. When stores are low and new red cells are being produced rapidly, iron absorption increases. Absorption is improved by the simultaneous absorption of ascorbic acid and of protein. Phytic acid and other phosphates inhibit the absorption of iron, due to the formation of insoluble iron phosphates and phytates. It is the high concentration of phytic acid in the cereal diets of north-west India and Pakistan and in the rice diets of South-East Asia which accounts for the prevalence of anaemia in the region.

The Joint FAO/WHO Expert Group (FAO, 1970b) recommends intakes on the basis of estimates of physiological losses from the body, and of increments in

TABLE 9/8

Malaysia: nutritive value of one day's menu suggested for pregnant woman

Food	Edible portion gm.	A.P. gm.	Calories	Protein gm.	Calcium mg.	Iron mg.	Vitamin A i.u.	Thiamine mg.	Riboflavine mg.	Nicotinic acid mg.	Vitamin C mg.	Cost cents
Rice (raw highly milled)	110	110	360	6·8	6	0·8	—	12	56	1·5	—	8
Margarine	30	30	216	0·2	6	—	594					2
Bread	55	55	138	4·0	6·8	0·4		14	24	0·4	—	4
Liver	55	55	74	11·8	10·2	4·6	15,310	170	1,416	8·6	18	25
Tow Gay (Bean sprouts)	110	110	46	6·2	48	1·0	180	23	20	0·8	13	3
Banana	90	120	88	1·2	8	0·6	430	0	0	0·7	10	2
Maize	85	170	297	8·4	10·2	4·2	84	282	111	1·2	—	5
Cuttle fish	110	110	84	18·4	24	1·2	0	240	0	0·8	—	10
Bayam (green)	110	170	20	2·6	108	5·2	9,072	104	124	—	100	8
Powder milk	30	30	138	7·2	255	0·2	397	85	326	0·2	2	10
Chilli (fresh)	15	20	7	0·5	3	0·6	65	27	—	—	20	3
Onions	30	35	14	0·4	34	0·3	Trace	46	28	Trace	4	2
Oil	55	55	510	—	—	—						3
Sugar	15	15	57	—	2·5	—	—	—	—	—	—	1
TOTAL			2,049	67·7	521·7	19·1	26,132	1,003	2,105	14·2	167	86

Source: Chan, Lee and Tan, 1967

body iron during growth, resulting in iron stores of 500 mg. or more in normal men and women. Many, especially young children and women of child-bearing age, have low iron stores. The Group also reviews information on absorption from different diets; their recommendations are made for diets with high, medium and low contents of animal foods (Table 9/4).

In diets with less than 10 per cent of calories derived from food of animal origin, absorption of iron is not above 10 per cent; diets with 10 to 25 per cent of calories from foods of animal origin, absorption rises to 15 per cent; where more than 25 per cent of calories are of animal origin, absorption of iron may attain 20 per cent.

Total daily iron loss (in faeces, urine and from the skin) for an adult man of 65 kg. is taken as 0.91 mg., for a woman weighing 55 kg., 0.77 mg. Menstrual loss in 95 per cent of women is less than 20 mg. daily, placing total iron losses at 2.8 mg. daily. Intakes recommended for children include allowance not only to compensate for basal losses, but also to provide for increase in haemoglobin mass, and iron content of body tissues associated with growth. The Group concludes that, for women whose iron intake has been adequate, increased amounts are not necessary during pregnancy and lactation, but notes that iron deficiency in women is common throughout the world, with a prevalence of 20 per cent in Asia, rising to 40 per cent during pregnancy. Thus no recommendations for pregnant and lactating women are made, since these would depend on knowledge of previous dietary practices.

TABLE 9/9

Indonesia: recommended food intakes

	gm. per caput per day
Cereals: Rice	300
Other	50
Roots and tubers	150
Legumes and pulses	40
Meat and poultry (excluding bones)	20
Fish	60
Egg	5
Milk	5
Fruits and vegetables	200
Sugar	25
Fats and oils	20

Note: These allowances provide 2,100 calories and 55 gm. protein per caput per day, and meet the recommended allowances for vitamin A and other nutrients.

Legumes and vegetable proteins may substitute part of recommended intake of meat, poultry, fish, eggs and milk.

It is desirable to reduce the intake of roots and tubers, while increasing that of cereals.

Source: Indonesian Institute of Sciences, 1968

BALANCE BETWEEN NUTRIENTS

The importance of ensuring balance between nutrients has been expressed by the Joint FAO/WHO Group on Vitamins (WHO, 1967):

The group deprecated programs which overemphasize the provision of individual nutrients (with certain exceptions such as iodine and fluorine). In particular, it drew attention to the potential harm inherent in the provision of protein supplements, which may stimulate growth and hence increase the requirement for other nutrients, unless due consideration is given to the need for ensuring adequate intakes of other nutrients at the same time.

Even a small increase in the concentration of certain amino acids can increase the need for others when the total protein intake is low (FAO, 1965). The utilization of one dietary amino acid may be depressed by the addition of another structurally related to it. Two examples are: the effect of an excess of leucine on the utilization of isoleucine and valine; and of lysine on the utilization of arginine. Large amounts of single amino acids added to diets may induce toxic reactions, including depression of growth. The most toxic are methionine, tyrosine and histidine, especially when added to a diet already low in protein. FAO and WHO consider that, pending the results of further research, these observations should be taken into account in

TABLE 9/10

Indonesia: recommended nutrient intakes

	Age yrs.	Body wt. kg.	Calo-ries	Prot. gm.	Ca. gm.	Fe mg.	Vita. A µg.	Thiamine mg.	Ribo-flavine mg.	Niacin equiv. mg.	Ascorbic acid mg.
Men	20–39	55	2,600	65	0·5	10	4,000	1·0	1·4	17	60
	40–59	55	2,400	65	0·5	10	4,000	1·0	1·3	16	60
	60 +	55	2,400	65	0·5	10	4,000	0·8	1·1	13	60
Women	20–39	47	2,000	55	0·5	12	4,000	0·8	1·1	13	60
	40–59	47	1,900	55	0·5	12	4,000	0·8	1·0	13	60
	60 +	47	1,600	55	0·5	12	4,000	0·6	0·9	9	60
Pregnant		extra	+300	+10	+0·5	+5	+500	+0·2	+0·2	+2	+30
Nursing		extra	+800	+25	+0·5	+5	+2,500	+0·4	+0·4	+5	+30
Boys	16–19	50	3,000	65	0·6	12	4000	1·2	1·7	20	60
	13–15	42	2,900	58	0·7	12	4000	1·1	1·6	19	60
	10–12	35	2,300	50	0·7	12	3450	0·9	1·3	13	60
Girls	16–19	45	2,100	57	0·6	12	4,000	0·8	1·1	14	60
	13–15	42	2,400	58	0·7	12	4,000	1·0	1·3	16	60
	10–12	35	2,300	50	0·7	12	3,450	0·9	1·3	18	60
Children	7–9	27	1,900	42	0·5	10	2,400	0·8	1·0	13	50
	4–6	18	1,600	30	0·5	10	1,800	0·6	0·9	9	40
	1–3	12	1,200	25	0·5	8	1,500	0·5	0·7	8	30
Infants	6–12 months	8	900	20	0·6	8	1,200	0·4	0·5	6	25

Source: Indonesian Institute of Sciences, 1968

TABLE 9/11

Philippines: recommended daily food intakes

	(1) Leafy & yellow vegetables		(2) Vitamin C-rich Foods		(3) Other fruits & vegetables		(4) Fats	(5) Protein-Rich Foods						(6) Energy Foods				
								Whole milk	Meat, poultry & fish		Eggs	Beans & nuts (dried)		Cereals	Kamote & potatoes		Sugar
	A.P. gm.	E.P. gm.	A.P. gm.	E.P. gm.	A.P. gm.	E.P. gm.	A.P. gm.	E.P. gm.	A.P. gm.	E.P. gm.	A.P. E.P. No.	A.P. gm.	E.P. gm.	A.P. E.P. gm.	A.P. gm.	E.P. gm.	A.P. E.P. gm.
Man—53 Kg.																	
Sedentary	125	80	120	80	125	100	30	—	140	100	1/3	10	20	350	60	50	35
Moderately active	125	80	120	80	125	100	35	—	140	100	1/3	10	20	450	90	75	40
Very active	155	100	150	100	185	150	50	—	140	100	1/3	10	20	550	120	100	55
Woman—45 Kg.																	
Sedentary	125	80	120	80	125	100	20	—	105	75	1/3	10	20	325	30	25	25
Moderately active	125	80	120	80	125	100	30	—	105	75	1/3	10	20	375	60	50	35
Very active	155	100	150	100	185	150	45	—	105	75	1/3	10	20	500	60	50	40
Pregnancy (latter half)	155	100	150	100	125	100	20	200	230	165	1	30	20	325	60	50	25
Nursing	155	100	150	100	125	100	40	450	230	165	1	30	20	350	60	50	45
Infant																	
Under 1 year (6 months)	30	20	45	30	25	20	—	200	15	10	1/2	15	—	10	25	20	20
Children up to 12 years																	
1–3 years	45	30	120	80	45	35	10	450	90	65	1/3	10	10	125	60	50	10
4–6 years	55	35	120	80	65	50	15	300	105	75	1/3	10	10	175	60	50	20
7–9 years	60	40	120	80	125	100	15	200	160	115	1/3	10	20	250	60	50	25
10–12 years	95	60	150	100	125	100	30	200	180	130	1/3	10	20	300	90	75	35
Children over 12 years																	
Girls: 13–15 yrs.	125	80	150	100	125	100	35	200	265	190	1	30	15	375	75	65	30
16–20 yrs.	125	80	150	100	125	100	35	200	230	165	1	30	15	300	75	65	30
Boys: 13–15 yrs.	155	100	150	100	125	100	35	200	265	190	1	30	20	450	75	65	30
16–20 yrs.	155	100	150	100	185	150	55	200	265	190	1	30	20	550	100	85	50
Per caput gm. A.P.	106		130		118		28	162	149			16	17	329	71		32

A.P.—As purchased
E.P.—Edible portion

Source: Philippines, FNRC, 1968

Note: This table will require modification to bring it up to date with Table 9/12.

TABLE 9/12

Philippines: recommended daily nutrient intakes

	Body wt. kg.	Energy Kcal.	Protein gm.	Calcium gm.	Iron mg.	Vitamin A activity i.u.	Thiamine mg.	Riboflavine mg.	Niacin equivalent mg.	Ascorbic acid mg.
Reference Man 25 yrs	56	2,500	63	0·5	8	5,000	1·3	1·3	16	75
30—49 yrs.	56	2,400	63	0·5	8	5,000	1·2	1·2	16	75
50—69 yrs.	56	2,200	63	0·5	8	5,000	1·1	1·1	15	75
70+ yrs.	56	1,950	63	0·5	8	5,000	1·0	1·0	13	75
Reference Woman 25 yrs.	49	1,900	55	0·5	18	5,000	1·0	1·0	13	70
30—49 yrs.	49	1,800	55	0·5	18	5,000	0·9	0·9	13	70
50—69 yrs.	49	1,600	55	0·5	7	5,000	0·8	0·8	13	70
70+ yrs.	49	1,450	55	0·5	7	5,000	0·7	0·7	13	70
Pregnant		2,300	65	1·0	18[1]	5,000	1·2	1·2	15	100
Nursing		2,900	75	1·0	18[1]	7,000	1·5	1·5	19	150
Infants 6—12 mths.	9	950	25	0·6	7	1,500	0·5	0·5	6	30
Children: 1—3 yrs.	12	1,300	26	0·5	7	2,000	0·7	0·7	9	35
4—6 yrs.	17	1,600	32	0·5	7	2,500	0·8	0·8	11	50
7—9 yrs.	25	1,900	38	0·5	7	3,000	1·0	1·0	13	60
10—12 yrs.	33	2,300	45	0·7	7	4,000	1·2	1·2	15	75
Boys: 13—15 yrs.	44	2,800	60	0·7	11	5,000	1·4	1·4	18	90
16—19 yrs.	55	2,800	65	0·6	11	5,000	1·4	1·4	18	100
Girls: 13—15 yrs.	44	2,300	60	0·7	13	5,000	1·2	1·2	15	80
16—19 yrs.	48	2,100	60	0·6	13	5,000	1·1	1·1	14	80

[1] It is assumed that the woman has adequate stores prior to this condition

Source: Intengan and FNRC, 1970

studies of the biological effectiveness of essential amino-acid patterns and in the supplementation of specific foods with amino acids.

Supplementation of *Sorghum vulgare* diets with L-lysine caused a marked increase in nitrogen retention and growth rates of children aged 7 to 12 years (Doraiswamy, Rao, Swaminathan and Parpia, 1968). However, increased growth supported by lysine supplementation is markedly inferior to that following dietary supplementation with green leaf protein, demonstrating that increased concentration of protein in the whole diet is required (Doraiswamy, Singh and Daniel, 1969). The merits of adding lysine in any amount may be questioned where diets are otherwise unbalanced. Where food grains are the principal source of protein, and if the lysine is raised to the level of reference protein, other amino acids, both essential and non-essential, will become limiting before this value is reached. Even if it were possible to induce a moderate improvement in the biological value of a protein by fortification with lysine, this may well cause a growth spurt in infants, children and adolescents. Thus a sudden increased demand will be created, not only for more protein, but also for vitamin A, calcium, iron and indeed all the nutrients essential for growth, so many of which are deficient in Asian diets.

What applies on the micro-scale with regard to amino acids is even more important on the broader canvas of the major nutrients. For example, full utilization of protein by the body depends upon the adequacy of essential fatty acids, certain vitamins and minerals. Riboflavine enhances protein utilization, and there is evidence that an increase in protein consumption increases the requirement for riboflavine. Protein deficiency affects the hepatic mobilization, transport and intestinal absorption of vitamin A, and even more so, intestinal absorption of carotene, leading eventually to xerophthalmia and keratomalacia (see Chapter 11) and the permanent blindness of young children which is so widespread in India, Indonesia and possibly China. Blankhart (1967) even found night blindness

TÁBLE 9/13

Japan: recommended daily nutrient intakes in relation to age and occupation

Age	Calories Male	Calories Female	Protein M (gm.)	Protein F (gm.)	Calcium M (gm.)	Calcium F (gm.)	Iron M (mg.)	Iron F (mg.)	Salt M (gm.)	Salt F (gm.)	Vit. A M (i.u.)[1]	Vit. A F (i.u.)[1]
Months 0 ~	120/kg	120/kg	3·4/kg	3·4/kg								
2 ~	110/kg	110/kg	2·8/kg	2·8/kg	0·4	0·4	6	6	1	1	1,300	1,300
Years 6 ~	100/kg	100/kg	3·0/kg	3·0/kg								
1 ~	950	950	35	30								
2 ~	1,200	1,150	40	40			7	7	3	3		
3 ~	1,350	1,300	45	40	0·4	0·4					1,500 (4,500)	1,500 (4,500)
4 ~	1,500	1,400	45	45								
5 ~	1,600	1,450	50	45			8	8	5	5		
6 ~	1,700	1,550	50	50								
7 ~	1,800	1,650	55	50	0·5	0·5					1,700 (5,100)	1,700 (5,100)
8 ~	1,900	1,750	55	60			9	9	8	8		
9 ~	2,000	1,900	60	65	0·6	0·6						
10 ~	2,100	2,050	70	70			10	10	10	10		
11 ~	2,250	2,200	75	75	0·8	0·8					2,000 (6,000)	2,000 (6,000)
12 ~	2,400	2,350	85	80								
13 ~	2,600	2,450	90	75	0·9	0·9	12	15	12	12		
14 ~	2,700	2,450	90	75								
15 ~	2,800	2,400	85	70								
16 ~	2,800	2,300	85	65	0·8	0·7	13	15	14	14	2,500 (7,500)	2,500 (7,500)
17 ~	2,800	2,250	75	65								
18 ~	2,700	2,200	75	65								
19 ~	2,650	2,150	75	65	0·7	0·6	13	15	15	15	2,000 (6,000)	2,000 (6,000)
(20) ~	2,550	2,100	70	60								
20 ~	2,500	2,000	70	60								
30 ~	2,400	2,000	70	60								
40 ~	2,300	1,900	70	60	0·6	0·6	10	15	15	15	2,000 (6,000)	2,000 (6,000)
50 ~	2,200	1,800	70	60								
60 ~	2,000	1,700	70	60								
70 ~	1,800	1,550	65	55				10³				
First half of pregnancy		2,100		75		1·0		15		15		2,200 (6,600)
Second half of pregnancy		2,400		80				20		15		2,400 (7,200)
Nursing mother		2,800		85		1·1		20		20		3,500 (10,500)
Light work	2,200	1,800	70	60	0·6	0·6	10	15	15	15	2,000 (6,000)	2,000 (6,000)
Ordinary work	2,500	2,000	70	60	0·6	0·6	10		15	15	2,000 (6,000)	2,000 (6,000)
Heavier work	3,000	2,400	70	60	0·6	0·6	10	10³	20	20	2,000 (6,000)	2,000 (6,000)
Very heavy work	3,500	2,800	70	60	0·6	0·6	10		20	20	2,000 (6,000)	2,000 (6,000)

Age	Thiamine M (mg.)	Thiamine F (mg.)	Riboflavine M (mg.)	Riboflavine F (mg.)	Niacin M (mg.)	Niacin F (mg.)	Vit. C M (mg.)	Vit. C F (mg.)	Vit. D M (i.u.)[2]	Vit. D F (i.u.)[2]
Months 0 ~	0·2	0·2	0·3	0·3	4	4				
2 ~	0·3	0·3	0·3	0·3	5	5	35	35	400	400
Years 6 ~	0·35	0·35	0·4	0·4	6	6				
1 ~	0·4	0·4	0·5	0·5	8	8				
2 ~	0·6	0·5	0·6	0·6	10	9				
3 ~	0·6	0·6	0·7	0·7	11	11			400	400
4 ~	0·7	0·6	0·8	0·7	12	11				
5 ~	0·7	0·7	0·8	0·7	13	12	40	40		
6 ~	0·8	0·7	0·9	0·8	14	13				
7 ~	0·8	0·8	0·9	0·8	15	13				
8 ~	0·9	0·8	1·0	0·9	15	14				
9 ~	0·9	0·9	1·0	1·0	16	15				
10 ~	1·0	0·9	1·1	1·0	17	17			400	400
11 ~	1·0	1·0	1·1	1·1	18	18				
12 ~	1·1	1·1	1·2	1·2	19	19	45	45		
13 ~	1·2	1·1	1·3	1·2	20	20				
14 ~	1·2	1·1	1·4	1·2	22	20				
15 ~	1·3	1·1	1·4	1·2	23	19				
16 ~	1·3	1·0	1·4	1·2	23	19	55	50		
17 ~	1·3	1·0	1·4	1·1	23	18				
18 ~	1·2	1·0	1·4	1·1	22	18				
19 ~	1·2	1·0	1·3	1·1	21	17	60	50	—	—
(20) ~	1·2	1·0	1·3	1·1	21	17				
20 ~	1·1	0·9	1·3	1·0	20	16				
30 ~	1·1	0·9	1·2	1·0	19	16				
40 ~	1·0	0·9	1·2	1·0	19	15	60	50		
50 ~	1·0	0·8	1·1	0·9	18	15				
60 ~	0·9	0·8	1·0	0·9	16	14				
70 ~	0·8	0·7	0·9	0·8	15	13				
First half of pregnancy		1·1		1·2		18		55		400
Second half of pregnancy		1·2		1·3		20		60		
Nursing mother		1·5		1·7		23		90		400
Light work	1·0	0·8	1·1	0·9	18	15	60	50	—	—
Ordinary work	1·1	0·9	1·3	1·0	20	16	60	50	—	—
Heavier work	1·4	1·1	1·5	1·2	24	19	60	50	—	—
Very heavy work	1·6	1·3	1·8	1·4	28	23	60	50	—	—

Source: Japan, Ministry of Health and Welfare, 1969

[1] Figures in brackets refer to carotene

[2] Some intake of vitamin D is necessary for adults; 400 i.u. or less are adequate, since this vitamin is synthesized in the presence of sunlight.

[3] After menopause requirement 10 gm.

occurring in Javanese children who were receiving milk powder containing 400 i.u. vitamin A daily; the protein had induced a growth spurt with an increased demand for vitamin A not fully met by the milk powder.

Haemoglobin synthesis requires iron, protein, vitamin E, folic acid, vitamin B_{12}, pyridoxine and ascorbic acid; iron absorption is facilitated by the presence of ascorbic acid and proteins, while phytic acid in cereals prevents absorption of iron unless adequate calcium and vitamin C are available. The relation between the absorption of calcium and the simultaneous presence of vitamin D and protein has been noted, as also that between the requirement of thiamine in relation to calorie intake. Adequate fat, particularly of animal origin, helps to ensure the availability of the fat-soluble vitamins, A and D, as well as of adequate essential fatty acids, which has been related to protein absorption (El Maraghi and Stewart, 1963).

Davidson and Passmore (1966) state that in many tropical countries it is impossible to over-emphasize the improvement of health that is likely to arise from even a small increase in the vegetable supply. A poor anaemic woman with insufficient iron, vitamin A and ascorbic acid in her diet may find immeasurable improvement in her health as a result of taking one helping of vegetables a day.

Thus it is clear that attempts must be made to introduce greater variety into many Asian diets, and to increase the proportions of the protective foods. Recommended intakes of individual nutrients may be useful for nutritionists and medical workers. What the agricultural planners need to know, for each basic food pattern within the region, are the approximate amounts of foods which should be produced to ensure health and growth for all members of the community.

ANTHROPOMETRIC STANDARDS

Most nutrient requirements are calculated according to a theoretical average height and weight of Reference Man and Reference Woman. Work is being done in most Asian countries aimed at acquiring a more precise definition of optimal height and weight of healthy adults, and of the rate of maturation of children at different ages — height, weight, bone formation, etc. Some examples are:

General: Meredith (1968, 1969a, 1969b, 1970a, 1970b).
Cambodia: Nouth-Savouen (1966).
India: Agarwal, Manwani, Khanduja, Agarwal and Gupta (1970);
     Banik, Krishna, Mane, Raj and Taskar (1970);
     Banik, Nayar, Krishna, Raj and Gadebar (1970);
     ICMR (1968);
     Raghavan, Singh and Swaminathan (1971);
     Sharat, Khanduja, Agarwal, Saha, Gupta and Bhardwaj (1970);
     Shirole and Phadke (1970).
Malaysia: Chen and Dugdale (1970).
Hong Kong: Crooke-Fry, Leverton and Suna (1967);
     Field and Baber (1973).
Philippines: Bulato-Jayme, de la Paz and Gervasio (1971);
     Camcam (1969);
     Matawaran and Gervasio (1971).
Korea: Yonsei University (1967-8).
Japan: Japan, Ministry of Health and Welfare (1969);
     Japan, Ministry of Health and Welfare (1972);
     Hayami, Tamura, Chikaraishi, Shirai and Okabe (1970).

THE LAND AND THE NUTRITIONAL TARGETS

The dietary and nutritional recommendations, if they are to have any practical reality, must ultimately be expressed in terms of the capacity of the land and its cultivators and animal husbandmen to meet these demands. It is only when we multiply individual recommendations for the different age groups by the numbers of population involved that the enormity of the targets is revealed. This calls for refinement and co-ordination of present techniques for the analysis of individual components of the land and the assessment of maximum potential production within the innumerable economic ecosystems which are to be found in Asia. As long as the present serious imbalance between population and land resources is permitted to continue, there can only be an aggravation of the stress on the vulnerable groups (Chapter 10), and the continued presence of under-nutrition and malnutrition described in Chapter 11.

10 The Vulnerable Groups

AMONG the rural people, the correct nutrition of the vulnerable groups within the community must receive priority if the children of the present are to become capable citizens of the future, fully developed and strong in body and brain capacity. The vulnerable groups are usually defined as including infants and children of pre-school age (1 to 6 years), pregnant and nursing mothers, and the sick. Where diets are known to be unsatisfactory, probably all women of reproductive age should be included. School children and adolescents also have special needs. Increasingly it is being recognized that these groups need particular consideration in nutrition policies, especially where resources of plant and animal protein are in deficit; the welfare of the present and future generations of children demands that limited supplies of the acceptable forms of protein, particularly those of animal origin, should be reserved for the vulnerable groups.

Environmental factors in addition to nutrition affect the general well-being of the child. Poor environmental sanitation and overcrowding expose Asian children to diseases against which their low nutritional status gives them little resistance. If the mother returns to work in the fields after the first few months of giving birth, the infant may not be breast-fed as frequently as it requires. In this respect, infants in the Far East seem to be favoured, since the method of carrying them does not interfere with the mother's activities, and they are frequently taken along on her back, until they become too heavy. Infants are soon left with older siblings, who, though they quickly learn to accept the responsibility and to pacify their charges, cannot be expected to care for them properly, or to provide cooked food. When a child falls sick, poverty and ignorance prevent suitable remedial measures.

Asian children are rarely without the company of their peers, and do not lack stimulus to play; they learn quickly to become members of their social community. Intellectual stimulus from illiterate parents in surroundings devoid of printed matter, and without the necessary light to read after dark, is minimal. The complex interrelations of these handicaps fall within the field of specialization of the child sociologist and the child psychologist (Whiting, Child and Lambert, 1966).

The vulnerable groups in the population of Monsoon Asia alone represent about one-third of the total world population. Although population statistics and the breakdown of total figures into groups are notoriously unreliable, one may probably accept the common generalization that some 50 per cent of the population of Monsoon Asia is below 15 years of age. Add to this the number of mothers of child-bearing age, and it will be seen that a considerable proportion of the total population is included in these three groups. It cannot be said that the recommended standards of nutrition are achieved, particularly among the 80 per cent of the total Asian population living in rural areas. On the other hand, it must be realized that, if they were, Asia and the world would be faced with a population explosion of unprecedented dimensions.

THE CRITICAL PHASES

There are four critical phases in the early life of the human organism when the Asian child is particularly subject to nutritional stress:

from conception to birth;
from birth to weaning;
from weaning to about six years of age; and
adolescence.

Inadequate nutrition at any time before maturity is expressed in impaired growth and reduced resistance to disease; inadequate nutrition during the first three stages results in impaired neuromotor development in the short term, and reduced mental capacity in the long term. The nutritional status of the infant is, of course, largely governed by the nutrition and health of the mother.

By the time the child has reached 5 or 6 years, it is usually obtaining a share of the adult diet, and becomes adapted to this level of intake, though disease and other stress will often give rise to parallel signs of nutritional deficiency. The higher nutrient demands of adolescence, however, are frequently not met in Asia, and this may again be a period of critical deficiency; this age-group has been little studied.

NUTRITION DURING PREGNANCY AND LACTATION

The WHO Expert Committee on Nutrition in Pregnancy and Lactation (1965a) assessed the physiological cost of pregnancy and lactation as far as was possible from available evidence. There are extensive changes in maternal body composition and metabolism during pregnancy and a probable increased efficiency in absorption of iron, vitamin B_{12}, calcium and other nutrients during both pregnancy and lactation. The Indian Council of Medical Research (1969) notes there is increased absorption of dietary iron and calcium with the advance of gestation. Increase of dietary iron is largely independent of the iron nutritional status of women. While it is possible to assess physiological cost for some nutrients, there are difficulties in making recommendations for dietary intake. Requirements may be met from maternal reserves. It is difficult to assess losses during absorption.

The FAO Committee on Calorie Requirements (1957), estimating the physiological cost of pregnancy with an average weight gain of 12.5 kg., suggests an additional requirement of 80,000 kcal., of which more than half is for fat storage. Mothers in developing countries may gain only 6 kg. or less, without a corresponding drop in birth weight; in this case, the additional calorie requirement is also halved. An average daily milk secretion of 850 ml., using an efficiency coefficient of 60 per cent, would involve a physiological cost of 1,000 kcal., an efficiency coefficient of 80 per cent, 750 kcal.

Research suggests that 0.5, 3.0, 4.5 and 5.7 gm. protein daily are laid down in the foetus and foetal membranes during the four semesters of pregnancy, giving a total of 950 gm. For women with low protein intake, the FAO/WHO Expert Group on Protein Requirements (FAO, 1965) recommends an additional 6 gm. reference protein per day during the last half

of pregnancy. There is pronounced retention of nitrogen during pregnancy, two-thirds outside the products of conception and maternal reproductive tissues, considered to be a reserve for lactation (Toverud, Stearns and Macy, 1950). Human milk contains an average 1.2 gm. protein per 100 ml.; even in areas of chronic malnutrition this rarely falls below 1 gm. The Expert Group assumes tentatively that 2 gm. food protein will be necessary to produce 1 gm. milk protein, and calculates that 15 gm. additional reference protein daily would be adequate for nearly all women.

The WHO Expert Committee on Nutrition in Pregnancy and Lactation considers that 2 to 3 mg. iron should be supplied daily in the latter half of pregnancy. It estimates that the physiological cost in terms of calcium deposited in the foetus, mostly during the latter half of pregnancy, is 30 gm. They accept the findings of the Joint FAO/WHO Expert Group on Calcium Requirements (WHO, 1962) which recommends 1,000 mg. daily during pregnancy, and 1,200 mg. daily during lactation; there is, however, little evidence of adverse effects over much of the world where intakes are far lower. The WHO Expert Committee on Nutrition in Pregnancy and Lactation considers the evidence to be inadequate for estimations with regard to other nutrients, although requirements for several are certainly increased.

The WHO Expert Committee finds a general association between low birth weights, high foetal and infant mortality rates on the one hand, and diets of poor nutritive value on the other: 'It seems reasonable to conclude that undernutrition and malnutrition among mothers, especially in the developing countries, contribute towards impaired maternal, foetal and infant health and vitality.'

A higher stillbirth and neonatal death rate is found within different ethnic groups among low-income mothers, whose dietary intakes are inadequate and who are invariably working. Chronic subnutrition is doubtless responsible for lower heights and weights of women in lower socio-economic groups. Infant and maternal mortality rates for Malays are higher than for other ethnic groups in Malaysia and Singapore, and greater in rural than urban areas (Millis, 1958b). Undernourished women produce smaller babies, which have a higher death rate. A precarious adaptation to low intakes of major nutrients may be disturbed by the stress of pregnancy and lactation, which are achieved at the expense of maternal tissue. A long succession of pregnancies results in premature ageing, which is aggravated by poor environmental conditions and by disease. During successive pregnancies with little or no respite between periods of nursing, women draw upon their own body reserves, which become progressively depleted. In south India, 20 per cent of the women become pregnant within one year of the previous birth (Rao, Swaminathan, Swarup and Patwardhan, 1959). The WHO Scientific Group on Nutritional Anaemias (1968a) considers that anaemia exists in a pregnant woman whose haemoglobin level is lower than 11 gm. per 100 ml. venous blood, and in a non-pregnant woman whose haemoglobin level is lower than 12 gm. per 100 ml. venous blood. Concentrations lower than these are common in all developing countries.

There is little information to indicate how mothers, who are usually working while nursing, meet the energy costs of lactation. The WHO Expert Committee on Nutrition in Pregnancy and Lactation considers that sustained production of milk is probably achieved at the expense of the mother's health. Milk secretion does not appear to fall below 750 ml. per day, although Bailey (1962b) found a daily production of only 400 to 500 ml. in the cassava areas of Java where malnutrition is endemic. The volume of breast milk produced by Indo-Chinese mothers diminishes early in lactation (Jelliffe, 1968a). Diets in the developing countries are likely to be low in vitamin A, the B complex, ascorbic acid and calcium (WHO, 1965a). Jelliffe (1968a) considers avitaminosis to be prevalent throughout Asia, describing findings in India, Indonesia, Burma, Philippines, Ceylon and China; it is common in Korea (Haw, Yu, Lee, Sung, Tchai and Cha, 1970). Most Indian women in lower socio-economic groups are able successfully to breast-feed children in the first half of infancy, despite the prevalent poor diet; there is, however, a direct relation between the protein and fat intake of mothers and the concentration of these constituents in milk on lower levels of intake (Belavady, 1963). Histidine, methionine, cystine and tryptophan show a direct relation with intake. All the vitamins in milk show a positive and significant relation with intake. Yield starts to decline after twelve to sixteen weeks of pregnancy, and is considerably reduced after thirty to thirty-two weeks. Only iron and calcium seem to remain constant in breast milk, regardless of diet.

Deficiency of vitamin A is characteristic of all ethnic groups in Malaysia (Thomson, Ruiz and Bakar, 1964). The nutritional intake of pregnant women in low-income groups is deficient in both protein and vitamin A, according to studies of blood samples taken at delivery.

The Joint FAO/WHO Expert Group on Protein Requirements states that, in the absence of sufficient dietary protein to sustain satisfactory lactation, especially in a mother who has had several closely-spaced pregnancies, the protein needed for milk secretion must be derived from her own tissues. There is evidence that in developing countries the body weights of women of low-income groups may decrease progressively with each successive pregnancy (Venkatachalam and Rebello, 1966).

Jelliffe (1968a) has stressed that:

the importance of ensuring optimal stores is even greater in tropical mothers than it is in the temperate zone, the mother acting as a refinery for the coarse foods usually obtainable, which the infant would find difficulty in digesting in the early months of life. The effect of poor foetal storage is usually only manifested later in the first year of life, when rapid growth is unsupported by adequate supplementation of breast milk.

Stores are laid down chiefly during the last three months of pregnancy.

Asian Diets during Pregnancy and Lactation

Little information is available on dietary intakes among pregnant and nursing women in rural areas. The Institute of Medical Research and the Maternity Hospital in Kuala Lumpur have investigated nutritional status of one hundred Malayan pregnant mothers from lower-income urban groups. Thiamine, iron and riboflavine were most deficient, with niacin, ascorbic acid and calcium also inadequate. It was expected that greater dietary deficiencies would be found among pregnant women in the rural areas (Chong, Lourdenadin, Thean, Lim and Lopez, 1968).

Millis (1958b) studied modifications of food selection by the wives of 358 lower-income women, wives of policemen, who returned to their kampong for confinement and remained until the baby was four to six weeks old. The usual diet in urban areas was highly milled rice, white bread, up to 45 gm. sugar, root vegetables, and fish as the most important source of animal protein. Most claimed to eat meat, but in small quantities. Most used sweetened condensed milk; 9 gm. egg, and 3 gm. liver, with 9 gm. legumes were taken per head per day. The average total protein intake was 23 gm. daily. The popularity of small fish ensured adequate supplies of calcium, while vegetables probably provided sufficient vitamins A and C. The vitamin B complex, especially riboflavine, was low.

No special increases were made for pregnancy or lactation, but few foods were avoided (Millis, op. cit.). After confinement, however, when the mother moved to her family kampong, taboos were observed, with shellfish, fish, fruits and vegetables avoided by most. Many refused fats and dried foods. Ginger, black pepper, turmeric and garlic were increased to promote milk production. After forty-four days, most mothers had returned to the town and resumed a normal diet, though modifications were made by some. 'Cooling' vegetables and fruit were still avoided by some mothers. The diet failed to supply the additional nutrients, particularly vitamins A, the B complex and C, necessary for the production of good milk, causing depletion of maternal tissue; 70 mothers had weaned by the third month, because of failure of lactation, and 90 before one year, for the same reason.

Among poor, pregnant and lactating women in south India, there was a direct relation between intake of nutrients and family income; a woman's diet actually deteriorates during pregnancy, since she can no longer work and contribute to the total budget (Pasricha, 1958). Table 10/1 reveals the discrepancies in consumption concealed by the averages given for each group.

In West Bengal, women do not eat extra food during pregnancy, while family diets are high in carbohydrates and low in protein. Milk yield falls during the third month, and among many has diminished or stopped altogether by six months (Bagchi, Halder, Choudhury, Sanyal and Sen, 1960).

A survey of diets of nursing mothers made before beginning an applied nutrition project in three villages in Coimbatore District, south India, showed negligible consumption of milk and leafy vegetables, but fair amounts of flesh foods. Diets were deficient in protein, calcium, vitamin A and riboflavine (Devadas and Prema, 1965). (See Table 10/2).

In Tokushima Prefecture, Japan, pregnant women during summer in a mountain village and a fishing village lacked vitamins A and C, protein and calories, while women in a farming village lacked protein and vitamin C. In winter, women in the mountain village lacked protein, iron, vitamins A and C (Yoneda, Omi,

TABLE 10/1(a)

India South: calorie and protein intake of pregnant and lactating women
from lower socio-economic groups

	Calories			*Protein (gm.)*			*Animal protein as percentage of total protein*		
	Maximum	*Minimum*	*Mean*	*Maximum*	*Minimum*	*Mean*	*Maximum*	*Minimum*	*Mean*
Pregnant	3951	789	1815	99·1	17·5	44	71·6	0	14·9
Lactating	2936	805	1858	68	16	42·7	49	0	12·2
Before pregnancy	4291	1133	2152	108·9	26·4	49·8	60·7	0	13·4

The diet of 100 women prior to and during pregnancy, and that of 70 lactating women, was studied

Source: Pasricha, 1958

TABLE 10/1(b)

India South: number in family and income per caput

	Number in family	*Income per caput per month (Rs.)*		
		Maximum	*Minimum*	*Mean*
Pregnant	4 to 5	47·4	3·4	17
Lactating	5	32·6	4·5	15

Source: Pasricha, 1958

TABLE 10/2

India: Coimbatore: average quantities of foods consumed daily by nursing mothers
in three villages

	Quantity consumed (gm.)			
	Rajannagar	*Basuvapalyam*	*Kothamangalam*	*Recommended intake*
Cereals	500	473	455	312
Pulses	40	24	35	85
Leafy vegetables	4	Nil	1	85
Other vegetables	25	14	18	142
Fruits	Nil	Nil	Nil	85
Milk and milk products	11	87	Nil	91
Flesh foods	90	Nil	30	85

Source: Devadas and Prema, 1965

Oe, Kishi, Yamanashi, Sako, Yumura, Sano, Otsuka, Tomida, 1966). The diets of a group of housewives aged 30 to 49 in a rural mountain district of Kyoto were found to be deficient in total protein, animal protein, thiamine, riboflavine, vitamin C, vitamin A and calcium; only carbohydrate intakes were satisfactory, and there was a high incidence of fatigue (Matsudaira, 1969).

In the cassava areas of Java, Bailey (1961b) reported hunger oedema in 55 per cent of lactating women during the first year, with a lower incidence thereafter. There is a trend towards higher incidence of this oedema when calorie intake is relatively adequate and protein intake low, while physical exertion is maximal, for example during the planting season. Oedema in lactation demonstrates the inadequacy of diet and the failure of compensatory metabolic adjustments during pregnancy and lactation.

CHILDREN: BIRTH TO WEANING

When the mother is healthy, breast-feeding is considered sufficient in terms of nutrient intake for her child up to the age of about 6 months. If the mother is malnourished, supplementation will be required earlier. Malnutrition in the mother may be a continuous condition, or may be due to seasonal variations, particularly in the supply of vegetables (see Chapter 3). A reflection of seasonality of food supplies is found in birthweights of children in west China. While severe deprivation of essential nutrients in the preceding eight years had had little effect on the yearly average of birthweights, there was a statistically sig-

nificant seasonal variation; the lightest babies were born in September, the heaviest in January (Lee, 1948).

It is common practice for mothers to deny the breast to the newborn for the first two to five days, until colostrum is replaced by milk. During this time, infants are given a variety of substances, many of which may be contaminated and carry the risk of infection. In Gujarat, India, diarrhoea occurs among some 10 per cent of newborn babies given jaggery or honey on the mother's finger, or on a cotton plug (Lala and Desai, 1970). As birth itself is regarded as an unclean process, both mother and child are often purged. The Chinese consider purging the newborn drives out heating substances. In south India it is common practice to purge children from birth to 18 months as frequently as every second day, a practice which leads to chronic gastro-enteritis (Rao, 1962).

Beyond 6 months, breast milk becomes progressively inadequate to meet the needs of the growing child. Ideally, the infant's diet should be supplemented with vitamins, minerals and animal protein, and with carbohydrates to provide additional calories. Jelliffe (1968a) considers that giving supplements before 6 months of age carries a serious risk of infection. WHO, however, recommends the addition of suitably prepared rice, legumes, fish, eggs and yellow vegetables from 3 months, and leafy vegetables and dried fish from 7 to 12 months (WHO, 1968b, FAO, 1967b). The Western Pacific Regional Office of WHO advises banana with yellow core and the staple food, suitably prepared, from 3 months, followed by papaya or mango, yellow sweet potato or pumpkin and dried beans, fish flour, fresh fish or soft-boiled egg at 4 months (WHO, 1969). Rajalakshmi (1969) refers to the importance of giving boiled water to the infant during the first few months of life.

Where protein deficiency in the weaning diet is suspected, and especially where the drinking of cow's milk is not traditional, nutritionists emphasize the importance of ensuring a balanced diet for the mother in order that lactation may be sustained, and weaning from the breast delayed. Paediatricians recommend the prolonging of lactation into the second or even the third year, with appropriate feeding of the mother to sustain this. Platt calculates that only half a litre of milk per day is necessary to make an African child's diet of 1,000 calories sufficient for growth (Jelliffe, 1968a). However, the increased production and consumption of vegetables and grain legumes by the rural mothers that these proposals entail present formidable problems of agricultural extension and nutrition education.

In actual practice, while supplementation of breast milk with the staple or mashed banana may take place from the first few days of life in South-East Asia, other foods are added by most mothers only when the child is withdrawn from the breast.

Supplements and Infant Nutritional Status

Pakistan. More than half the children in both Pakistan and former East Pakistan (now Bangla Desh) are breast-fed until they are 2 years old or more. Principal supplementary foods are carbohydrate, with little meat, fish or egg (Tables 10/3 & 10/4).

Nepal. The Vaisya caste breast-feed for longer periods than other groups, most ceasing when the child is two years old or more. Most give supplements before the first year, starting from 3 to 6 months, or from 6 to 12 months. All groups choose rice in some form as the first food, though Vaisyas tend to mix it with milk. Additional supplementary foods are meat, or dhal, while other groups use bread (Brown, Worth and Shah, 1968a). No clinical evidence of protein-calorie malnutrition was found in health surveys in nineteen villages throughout Nepal, but infant mortality of 150 per 1,000 and 39 deaths per 1,000 in the 1 to 4 age group suggest some degree of malnutrition (Brown, Worth and Shah, 1968b).

India. Breast-feeding continues until at least 18 months; one in five is still breast-fed at 2 years, and one in eight at 3 years of age (Rao, Swaminathan, Swarup and Patwardhan, 1959). Supplementation with solids takes place very late; after one year in north India, and at about 18 months in the south, when children are able to pick up their food (Rao, 1962).

Great variations in practice occur, however. Rao *et al.* (1959) found that in Andhra Pradesh, 90 per cent received rice gruel, 9 per cent milk, mostly in the first year of life. In Madras, Mysore and Kerala, from 25 to 50 per cent received some form of milk food,

TABLE 10/3

Pakistan (before secession of Bangla Desh): infant feeding supplements and age started

Type of food	*Age of child in months*				
	6-9	*9-12*	*12-15*	*15-18*	*18 & above*
	Per cent of mothers reporting				
Biscuits	41·1	22·3	10·8	17·9	7·8
Banana	39·7	19·6	12·1	14·0	13·9
Rice	16·3	12·3	14·9	38·9	18·2
Other cereals (barley)	19·4	21·8	12·7	24·3	21·5
Meat or fish	8·2	4·1	10·2	47·0	26·5
Other foods	20·7	14·4	14·5	28·0	21·6

Source: Rahman, 1968a

TABLE 10/4

Pakistan: age, number and percentage of infants receiving supplements

Number of mothers	Food items	6-9	9-12	12-15	15-18	18 months & above	Total
1,583	Biscuits	193 (10·7)	146 (13·3)	55 (11·8)	6 (1·3)	67 (14·3)	467
	Banana	—	1 (100·0)	—	—	—	—
	Rice	85 (11·4)	272 (36·4)	197 (26·3)	24 (3·2)	170 (22·7)	748
	Roti	167 (15·8)	372 (31·4)	345 (29·1)	46 (3·9)	234 (19·8)	1,184
	Other fruits	19 (17·3)	31 (28·2)	30 (27·3)	2 (1·8)	28 (25·5)	110
	Other foods	14 (10·7)	25 (19·1)	28 (21·4)	3 (2·3)	61 (26·6)	131

Note: Figures in parentheses show the percentages

Source: Rahman, 1968a

while in Madras and Kerala less than 10 per cent received other solid or liquid foods, such as tapioca, banana, congee, tea or coffee. The high average number reported to be giving milk to infants in Mysore is explained by a particularly high figure in one locality, where milk could not be sold due to distance from market. Milk when given is always in small quantities — from 10 to 300 ml. per day, and heavily diluted with an equal quantity of water. Mortality up to the age of 1 year is 162.5, and from 1 to 4, 33.5 per 1,000 in south India.

In a village in North Kanara, Mysore, supplementary feeding starts at 8 months (Swaminathan, Apte and Rao, 1960), while breast-feeding continues to 2 or 3 years of age. Supplements given are usually rice gruel. Brahmans and Vaisyas prefer to use milk, but this is extremely diluted. The weaning diet is thus most inadequate (Table 10/5a).

Tribal groups throughout India (Roy and Roy, 1962) usually use a soft gruel made of rice as a supplement to breast milk. The Padan Abors of northeast India add a home-fermented beer to this.

In Calcutta, Bose (1966) notes that mothers wish to continue feeding their children, but that milk flow often ceases almost entirely by 6 months, probably due to poor dietary intakes, especially of protein. Most mothers choose sago or barley as supplementary

food as they cannot afford milk. A gruel, composed of 110 to 170 gm. sago, 30 to 55 gm. cow's milk, 30 gm. sugar with water, is given six to eight times daily up to 18 months; then small quantities of puffed or cooked rice and boiled, mashed green plantains may be given. Protracted diarrhoea precedes the development of clinical signs of protein malnutrition. When diarrhoea commences, mothers immediately stop putting milk in the gruel (Bagchi *et al* 1960).

In Bikaner, Rajasthan, prolonged breast-feeding without supplements is common practice among poor groups and uneducated middle classes. The first feed is delayed from twelve to twenty-four hours, and a decoction of nutmeg, cardamom, raisin, black salt, pomegranate skin and dry ginger given to the infant (Saxena and Garg, 1968).

Cambodia. Infants are fed banana from 3 months, and supplements continue until weaning, which takes place from 1 to 2 years or later (Hong, 1968). Should the mother become pregnant again, the infant is given rice water or possibly some form of milk from 6 months. There is no introduction of meat, egg or soybean. Supplementation with vitamin A (despite the use of banana) and of iron is too late. The files of sick children admitted to the Centre de Pétiatrie Kantha Bopha, Phnom Penh, show 3.5 per cent suffering from malnutrition, of which 6.45 per cent are below

TABLE 10/5(a)

India South: amounts of proteins and calories per day
supplied by supplementary weaning foods, and recommended intakes

| Age in months | Weight of child kg. | Supplements per head per day | | Recommended levels | | |
		Protein gm.	Calories	Nutrition Advisory Committee (India) gm.	Calories	FAO gm.
0—6		3·0	90	20	650	
7—9	6·5	3·3	110	23	750	
10—12	7·0	5·8	195	25	800	19·1
13—18	7·5	7·1	265	26	900	
19—24	8·3	10·6	380	29	1,000	17·9
25—30	9·4	12·7	490	33	1,050	
31—36	10·1	16·9	680	35	1,100	19·7
37—42	11·0	18·1	715	39	1,150	
43—48	11·6	18·7	740	41	1,200	20·4
49—54	12·3	19·3	775	43	1,250	
55—60	12·8	20·6	830	45	1,300	20·0

TABLE 10/5(b)

India South: amounts of proteins and calories
per day supplied by breast milk

Age in months	Protein gm.	Calories
5—6	9	490
7—8	8	440
9—10	7	400
11—12	6	350
13—15	6	350
16—18	5	300
19—24	5	270
25—36	5	280
37—48	4	230

Source: Rao, Swaminathan, Swarup and Patwardhan, 1959

3 years of age. Children from the country have a higher degree of parasitic infestation than the urban children. Malnutrition increases in the dry season when there is increased concentration of sources of infection from evaporation from stagnant water, and more flies. Infants whose thermal regulation has not yet formed show high temperatures. The rainy season favours malaria and hookworm infection.

Malaysia. In 1950, rice was being given to infants — in one case 110 gm. boiled rice and 28 gm. sugar daily to a month-old child (Burgess and Laidin, 1950). Cornflour and wheat flour made into a soft porridge now replace rice gruel in most areas; also softened bread and biscuits. Supplement may be given before 6 weeks. Health staff object to this practice, because it is too early, and virtually always the wrong food is given. Substitution of breast milk takes place if the mother goes to work or if her milk fails; this is done generally with sweetened condensed milk, more rarely Lactogen (McArthur, 1962). Sweetened condensed milk, with its high proportion of carbohydrate and comparatively low protein can have harmful results, particularly as it is usually overdiluted. An open tin easily becomes infected with staphylococci. In a coastal fishing village in Trengganu, rice gruel and sugar continue to be used as supplements from the first week of life (Wilson, 1970a & b). This is moistened later with a little sauce from the family curry. Other supplements are banana, sweet biscuits or softened bread, and more rarely dry skim milk or commercial baby foods.

Among the Melanau, in Sabah, a gruel made of sago or wheat flour is introduced at the end of the first month of life; sometimes cooked rice mixed with condensed milk and sugar. Bananas are introduced at the end of the second month, and later, sago jelly and small portions of dried fish (Morris, 1953). Among the Semai aboriginal peoples in West Malaysia, those in the east suckle for longer than those in the west, where they are more open to modern Chinese and Malay influences. In the east, solid, prechewed food is given at about one year, and the child may breast-feed until it is 4 or 5 years old, unless another pregnancy intervenes. In the west, weaning is usually complete by 2 years (Dentan, 1968). Practices similar to those of the east Semai are reported from Iban communities in Sarawak (McKay and Wade, 1970).

Indonesia. In central Java, supplementation may begin before 10 days of age, or between 10 days and 3 months. In some cases, the infant is given a piece of thick rice porridge in the form of a stick to suck, to 'clean him out'. This is discontinued after a few days, and no further solids given until he is several months old. In a village with a health centre, supplements are not given until three months. Congee is the first food, followed by a piece of sweet or fried cassava cracker when he reaches for it. After one year, small amounts of beans, eggs and fish are added to congee or rice. The most common soybean preparations are tempe and tahu. Fish is given dried and salted, for the taste of the salt only; eggs and meat hardly ever, at most once or twice a month, because of the high cost (Tie, Lian, Ong and Rose, 1967). Eighty-nine per cent of the children were breast-fed up to 2 years of age, half of the children in some villages studied continued up to 3 years, and a considerable number beyond 3.

Philippines. A base-line dietary survey shows that infants, toddlers, pre-school children and school children and pregnant and nursing mothers are generally more deficient in calories and nutrients than other groups (Bulato-Jayme, Ramilla, Aleid and Bailey, 1966). The most critical groups are the 6 to 11-month age group, and then the toddlers. Evaporated milk is used for transitional feeding, but diluted with an equal amount of water, or even one part of milk to eight parts of water (Guthrie H.A., 1964); some 88 per cent of barrio mothers use rice gruel as the first supplement, only 33 per cent in urban areas. Only 4 per cent of barrio infants receive supplements by 6 months of age.

Supplements are mashed bananas or rice and water gruel, given sometimes only a few times per week, but usually two or three times daily. If the mother can afford it, egg or milk may be added to the porridge.

Fruits other than bananas and vegetables and fish are avoided. Cracker biscuits are also given. Supplementary feeding is generally introduced around 8 months of age. Further improvements in diversification are unlikely while the conception of rice as a whole and perfect food continues to have the wide credence it has. Such a conception of the completeness and wholesomeness of the basic staple in the Philippines is particularly obdurate and has proved most difficult to supplant (Nurge, 1957). Not more than 1 per cent of infants in northern Luzon, southern Tagalog and Western Visayas are given vegetables (Bulato-Jayme and Madlangsacay, 1965). Supplementation starts around 6 months. Fruit juice is often given, but animal protein is used only by a very few.

Thailand. Breast milk is the primary source of food for the first 18 months, with the addition at one month of pre-chewed glutinous rice and mashed banana in north Thailand (Thanangkul, Whitaker and Fort, 1966). About 60 per cent of village families start feeding glutinous rice on the third day of life, and 90 per cent in the first four weeks (Valyasevi, Halstead, Pantuwatana and Tankayul, 1967). The rice is sometimes mixed with mashed banana and a few drops of breast milk. In Ubol town, mothers do not generally introduce supplements until after 3 months, and then only boiled rice. This is thought to reduce intake of breast milk, and therefore of protein, and the practice may thus be a cause of bladder stone, which is common in north Thailand and also in India, Pakistan, Indonesia and China.

Laos. Pre-chewed rice and banana are given a few weeks after birth; by 1 year the diet is generally the same as that of adults (Gerhold, 1965).

South Korea. In a rural area 220 infants showed growth comparable with American infants up to 6 months of age, after which there was a steady decline, due to lack of adequate supplements. Anaemias were observed up to 18 months. While clinical signs of nutritional deficiency were not observed, 43 per cent had a history of gastro-intestinal disorders (Lee, Bang and Yun, 1963). Rice gruel supplements are fed from 3 months, boiled rice from 6 months in mountain, coastal and plain villages, and rice gruel is given during attacks of diarrhoea (Yonsei University, 1967—8). Infants up to 5 months from plain, mountain, island and town areas were superior to or level with WHO standards, but many between 6 to 11 and 18 to 23 months were underweight and showed signs of both energy and protein deficiency. Diarrhoea was most frequent during the second year of life. The first supplement was invariably boiled rice, other carbohydrate foods coming later, and rarely animal protein (Yoon and Kim, 1970).

China. Shensi (Myrdal, 1966). Mothers breast-feed until the child is 2, 3 or more years. If a woman cannot feed her own child, she will not seek a wet nurse, but gives the infant goat milk. At 7 months, a thin porridge of millet, rice and water is introduced; this is followed by a thin porridge of millet and water alone. At 1 year, the porridge is thicker; subsequently noodles and steam-baked bread soaked in gruel are given. No vegetables are given until 3 years ('vegetables are too difficult for children's stomachs to digest'). Egg also is given only at this stage.

PRE-SCHOOL CHILDREN: WEANING TO 6 YEARS

Weaning is a period of critical protein deficiency in all developing countries. It is a slow process, which may be divided into three stages: the introduction of supplementary foods (see preceding section); denial of the breast, and finally, full participation in adult meals.

When children participate in adult meals, it is common in Asia to deny them fish and egg, in the belief that these are harmful. They are generally given an inadequate share of the available grain legumes. There is an added problem, particularly in India, Pakistan and Malaysia, where the side dishes or supplement to the cereal staple are highly spiced and unpalatable, even harmful to children. Mothers say that they have not the time to cook separate dishes. Animal protein is invariably withdrawn during illness. Vegetables in season are available only in small quantities as a relish to the main dish, and are often refused by children. Fruits in season are eaten infrequently as snacks. There is a great need throughout the region for more knowledge and promotion of correct feeding after weaning, with protein-rich foods of animal and plant origin, and more vegetables.

Chinese mothers do use small amounts of animal protein — fish, meat, egg — in cooking food for toddlers, though this is often removed before feeding. In Thailand the proportion of hospital admissions suffering from kwashiorkor who were of Chinese origin was low. This was attributed to the Chinese custom of using minced pork quite early in infant feeding, as well as the generally higher protein quality of Chinese diets (Netrasiri and Netrasiri, 1955). Dean (1961) found kwashiorkor among Malay children, but not in Chinese and Indian children. Chinese mothers breast-feed less continuously, since they are employed away from the home, but they provide milk substitutes for their children. Tamil workers on plantations leave their children in crêches, the conduct and nutrition of which are controlled by law; a number of tins of milk are provided per child per month.

Growth rates of Asian children are lower than those of western children after six months. Pre-school Malay children in Singapore show continuous gains in height and weight, though these are slower than those of western children (see Table 10/6). Differences increase with age (Millis, 1957). Pre-school Chinese and south Indian children record greatest gains in the first year, with weight gains tending to decrease with increasing age (Millis, 1958a). At five years, Malays have made better progress than Indians, and Indians than Chinese. Although diets of the three groups differ considerably, none would meet the physiological requirements for growth.

In Asia, weaning from the breast does not generally take place in rural areas until the next pregnancy begins or is advanced. The child may be aged 13 months, 2 years or more, a time when physical growth and development are seriously impaired by sudden defi-

TABLE 10/6

Singapore: increases in growth of Malay infants, compared with British and American infants, from three months to five years of age

| | Malay | | British | American | |
	Height cm.	Weight kg.	Weight kg.	Height cm.	Weight kg.
Male	40·9	9·6	12·5	48·5	12·7
Female	41·4	9·5	12·4	48·5	13·1

Source: Millis, 1957

ciency of protein. The brain reaches its full size at 5 years of age, and impaired nutrition up to that age almost certainly results in reduced intellectual capacity (Chapter 11).

A supply of clean, good-quality milk is of great significance, when acceptable, in the diets of Asian children in this age group, to provide:

(a) readily assimilable animal protein for growth and development;

(b) a good source of vitamin A, to counteract inadequate vegetable intakes and prevent those extreme forms of vitamin A deficiency which cause permanent blindness; and

(c) a rich source of calcium for skeletal development.

Milk is also a good source of other nutrients in high demand at this stage of growth. Dried skimmed milk supplied through UNICEF and other agencies is generally fortified with vitamins A and D. When available on the market, it is often the cheapest milk obtainable. WHO (1969) recommends that it be used in the dry form to supplement weaning foods, added to mashed banana or rice porridge, rather than as liquid milk. The value of the four-decade tradition of consumption of condensed milk in Malaysia should not be exaggerated, in view of its high carbohydrate content. In the Philippines there is a small intake of various forms of processed milk.

Actual milk consumption, as distinct from national figures for average availability per caput, is hard to assess. Milk has traditionally had an honoured place in the dietaries of Pakistan and north-west India, but this has been greatly disturbed by the creation of an attractive market in urban milk-collection centres. It is perhaps true that Indians and Pakistanis, wherever they are, will give their children milk if there is no overriding financial advantage in disposing of it. In north-east Uttar Pradesh, if families can afford it, they purchase or save milk for their children (Minturn and Hitchcock, 1966). Those who do not have a buffalo or cow in milk cannot afford to buy milk for children, although they will try to do so for the sick. The degree of retention of milk in the rural areas is related to tradition and the economic attractions of selling milk to processing plants. Far less milk is produced in south than in north India, and up to 90 per cent of this is sold (Rao *et al*, 1959).

The Protein Advisory Group *Ad Hoc* Working Group on Feeding the Pre-School Child (FAO, 1969) recommends that infants' diets should provide 35 to 50 per cent of calories from fat sources, while linoleic and arachidonic acid should represent 1 per cent of calorie intake. The Group recommends the addition to low-fat or fat-free cow's milk of vegetable oils rich in linoleic acid, such as maize, groundnut, soybean or sunflower oils.

In *Pakistan,* diarrhoea, infection of upper respiratory tract and intestinal infestation are major factors associated with malnutrition, with a higher rate of prevalence in East Pakistan: Bangla Desh. About 50 per cent of children under 5 years of age are below the borderline of optimal nutrition, and 35 per cent are in poor nutritional status (Rahman, 1968a). Anaemia, clinical manifestations of vitamin A deficiency (especially in East Pakistan: Bangla Desh), kwashiorkor and marasmus are found in this age group. Classical deficiency diseases with the prevalence of a dominant manifestation of one deficiency are less common than a combined form of deficiency diseases. Protein-calorie malnutrition affected 85 per cent of all children examined (Rahman, 1968a).

In south *India,* about 1 per cent of children aged 1 to 5 years showed signs of kwashiorkor (which in the region covered meant 120,000 cases). The true incidence was probably more than 1 per cent, and even this did not give the whole picture. For every case of kwashiorkor, there were two of marasmus, three to five of vitamin deficiency, five with low serum albumin, and as many with low haemoglobin (Rao, 1962). Twenty per cent of all children die before 5 years of age.

In *Ceylon* (now Sri Lanka) in 1954, 45 per cent of all deaths were children under 5 years, and 49 per cent children under 10 years, a figure which, despite successful eradication of malaria at that time, had remained unchanged since 1931; this was due primarily to under-nutrition and malnutrition, particularly of protein, vitamin A and riboflavine, first in the mother and then in the child (de Silva, 1956).

In Shensi, *China*, steamed millet bread, bean stuffing and some egg and vegetables are given after 2 years of age (Myrdal, 1966). The child's food is not spiced.

In *Hong Kong*, Chinese mothers, many of whom come from rural areas in Kwangtung Province, China, begin weaning their infants from about the 4th month; usually congee is given first, and milk slowly reduced. A cereal may be introduced around the 7th month, and fish, vegetables and eggs slowly introduced. By about 9 months of age, milk is suddenly withdrawn completely. At this stage protein intake is inadequate; the whole process of growth and development slows down, and in some cases appears to be arrested for some time. Infections are contracted, undermining health. Not until 18 months or 2 years does improvement begin (Field, 1971; Field and Baber, 1973).

In northern *Thailand,* urban children are fed some vegetables and meat in small quantities much earlier than those in rural areas, where the majority begin after 1 year, many after 2 years of age. A higher proportion of the urban children are weaned by 2 years of age.

Malay mothers in *Malaysia* do not give vegetables to children until their molars appear, 'otherwise they might choke' (McArthur, 1962). However, even when permitted, children refuse many or all vegetables. They do, however, soon start insisting on receiving a little fish, despite parental fears that this is bad for them. Objections to the use of fish or egg for toddlers are not found in a fishing village in Trengganu, where the child receives small quantities of the side-dishes, chiefly fish (Wilson, 1970a and b, 1971). The diet at this period is high in carbohydrate and low in most other nutrients (see Table 10/7).

TABLE 10/7

Malaysia: nutrient intake of a Malay toddler in Trengganu fishing village

Calories	833
Protein (gm.)	20·5
Calcium (mg.)	228
Iron (mg.)	2·5
Vitamin A (μg)	119
Vitamin C (mg.)	35·8
Thiamine (mg.)	0·26
Riboflavine (mg.)	0·37

[1] Aged 22 months, displaced at breast three months previously. Weight 8·6 kg.; height 74·5 cm.

Source: Wilson, 1970b

In a *Philippines* barrio mothers are unable to afford milk for children upon weaning, although dried fish might be used; only urban mothers can afford eggs. There are fewer taboos against giving children animal protein; socio-economic factors are the main reason for its omission (Guthrie, H.A., 1964).

Weaning in a Minangkabau village in *Sumatra* takes place from about seven months; the food is rice porridge, water and sugar; no fish or meat until 2 years, rarely egg and no milk. Most Indonesian children dis-

like vegetables; girls take more than boys (Postmus and van Veen, 1949). In *Java,* boiled rice with a leaf or two of spinach are given early in the second year; it is not customary to give children fish, dried or fresh, or bean shoots (Freedman, 1954). In five villages in central Java, 500 children under 5 years of age were smaller and lighter than Djakarta children, and motor development was poor compared with western standards. The diet was adequate only during the first months, and then became deficient in protein and vitamin A. Physical condition was good among 34 per cent of children under 1 year of age, and only among 21 per cent between 1 to 5 years (Tie, Lian, Ong and Rose, 1968).

SCHOOL-AGE CHILDREN

So far we have been dealing with children who are difficult to reach for the introduction of improved foods and dietary practices. Once children are assembled at school, even in remote areas, it becomes easier to introduce items into their daily diets as supplements to meals brought from home, or as school meals. This approach has to some extent proved the means for overcoming lactose intolerance in East Asia.

Weights and heights of Asian school children are often considerably below international averages. WHO (1969) has noted a number of reasons for this; droughts, floods or failures of crops due to other causes, or socio-economic reasons, lead to impaired growth; a period of severe deprivation may leave a permanent mark. Growth rates and overall nutritional status of school children in China were worse in the late 1940s than they had been at the beginning of the decade, due to serious disruption of food production and distribution. There may be periods of stationary weight during the season of scarcity before harvest. In its Western Pacific Region, WHO considers nutritional inadequacy to be caused chiefly by chronic calorie deficiency. This is also the conclusion of the Nutrition Research Laboratories for India. A decreasing growth rate has been observed during the school term; many children have insufficient or no breakfast, and often have to walk a long way to and from school.

School-age Children: Diets and Nutritional Status

Pakistan. 4,991 schoolchildren between 5 to 19 years of age were examined in Lahore, first between 1961–2 and 1962–3. Growth curves were well below those of American children. Mean height and weight of a Pakistani boy of 19 were about those of an American boy of 14. Girls of the same age correspond with an American girl of 13. There were clinical signs of marginal vitamin A deficiency, particularly from 5 to 12 years. Early signs of vitamin C deficiency were particularly common among boys (11.2 per cent from 5 to 12 years; 7.3 per cent from 13 to 19 years). Six per cent of girls from 5 to 12 years, and 6.6 per cent of those from 13 to 19 showed similar signs. Multiple deficiency of the B complex vitamins, especially riboflavine, was noted; 12 per cent of girls from 13 to 19 years showed signs of riboflavine deficiency (Rahman, Ikramul and Maqsood, 1968).

India. From October 1964, to March 1965, 8,360 children from 6 to 16 years of age were studied in 57 schools in twenty-three towns and villages of Palghar Taluk (covered by Rural Health Units from Bombay) (Shah and Udani, 1968). Children weighed less than some urban Bombay children and children in the United Kingdom and America, but more than those in other rural areas of India and from lower socio-economic groups in Bombay. Head circumference was greater than that of Bombay children, less than that of American children. As with weights, these children were 3 to 4 years shorter than American children of the same age. One-third were considered well-nourished, 10 per cent had poor nutritional status, and 1.4 per cent very poor nutritional status. Two frank cases of kwashiorkor were found. Malnutrition was noted more frequently among younger children, but varied according to locality. 28.8 per cent were anaemic, more girls than boys, particularly after 11 years of age. The proportion of those with anaemia varied from 20 to 62 per cent of children in any one school, due to the presence in some areas of ankylostomiasis. Eight per cent showed signs of hypovitaminosis A, mostly younger children, with variations from 2.9 to 14 per cent in different schools; 2.4 per cent of boys and 1.7 per cent of girls showed signs of riboflavine deficiency, varying among schools from 0.7 to 16.9 per cent. (Deficiency findings of other workers range from 0.5 per cent in Assam to 32.5 per cent in North Arcot, Tamil Nadu). No evidence of thiamine or niacin deficiency was found. Clinical scurvy ranged from 0.2 to 1 per cent among schools; 9.4 per cent showed signs or stigmata of rickets.

In a survey of rural primary school children near Lucknow, Uttar Pradesh, heights of boys were above the Indian average, except from 13 to 14 years of age, and weights above average except from 14 to 15; girls were below average Indian heights from 8 years onwards, and below average weights from 9 years. One or more nutritional deficiencies were noted in 78.65 per cent of the children; 54.65 per cent had vitamin A deficiency; 14.34 per cent had past signs of rickets (more boys than girls); no thiamine deficiency; only 1.93 per cent had signs of riboflavine deficiency; 4.48 per cent early signs of niacin deficiency; 11.29 per cent suffered spongy and bleeding gums. A dietary survey was undertaken of 45 families, with an average monthly income of Ind. Rs. 58.30. Diets were deficient in calories, animal and vegetable protein (pulses), calcium, vitamin A, ascorbic acid and, to a lesser extent, niacin and riboflavine (Malaviya, Sen Gupta, Srivastava and Prasad, undated).

School children in a North Kanara village (Swaminathan *et al*, 1960) showed gross retardation in growth compared with western children, but rates comparable with others in south India. The children had poor musculature and deficient subcutaneous tissue, particularly boys, due to vitamin B complex deficiency; glossitis and angular stomatitis were found, indicating riboflavine deficiency; anaemia was common, particularly among girls.

The home diet of school children in a Tamil Nadu village was deficient in calories, protein, vitamins A, C and D, and calcium (Devadas, Anandam, and Bhanumathi, 1967). Some diets contained no green leafy vegetables; their daily inclusion in a school lunch appeared to have made a substantial contribution to the supply of vitamins A and C. Indian Multipurpose Food made from vegetable sources (75 per cent low-fat groundnut flour, 25 per cent bengal gram flour, fortified with calcium, phosphate, thiamine, riboflavine and vitamins A and D) is supplied free by the State Government of Tamil Nadu, at 11 gm. per child per day. This food is as effective in maintaining growth as is a supplement of skim milk, although inferior to a mixture of Multipurpose Food and skim milk, with the staple, rice.

The influence of socio-economic factors on the food intake and nutritional status of pre-school children from 82 selected rural families in south India was studied. Factors such as caste, occupation and educational level of the parents do not have much influence on the food practices of the children; income appears to have a decisive influence; the low-income group has a predominantly cereal diet from the post-weaning stage. Middle-income families include cereals, pulses, vegetables and negligible amounts of milk and flesh foods in the children's diet. Upper-income families have more protective foods, although leafy vegetables still do not find a place. Clinical assessment showed that the nutritional status of the upper-income group was better than the middle and low-income groups, the last showing the poorest picture (Devadas and Easwaran, 1967).

Children in an Indian orphanage from 2 to 5 years of age were given lysine-supplemented diets; while there was significant increase in height, differences in haemoglobin value, packed cell volume, total serum protein, serum albumin or nitrogen retention were not significant (Pereira, Begum, Jesudian and Sundararaj, 1969).

Ceylon (now Sri Lanka). 300 middle- and upper-class Ceylon Tamil schoolboys, aged from 8 to 19 years, were examined and their diets studied. Energy intake was expressed as calories per unit height and weight; values obtained were much less than for British boys. Intake of dairy products, meat, fruit, green vegetables, sugar preserves and sweets was also less, cereals, fish, nuts, vegetable fruits and pulses greater. These boys appeared to be in good health. A survey of low-income groups, however, showed low intakes of fat, calcium, phosphorus, iron, vitamin A, the B complex vitamins and vitamin C, with a high incidence of clinical signs of under-nutrition and malnutrition (Cullumbine, 1951). More than half the families at three socio-economic levels did not have sufficient calories (Bibile, Cullumbine, Watson and Wickremanayake, 1949).

Malaysia. The survey team of the Interdepartmental Committee on Nutrition for National Defense investigated the status of Tamil, Chinese and Malay children attending school (ICNND, 1964). All nutrients, including calories, were below recommended levels for Malaysia. Many of those attending morning classes did not have a meal before leaving home, others only bread and tea or coffee with sugar.

Indonesia. A group of 90 Indonesian children whose nutritional status had been studied over a two-year period from 1957 to 1959 were again examined in 1964. The classification of healthy, malnourished, and malnourished with vitamin A deficiency made in the first examination was clearly reflected in the results of the second. Children of the malnourished group were smaller and in poorer physical condition than those of the healthy group, and were more susceptible to infection. Those who had suffered vitamin A deficiency were most seriously affected.

Serum vitamin A and carotene were very low, lower in the malnourished than in the healthy children.

The dietary study showed a low food intake with deficiency of protein, particularly animal protein, and vitamin A. Of the major nutrients, only the intake of vitamin A was much lower among children than among mothers. Almost all vitamin A was supplied as carotene, which may be less efficiently utilized than preformed vitamin A (Giok, Rose and György, 1967).

Thailand. The children of labourers, skilled craftsmen and clerical workers in a village 15 km. north of Bangkok, and children of clerical workers in Bangkok, were found to be taller and heavier than in previous surveys, but there was biochemical and clinical evi-

TABLE 10/8(a)

Indonesia: daily food intakes of Javanese children in 1964

Condition in 1957-9	Age	Calories	Protein Total gm.	Animal gm.	Fat gm.	Calcium mg.	Iron mg.	Vitamin A i.u.	Thiamine mg.	Vitamin C mg.
Healthy	6—12	1075 ± 230	29·1 ± 9·5	5·0 ±3·5	12·3 ± 5·9	174 ± 85	6·4 ±2·4	765 ±1010	578 ±178	19 ±16
Malnourished	6—12	1172 ± 285	30·3 ± 6·5	5·9 ±4·5	13·8 ± 7·3	223 ±147	7·1 ±2·7	720 ±480	582 ±268	24 ±23
Vitamin A-deficient	7—11	1053 ± 295	25·9 ± 9·5	5·0 ±3·4	9·4 ±5·3	204 ±186	6·2 ±3·8	460 ±430	544 ±218	16 ±11

TABLE 10/8(b)

Indonesia: same children: intakes of some nutrients, 1957-9

Condition	Age	Calories	Total protein					Vitamin A
Healthy	2—4	950	25					1625
Vitamin A-deficient and malnourished	2—4	845	25					935

Source: Giok, Rose and György, 1967

dence of deficiencies of riboflavine, thiamine and vitamin A, and of anaemia (Chandrapanond, Rajatasilpin, Tunsupasiri and Pungpapongse, 1969).

Philippines. Following an Applied Nutrition Program in Bayambang, there were significant increases in serum albumin and total protein levels, improvement in vitamin A nutrition, and a fall in drop-outs and sporadic school absences (Roxas, Dominguez and Kuizon, 1970).

Taiwan. Some schools prepare hot soups at a nominal charge to supplement meals brought from home. Others provide 300 cc. hot, liquid, non-fat milk to lower-grade pupils (UNICEF milk). Various societies donate wheat flour, butter oil and non-fat milk powder for schools in indigent and aboriginal areas, which are also required to grow vegetables and fruits. Yeast is being used in soups.

South Korea. Studies of basal metabolism and energy expenditure from 1963 to 1968 show that average daily expenditure of calories of a high-school boy is higher (2,362) than that of a middle-school boy (2,280), or a college boy (2,306). The comparable figures for girls are: college girls, 2,133; middle-school girls, 1,870; high-school girls, 1,928 (Kim, 1968). Although contents of lunch boxes are deficient in calories, protein and animal protein, calcium, vitamin A, riboflavine and vitamin C, the academic achievement of those bringing lunch boxes was better than those with none, and these differences increased with age (Yonsei University, 1967–8).

Japan. Among school-children (83,850) in Tokushima Prefecture, Shikoku, from small towns, cities and coastal villages, 1.55 per cent obesity was found; none occurred among farm or mountain children; 0.55 per cent of mountain children suffered from malnutrition. Obesity was more marked in children above average height (Mizui, Kochi, Kato, Ishikawa, Hamaguchi and Kurobe, 1968). Heights and weights of children in primary schools are lowest in mountain areas, best in urban and coastal areas, with farm children intermediate (Fukui, Fukui, Sasaki and Murakami, 1961). This relates directly to intake of protein, especially animal protein. In groups aged 4 to 14 years given 0.5 or 1.5 gm. lysine per day for 6 to 12 months, there is a significant increase in height over the controls. In Ehime Prefecture, town children received more and hill children less than recommended food intakes, while total and animal protein was adequate for children on coasts and islands. Inland children received less calcium, thiamine, riboflavine and less protein, with insufficient lysine, tryptophan and sulphur amino acids. In all districts lysine was the first and threonine the second limiting amino acid (Naruse, 1969). In Kagawa Prefecture, the physique of children in municipal, coastal and island areas was superior to that of those in agricultural areas, while that of mountain-dwelling children was poorest of all (Kambara, 1970).

A Protein Resources Research Group was established in 1956, subsequently reorganized as the Research Committee on Essential Amino Acids, staffed by leading academic nutritionists. A Sub-Committee on Amino Acid Supplementation studied the effect of lysine enrichment in school lunch programmes on 3,000 children, mainly in second- and third-year classes, aged 8 to 10 years, in representative urban and rural areas. Since the children in the better socio-economic conditions of the urban areas (Tokyo and Osaka) have a better intake of protein, especially animal protein, no marked effect is obtained with lysine enrichment. But in general, there are improvements in height, weight and 'grasping power'. The effect of lysine enrichment is most marked in the rural areas of Yamanashi, Shikoku and Aomori. The value of these findings is reduced, however, by the fact that the diet before and during supplementation is not given, and possible alternative sources of lysine are not known (Japan Essential Amino Acids Association, 1966).

ADOLESCENTS

It is only in recent decades that the advanced countries have come to give possibly an exaggerated attention to the adolescent, who has a maximum liberty of action with a minimum of responsibility. Asia cannot afford this luxury. Childhood ends early and abruptly at maturity, with all its responsibilities. For the boys, this means increasing participation at an early age in heavy labour in the fields, fishing, hunting and other work. For the girls, it means early marriage and thus the bearing of children while the nutritional requirements for their own growth are still high. The mortality of infants from 13-year old mothers in Malaysia is 40 per cent (Thomson, 1960).

In a village six miles from Coimbatore, Tamil Nadu, 50 per cent of the adolescents were found to be in poor condition; 25 per cent had vitamin A deficiency; 40 per cent of the girls were anaemic (Devadas, Usha, Shankari, Rajalakshmi, Patrath and Babtiwala, 1965). In Gujarat, clinical symptoms of vitamin A and riboflavine deficiency are more common among adolescents than in younger children. It is at this age that

TABLE 10/9

Nutrient intakes for vulnerable groups recommended by international and national authorities
(for Japan, see Table 9/13)

	Under 1	1 to 3	4 to 6	7 to 9	10 to 12	13 to 15 Boys	13 to 15 Girls	16 to 19 Boys	16 to 19 Girls	Pregnant	Lactating
CALORIES											
F A O	1000	1150-1450	1700	2100	2500	3100	2600	3600	2400	2750[1] (latter half)	3000[1]
India	120/kg.	1200	1500	1800	2100	2500	2200	3000	2200	2500	2900
Indonesia	1120	1200	1570	1940	2310	2860	2400	3000	2100	2300	2800
Malaysia	110/kg.	1180	1550	1910	2280	2820	2370	3280	2180	2000	2700
Philippines	950	1300	1600	1900	2300	2800	2300	2800	2100	2300	2900
PROTEIN (gm.)											
F A O		0·88/kg.	0·81/kg.	0·77/kg.	0·72/kg.	0·70/kg.	0·70/kg.	0·64/kg.			
India	1·5/kg.	16·5-20·0	22·0	33·0	41·0	55	50	60	50	55	65 (Vegetable protein, NPU 50-65)
Indonesia	1·7/kg.	12·72	17·46	24·84	30·10	35·28	35·28	38·50	34·65	39·37	48·37 (reference protein)
Malaysia	2·3-1·2/kg.	20	25	35	44	59	55	61	55	60	71 (NPU—70)
Philippines	1·7/kg.	12·72	16·49	23	28·38	36·96	36·96	42·35	36·96	40·79	47·29
VITAMIN A											
W H O µg.	300/800	250/675	300/800	400/1075	575/1530	725/1950		750/2000		750/2000	1200/3194 (Vitamin A/carotene 25/75%)[2]
India µg.	300/1200	250/1000	300/1200	400/1600	600/2400	750/3000		750/3000		750/3000	1150/4600 (Vitamin A/carotene)
Indonesia µg.	1200	1500	1800	2400	3450	4000		4000		4500	6500 (100 per cent carotene)
Malaysia i.u.	1000	2500	3000	4000	5500	7000		7500		7500	12000 (80 per cent carotene)
Philippines i.u.	1500	2000	2500	3000	4000	5000		5000		5000	7000 (two-thirds carotene)
CALCIUM (gm.)											
W H O	0·5-0·6	0·4-0·5	0·4-0·5	0·4-0·5	0·6-0·7	0·6-0·7		0·5-0·6		1-1·2	1-1·2
India		0·4-0·6	0·4-0·6	0·4-0·6	0·6-0·7	0·6-0·7		0·5-0·6		1	1
Malaysia	0·55	0·45	0·45	0·45	0·65	0·65		0·55		1·2	1·2
Philippines	0·6	0·5	0·5	0·5	0·7	0·7		0·6		1	1
Indonesia	0·6	0·5	0·5	0·5	0·7	0·7		0·6		1	1
VITAMIN C (mg.)											
India				30 to 50 (under 1 to 19 years)						50	90
Indonesia	25	30	40	50	60	60		60		90	90
Malaysia	30	30	30	30	30	30		30		60	60
Philippines	30	35	50	60	75	90	80	100	80	100	150
IRON (mg.)											
India	1/kg.	15-20	15-20	15-20	15-20	25	35	25	35	40	30
Indonesia	8	8	10	10	12	12	12	12	12	17	17
Malaysia	7	8	10	12	15	15	15	15	15	15	15
Philippines	7	7	7	7	7	11	13	13	18	18	18

Sources: all entries under:
    India (Rao, 1969)
    Indonesia (Indonesian Institute of Sciences, 1968)
    Malaysia (Chong, 1969)
    Philippines (Intengan and Food and Nutrition Research Center, 1970)

[1] recommendations made by Davidson and Passmore, 1966

[2] Vitamin A = crystalline vitamin A_1 alcohol (retinol). Carotene = β-carotene

Also:
    CALORIES   FAO (1957)
    PROTEIN   FAO (1965)
    VITAMIN A   WHO (1967)
    CALCIUM   WHO (1962)

TABLE 10/10

Recommended intakes of thiamine, riboflavine and niacin in relation to calorie intake

| Calories per day | | Thiamine | Riboflavine | Niacin |
Age	Calories	(mg.)	(mg.)	(mg.)
7–12 months	1,000	0·4	0·6	6·6
1 year	1,150	0·5	0·6	7·6
2 years	1,300	0·5	0·7	8·6
3	1,450	0·6	0·8	9·6
4–6	1,700	0·7	0·9	11·2
7–9	2,100	0·8	1·2	13·9
10–12	2,500	1·0	1·4	16·5
13–15	Boy 3,100	1·2	1·7	20·4
	Girl 2,600	1·0	1·4	17·2
16–19	Boy 3,600	1·4	2·0	23·8
	Girl 2,400	1·0	1·3	15·8
Man (65 kg.)	3,200	1·3	1·8	21·1
Woman (55 kg.)	2,300	0·9	1·3	15·2

Note: Requirements for these vitamins are related to energy expenditure. Individuals should be in calorie balance, to ensure that energy expenditure and calorie intake are equal.

Source: WHO, 1967

the difference between poorly and well-nourished children is most evident, in both height and weight gain (Rajalakshmi, 1969).

An evaluation has been made of the dietary adequacy of food intake of selected female adolescents of the high school department of the University of the Southern Philippines at Cebu City (Perillo-Dia, 1968). This, of course, is a survey of girls living under urban conditions, and coming from families with an income level permitting attendance at university. But no girl has an adequate diet, only eggs and cereals being above the recommended levels. Less than 49.9 per cent of the recommended level of yellow, leafy and vitamin C-rich vegetables is consumed; calcium intake falls below 50 per cent of recommendation. Protein, thiamine and nicotinic acid reach 90 per cent of the recommended levels.

Systematic surveys of the nutritional status and diets of adolescents in rural areas in Asia are lacking. Much nutritional research relating to this group in developed countries is devoted to the problems of obesity, and to the emotional problems of adjustment into adult society. It is in this group that circum-stances in developed and developing countries diverge most markedly. Little attention appears to have been given to the special requirements of adolescents under Asian conditions.

RECOMMENDED NUTRIENT INTAKES FOR THE VULNERABLE GROUPS

This chapter has discussed the special requirements of the vulnerable groups and has shown dietary practices which are common in the nutrition of children and pregnant and nursing women in Asia.

The UN Agencies, WHO and FAO, and a number of national authorities in the region have made specific recommendations for optimal nutrient intakes for these vulnerable groups. Table 10/9 gives the recommendations made by WHO and FAO and by authorities in India, Indonesia, Malaysia and the Philippines. Recommendations for Japan are included in Table 9/13. The special requirements for thiamine, riboflavine and niacin are given separately in Table 10/10, since the age groupings do not correspond to those in Table 10/9.

11 Malnutrition

NUTRITIONAL deficiencies are usually multiple, particularly where calories are deficient and the diet is monotonous. It is often difficult to diagnose the consequences of malnutrition in terms of disease or other manifestations in these circumstances. The presence of clinical signs of deficiency of one nutrient does not necessarily presuppose a sufficiency of other nutrients. The poor sanitation of the environment in which most rural Asians live leads to infestation by intestinal parasites or hookworm, and to infectious diseases which exacerbate and are exacerbated by malnutrition. The appearance of signs of deficiencies is frequently seasonal, rather than permanent, coinciding with lowest annual availability of food, heavy expenditure of energy by adults and, in children, with 'the months of diarrhoea' which reduces absorption of nutrients already deficient in the diet.

MARGINAL MALNUTRITION

It has been demonstrated throughout the region that adults and even children can maintain apparent health, and mothers sustain pregnancy and lactation without ill-effects to their infants, on diets which are considerably below recommended levels. It is believed that the lower height and weight of many Asian peoples is a form of adaptation to a lower plane of nutrition, necessitating lesser amounts of calories and nutrients. In addition, there is evidence of increased efficiency of utilization of some dietary nutrients. A reduction in basal metabolism of up to 25 per cent has been observed (Rajalakshmi, 1969). The appetite may be so affected in chronically under-nourished individuals that their food intake is limited even when there is no restriction in supplies. Rajalakshmi (1969) found that a group of undernourished Bhils, when offered food *ad. lib.*, consumed only 1,800 calories daily. Waterlow and Stephen (1969) distinguish between the effects of a low level of protein nutrition

and protein depletion, or between adaptation and breakdown. Marginal malnutrition is a state of adaptation, involving metabolic regulations produced by enzyme changes.

In this condition, voluntary activity may be reduced. People do the tasks which must be done to earn a living, but will seldom exert themselves beyond this.... Individuals subjected to severe undernutrition are unable to concentrate long enough on a single problem, although their intellect is not impaired and they can function normally when adequately fed (Rajalakshmi, 1969).

This condition in Indonesia is vividly described by Napitupulu (1968):

... when malnutrition is endured from childhood, people appear lazy and enervated, their reaction becomes one of acceptance. The indolence characteristic of malnutrition is a familiar phenomenon in overpopulated areas of Java. Observe, for example, people assembling to await some event, say, a district meeting, or distribution of plantation wages. They squat, quiet and expressionless, hardly talking, let alone discussing anything.

It is within this large group of outwardly healthy people that there will be numbers living on the same nutritional intake, who will exhibit clinical signs of malnourishment. The vulnerable groups, the sick, those with a lower efficiency of absorption in digestion, those engaged in heavy labour — all who have higher nutritional demands are particularly prone to nutritional stress. Thus the status of these groups provides an indicator of the status of the entire community.

MATERNAL AND CHILD MALNUTRITION

There is thus certain evidence whereby malnutrition may be detected in a community without the presence of clinical signs of specific nutritional deficiencies. Reduced stature is the most prominent of these. A high rate of mortality, particularly among children and mothers, low birth weights and slow weight gain from about six months, are further signs. A high prevalence of disease and a high mortality from the diseases of childhood, such as measles, demonstrate reduced resistance.

It has long been known that malnutrition appears to increase susceptibility to disease. The WHO Expert Committee on Nutrition and Infection (1965b) stresses that infections are a major factor in precipitating acute nutritional disease in chronically malnourished populations, in particular the onset of protein-calorie disease, xerophthalmia and nutritional anaemias. Much of the retardation of growth and the malnutrition of children in developing countries is due to the loss of appetite, altered food habits, malabsorption and loss of nitrogen and other nutrients which result from infections and parasitism. In India it has been demonstrated that severe protein-calorie malnutrition results in impaired formation of antibodies and consequently reduced disease resistance (Srikantia, 1969). Thus peoples living in surroundings which are most likely to lead to infections are those least able to withstand them (Chapter 3).

The special requirements of pregnant and nursing mothers have been outlined in Chapter 10. The size of infants at birth is a reflection of the nutritional status of the mother. Evidence from all over the world shows that taller and heavier mothers produce larger infants. After 26 weeks' gestation, foetal growth in developing countries tends to slow down, with an increase in 'small-for-date' babies, greatly increased perinatal morbidity and mortality and a high incidence of sublethal damage with long-lasting effects. Such infants are more seriously affected by subsequent postnatal malnutrition (PAG, 1971).

In the developing world, size at birth is correlated with mental performance (see *Malnutrition and the Brain* below). The factors of height, weight, parity of the mother, as well as family income and sanitation, which govern her stature, health and personal hygiene, are all strongly related to the size of the infant at birth (Cravioto, Birch, de Licardie, Rosales and Vega, 1969).

Babies born of malnourished mothers may be partially depleted of nutrients such as iron, calcium, iodine and certain vitamins. In particular, it is frequently found that in a group of young children living on a diet with very low amounts of vitamin A, some will show clinical signs of deficiency, while others will not. This is believed to be due to inadequate storage in the liver before birth (Blankhart, 1967). Malnutrition of the mother may lead to permanently reduced efficiency of digestion in the offspring. Limitation of the diet of pregnant rats has induced not only stunting of the offspring, but also a derangement of their protein metabolism; limitation of protein in the maternal diet has produced the same effects, as well as diminished glucose tolerance (Chow, Blackwell, Blackwell, Sherwin, Hsueh and Lee, 1966). It has been calculated in Taiwan that, when a mother's diet is deficient in protein, the offspring requires up to 30 per cent more protein in its diet to maintain normal rates of increase in growth.

Malnourished mothers, particularly those who are anaemic and have inadequate protein in their diets, are likely to give birth prematurely; there is an increase in perinatal mortality and deaths of the mother herself (Lourdenadin, 1964). The national average maternal mortality in Malaysia is 1.7 per thousand, but 5.58 per thousand in the rural areas (Lourdenadin, 1969). In northern Thailand, maternal mortality is 6 per cent.

As with mothers and infants, so with young children, the death rate among those who are malnourished is very high. In India, where two-thirds of the children are said by leading authorities to be suffering from malnutrition, the death rate is 140 per thousand live births, and a further 200 per thousand die during the ensuing pre-school years. Some 45 per cent of all deaths in Ceylon (de Silva, 1956) are children under 5, and 49 per cent children under 10 years of age. A study of a community in Indonesia showed that 40 per cent of all children had died before 5 years. In Nepal, during one year, 55.5 per cent of all deaths occurred before 5 years of age, and 67.3 per cent before 15 years (Worth and Shah, 1969). The sudden spurt in growth characteristic of adolescents in the developing world is considered to be common only to those living on a low plane of nutrition.

UNDER-NUTRITION

The acute imbalance between population and land in parts of Asia leads to recurrent deficiency of cereal carbohydrates, and therefore of calories. This means that the diet is deficient in both calories and protein, and that much of the protein consumed is used for energy. A diet deficient in calories and proteins is usually deficient in other essential nutrients as well. Prolonged deficiency of all nutrients has been called *under-nutrition,* which in its extreme form is starvation. The WHO Expert Committee on the Medical Assessment of Nutritional Status (1963) has listed the clinical signs whereby under-nutrition may be recognized: lethargy, mental and physical (starvation); low weight in relation to height or other skeletal indices; diminished skin folds; exaggerated skeletal prominences; loss of elasticity of skin. Some of the clinical signs remain for some time, even after an improvement in the diet. There are indications that the body's capacity to benefit from an improved diet may be impaired following a period of severe malnutrition (Burgess and Laidin, 1950).

WHO (1968b) believes that, with the exception of beriberi, the classic nutritional diseases such as scurvy and rickets and the many clinical manifestations of deficiency, particularly of vitamins other than thiamine and vitamin A, are comparatively rare in the Western Pacific region. They are, however, more common in the Indian subcontinent and the Asian mainland in general where there is a more marked seasonal swing in the availability of vegetables. WHO would stress rather the importance of protein-calorie malnutrition, vitamin A deficiency and nutritional anaemias.

Reference has been made in Chapter 3 to the marked seasonality seen in Asian food production and rural dietary patterns. The period before the new crop has been harvested, when the previous year's stocks of grain have dwindled, and when few fresh foods of any kind are available, is known by Asian cultivators and their families as 'the usual hunger', the 'barley pass' (when rice is mixed with barley in Korea) and many similar expressions. This is also a time of growing heat, and of sickness, 'the months of diarrhoea', when field activities reach their peak.

This sequence of high and low levels of nutrition which is repeated every year may have a cumulative effect on human metabolism. This is a characteristic of human physiology in a monsoonal environment which does not appear to have been studied. It may be asked whether, after each successive period of under-nutrition and malnutrition, the organism revives with the return of more and better food to the same level as in the previous good season. Or is the peak of condition attained in each successive good season not slightly or markedly lower than the previous, leading in children to stunted growth, and to premature ageing? The seasonal cycle in nutrition is also important in relation to infestation with intestinal parasites. These will tend to have greater effect when the meta-

bolism of their human host is at its lowest ebb, i.e. towards the end of a period of 'usual hunger'.

The distribution of limited stocks of protein-rich foods by national or international agencies would best be concentrated during these critical months, to the extent permitted by difficulties of transport after the rains have begun.

PROTEIN-CALORIE DEFICIENCY

The most general and far-reaching deficiencies in Asia are undoubtedly those of calories and proteins. The terminology used to distinguish the different manifestations of these deficiency diseases is not wholly agreed upon by workers throughout the world. Originally it was thought that kwashiorkor and marasmus were two separate syndromes with different causes. Marasmus was considered to be due to deficiency of calories, and kwashiorkor to deficiency of proteins but with adequate calories. It was difficult to draw a hard and fast line between the two illnesses, symptoms of one often merging into the other; there were cases which were atypical of either extreme. Thus the term 'protein-calorie deficiencies' was adopted, and, more recently, protein-calorie malnutrition. Opening the Cambridge Colloquium on Calorie Deficiency and Protein Deficiency in 1967, McCance (McCance and Widdowson, 1968) considered that the early workers were perhaps correct, and that there were indeed two separate syndromes, with different causes and different metabolic consequences, demanding specifically different treatments.

At this same meeting, however, Gopalan (1968) stated that Indian research seemed to indicate that, at least as far as cause was concerned, the above hypothesis did not meet the facts. Nutritional dwarfism appeared to be a form of adaptation to mild protein-calorie malnutrition, while marasmus was attributed to acute protein-calorie malnutrition. Kwashiorkor appeared to be a lack of adaptation, a failure of the biochemical mechanisms usually invoked to protect the liver, pancreas and intestines at the expense of less essential muscle. Different children living on similar diets in the same community exhibited one or other of these symptoms:

It may be expected that in a poor community exposed to the stress of protein-calorie malnutrition, the great majority of the children will need to develop only a mild degree of adaptation, but a considerable number will show extreme results (marasmus) and a small number will show the effects of dysadaptation (kwashiorkor). This is the picture generally seen in poor Indian communities (Gopalan, 1968).

In this study, the terminology used by WHO and FAO — protein-calorie malnutrition — has been adopted.

The Joint FAO/WHO Expert Group on Protein Requirements (FAO, 1965) has stated:

Frank protein deficiency is common in the less developed countries and latent or subclinical protein deficiency is probably even more prevalent. Although protein deficiency may predominate, often calorie deficiency contributes important effects and the simultaneous insufficiency of other nutrients complicates the picture in varying degrees.

Protein-calorie deficiency occurs at all ages, but its incidence is greatest in the weaning and immediate post-weaning periods; deprived of a high-quality protein food, the child is not yet old enough to fend for himself in the family circle and is particularly subject to dietary taboos and prejudices. Milder forms of dietary deficiency, however, continue to occur among children and adolescents in low-income groups in developing countries. Available reports clearly indicate that the growth rates of children in developing countries deviate sharply from the normal at the time of weaning and continue at a low level throughout the entire period of growth, resulting in stunted adult stature.

Apart from the effect on growth, mild or moderate protein deficiency renders infants and young children particularly susceptible to respiratory and gastro-intestinal infections. The incidence of such diseases is much higher in malnourished than in well-nourished children, and mortality in the age group 1 to 4 is 20 to 50 times higher in the developing than in the developed countries; it is probable that this difference is due in large part to malnutrition.

Detection of Sub-clinical Malnutrition

The onset of protein-calorie malnutrition is insidious and the early stages are not usually recognized. The growth of a malnourished child may be retarded or may stop almost entirely months before any other sign of malnutrition is visible, and long before its parents suspect ill-health (Dean, 1961). This may occur during a time of social disorganization, especially during the wet monsoon, or in periods of epidemic illnesses when the nutrition of the children suffers badly. An acute condition is precipitated only by an attack of diarrhoea, infective illness or sudden weaning. Thus the prevalence of sub-clinical protein-calorie malnutrition is difficult to assess.

Various methods have been proposed. Those involving the collection of anthropometric data would obviously be simpler, less costly and require less highly skilled personnel than microscopic study of morphological changes in hair roots from the head, laboratory examination of buccal mucosa or biochemical analyses. However, most physical measurements are closely related to the age of the child, and this is rarely known accurately in the rural areas. It has been proposed (Fig. 11/1) that the mid-arm/head circumference ratio provides a measurement which is independent of either age or sex (Kanawati and McLaren, 1970), though doubts regarding the usefulness of this method have been expressed (Bradfield, Jelliffe and Jelliffe, 1972).

Whitehead and his associates have for many years been trying to find an accurate method of detecting sub-clinical protein-calorie malnutrition, a stage where adaptation to a low plane of nutrition is breaking down. Serum amino acid changes are helpful in detecting simple protein malnutrition, but only in the comparatively rare cases where kwashiorkor is caused simply by protein deficiency, not complicated by infection. Abnormality in the ratio of hydroxyproline to creatinine in urine and its relation to body weight are of value as an index of protein-calorie malnutrition, except in the presence of infestation with malarial parasites or hookworm. The aim of future work is not to evolve a test which will measure response to inadequate diet, but to prove that a change in tissue composition is actually significant in terms of essential body function:

FIG. 11/1   Relation between the mid-arm circumference/head circumference ratio and the percentage weight/age

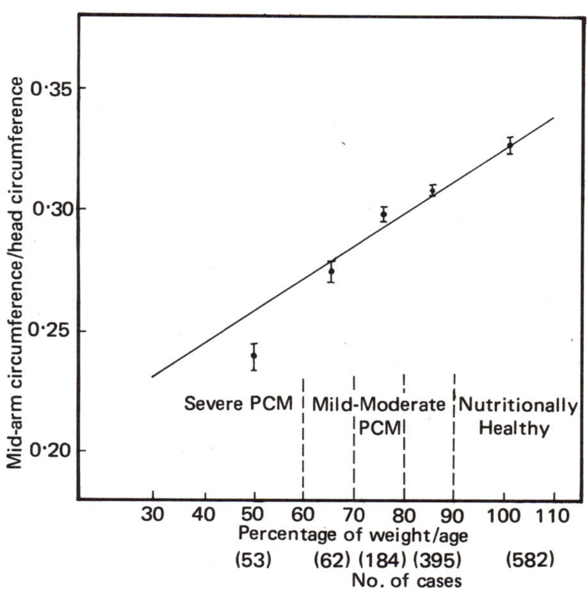

Source: Kanawati and McLaren, 1970

The evidence justifies the concept that many children in the world pass through a phase in which, because of the limited amount of protein in their diet, certain essential aspects of cellular function become abnormal. It is from this condition that clinical kwashiorkor may precipitate (Whitehead, 1969).

Complications and Evidence of Protein-Calorie Malnutrition

Bone malformations have been associated with severe protein-calorie malnutrition (Platt, Stewart and Platt, 1963; Dickerson and John, 1969). Children suffering from protein-calorie malnutrition frequently have anaemia, its severity increasing in proportion to the severity of the protein-calorie malnutrition (Allen and Dean, 1965; Woodruff, 1968). Vitamin A deficiency is the most serious and widespread complication of protein-calorie malnutrition. A form of congestive cardiac failure in Ceylon has been attributed to protein deficiency (Obeyesekere, 1968). The incidence of oral cancer in Asia is high. While a variety of factors is responsible — tobacco chewing and smoking and oral irritants such as the lime which is a component of pan or betel — dietary inadequacy of protein has also been implicated (Ungku Omar-Ahmad and Ramanathan, 1968). Bladder stones appear to coincide with early protein deprivation, induced possibly by premature introduction of carbohydrate foods and consequent reduction of milk intake (de Langen, 1934, ICMR, 1967, Halstead and Valyasevi, 1967b). Enlargement of the parotid gland (Klerks, 1959) and low blood pressure are also related to protein-calorie malnutrition.

The World Health Organization gives clinical signs for the recognition of protein-calorie malnutrition: oedema; muscle wasting; low body weight; psychomotor change; dyspigmentation and easy pluckability of the hair; thin sparse hair; moon-face; flaky paint dermatosis; diffuse depigmentation of the skin.

Biochemical changes include elevated total plasma protein concentrations, usually caused by increase in the gamma-globulin fraction indicating presence of infection; fall in serum albumin, becoming marked with severe deficiency; reduction of some plasma enzymes (WHO, 1963).

DEFICIENCY OF VITAMINS

Traditional Asian diets contain only small amounts of fruits and vegetables, and even less animal food. Intake of both water-soluble and fat-soluble vitamins is low. Absorption of calcium and iron may be inadequate as they may become insoluble in association with other items in the diet. Other minerals may also be deficient.

Vitamin A deficiency is severe in South and South-East Asia, constituting an important cause of preventable blindness (WHO, 1967). Remodelling of the bones is affected during vitamin A deficiency, causing damage to the spine and skull, while the limbs may become short and thick (Rajalakshmi, 1969). The presence of ocular manifestations implies depletion of liver stores and/or low serum levels. Irreversible damage is caused to the epithelial cells, the natural barriers to infection lining the intestines, respiratory, gastro-intestinal and urino-genital tracts, resulting in a high degree of infection and death. Infections may precipitate the clinical manifestations of vitamin A deficiency, while the deficiency may exacerbate the infection (WHO, 1967).

It is above all in the eyes that vitamin A deficiency is observed. An early sign is loss of the ability to see in the dark. Bitot's spots (white, foam-like patches on the surface of the conjunctiva) may occur. Drying of the conjunctiva is followed by drying of the cornea (xerophthalmia), and finally by acute ulceration of the cornea and opacity (keratomalacia) (WHO, 1969). Oomen (1963) states that 'the chosen victim is the toddler' from 1 to 5 years of age, with a preponderance among the males. A peak incidence of deficiency occurs in the third and fourth year, while the peak period of blindness caused by xerophthalmia occurs a little earlier. The younger the case, the graver the consequences. 'It is, in fact, the foulest variety of child malnutrition; it not only leaves graves in its wake, but also a number of pitiable invalids in a society that is rarely prepared to take good care of them.' Experience in India shows that deficiency of vitamin A can be wholly eliminated by one injection per year (Reddy, 1969). However, follow-up studies indicate that 6-monthly injections are advisable (Swaminathan, Susheela and Thimmayamma, 1970).

Vitamin A deficiency usually occurs in association with protein-calorie deficiency diseases, affecting the same age group. Fatality rates of those suffering from both protein-calorie malnutrition and keratomalacia are between 30 to 50 per cent; most of the survivors suffer from partial or complete loss of vision. In Indonesia, 75 per cent of those with severe protein-calorie malnutrition have xerophthalmia.

As with so many Asian nutritional deficiencies, the factor of seasonality is important. Most cases of night blindness occur in Java in the last five months of the year, at the end of the dry season and the beginning of the rainy season, when rice prices are highest, vegetables scarce and diarrhoea most prevalent (Blankhart, 1967). In North Vietnam (Ung Peang, 1966) the outbreak is at its worst in the hot months from April to July and during winter, when vegetables are scarce, and again during the months when diarrhoea is at its peak. In South Vietnam and Cambodia, clinical signs occur throughout the year, especially after weaning and measles, but above all during the 'months of diarrhoea' — July and August. Reports from South Korea are similar.

Chronic infections, such as tuberculosis and malaria, cause a gradual depletion of liver stores of vitamin A. There are, of course, many other infections which are endemic in Asia (Adams and Maegraith, 1964), all of which have the same effect on stores of this vitamin in the liver.

Beriberi is associated with a deficiency of thiamine; it occurs where highly milled rice is the staple food, and intake of vegetables and animal foods is low. Parboiled rice and legumes are good sources of thiamine for Asians. Deficiency in the diet of lactating mothers leads to the death of the infant. The varying syndromes of infantile beriberi have been described by Jelliffe (1968a). See also WHO (1963 and 1969). The greatest mortality rate in Thailand occurs in the second month of life, while a similarly high rate from 2 to 3 months is reported in Vietnam. This is associated with thiamine deficiency (Thanangkul and Whitaker, 1966).

Riboflavine deficiency is fairly common where intakes of animal foods and green vegetables are low, particularly in the Indian subcontinent and mainland East Asia. Clinical signs are changes in the lips and tongue, with ulceration of the corners of the mouth (angular stomatitis). The eyes become affected with conjunctivitis, and are abnormally sensitive to light. Some of these are also evidence of other deficiencies, but if several occur together, they may be attributed to lack of riboflavine (Rajalakshmi, 1969).

Pellagra, originally attributed to deficiency of niacin alone, is due rather to a generally unbalanced diet, involving lack of calories, protein, and certain amino acids, as well as excess of the amino acid, leucine. Changes in skin and tongue occur, and frequently diarrhoea and mental changes. Pellagra is found among maize-eating people of South-East Asia, and in India among those who subsist on jowar.

Despite the universally low intakes of vitamin C in Asia, scurvy is rare, though some cases have been reported from Malaysia among infants reared on sweetened condensed milk from early weeks of life (MacLean and Kamath, 1970). Sore and bleeding gums are common, but are attributable to causes other than deficiency of vitamin C.

OTHER NUTRITIONAL DISORDERS

Nutritional anaemia is common throughout Asia, particularly among women and girls, and in young children, especially during the second year of life. Folate deficiency is frequently found with anaemia (Marzan, Tantengco and Caviles, 1971). A systematic investigation of nutritional anaemia in South-East Asia is being made by the World Health Organization. Dietary inadequacy may be complicated by excessive blood loss, as with acute malaria and other causes, and by protein deficiency, when ability of bone marrow to remove iron from plasma is impaired. Chronic malaria and hookworm may also be contributory causes. Certain forms of anaemia are due to lack of vitamin B_{12} or folic acid (WHO, 1968a, 1969).

Endemic goitre is prevalent in mountainous areas where soil and water, and therefore local foods, are low in iodine. When the dietary supply is deficient or its utilization impaired, the thyroid gland is enlarged and goitre may result. Impaired thyroid function leads to a lowered rate of metabolism, arrested growth, and eventually mental changes. The condition is found in the northern submontane regions of India and Pakistan, in western China and in the mountains of Thailand, Indo-China and Ceylon. In Nepal, for example, leaching by glaciation and precipitation causes widespread iodine deficiency, and in Terai villages, the highest incidence of goitre is found in villages with the lowest water-table (Worth and Shah, 1969).

Jelliffe (1968a) has reviewed the effect on nutritional status of various infections during infancy; bacterial infection, measles, malaria, hookworm and ascariasis. A high degree of intestinal infection and infestation exacerbates malnutrition. Crowded, insanitary conditions are common to most villages throughout Asia, and there is a general absence of environmental sanitation. The degree of infestation and infection, and the relation between infestation and intestinal absorption of nutrients, have been studied in Singapore (Kan, Singh, Cheah and Siak, 1971); Vietnam (Colwell, Welsh, Boone and Legters, 1971); Thailand (Devakul, Chantachum, Boonyananta, Egoramaiphol and Viravan, 1971) and the Philippines (Tantengco, Salvosa, de Castro and Pantas, 1971).

Faecal contamination of the environment is widespread in Nepal, and multiple infection common, particularly with hookworm and *Ascaris,* though the latter appears to be limited somewhat by freezing winter temperatures (Worth and Shah, 1969). Infection with soil-transmitted helminths is much higher among Chinese children living in vegetable-producing farms in Malaysia where nightsoil is used, than among Malay children whose parents do not use nightsoil (Lie, Kwo and Owyang, 1971). In two villages on islands off Trengganu, more than 90 per cent of the population was infected with two or more helminth species, and the rate was particularly high among children under 14 (Balasingam, Lim and Ramchandran, 1969). A survey of 1,126 inhabitants of twenty-four villages in Bojolali Regency, Central Java, showed that 86.7 per cent had intestinal parasitic infections (Cross, Gunawan, Gaba, Watten and Sulianti, 1970). Many children had scabies, smallpox was endemic, but malnutrition was the most serious problem. The Provincial Health Department, Taiwan, reported in 1970 that three out of every four school children were affected with intestinal parasites.

The clinical signs of nutritional deficiencies, and the implications of different clinical manifestations, have been given by the WHO Expert Committee on Medical Assessment of Nutritional Status (1963).

TOXICITY OF FOODS

Toxin-producing organisms occur as moulds in foodgrains stored in tropic conditions. It is believed that the high prevalence of hepatic cirrhosis in certain parts of India may be attributed to aflatoxin in groundnuts (Tulpule, 1969). In both India and Pakistan the consumption of khesari dhal *(Lathyrus sativus)* during times of drought when there is a deficiency of all other foods, both cereals and vegetables, leads to a crippling nervous disease whereby the lower limbs become gradually immobilized (Nagarajan, 1969). The crop is a major standby in times of extreme deprivation and attempts at replacing it have not therefore been successful. The Nutrition Research Laboratories at Hyderabad have evolved a method for removing the toxin, involving either steeping (presupposing the availability of water, which is often most scarce at the time of highest consumption of khesari), or parboiling. The latter method unfortunately involves the loss of 15 per cent of the grain, and affects cooking quality. Screening is in progress in the hope of finding or developing strains with low toxin levels.

Other Asian legumes also have toxic properties, the most notable being the soybean. Where they are a regular part of the diet, safe methods of preparation have long been in use.

MALNUTRITION AND THE BRAIN

While nutritionists and paediatricians everywhere are seeking ways to combat the loss of life, impaired physical development and resistance to disease associated with malnutrition, a subject of even greater concern is the effect of malnutrition on mental development.

It is understood that an impoverished environment undoubtedly fails to provide the stimuli which are necessary for mental development in early life; such circumstances have been termed sociogenic malnourishment (Montagu, 1972). However, it seems inconceivable to the human ecologist that the poverty which leads to this sociogenic malnourishment does not at the same time involve defective nutrition.

Evidence from experiments with both animals and humans is accumulating to demonstrate that malnutrition in early life seriously limits the individual's capacity for intellectual development, and that severe early malnutrition causes irreversible damage.

There are difficulties, which some believe cannot be overcome even in the most carefully conducted studies, in establishing beyond doubt the precise nature of cause and effect of early malnutrition (Eichenwald and Crooke-Fry, 1969). The environment in which children suffer malnutrition — poor housing and sanitation, parental illiteracy and consequent lack of awareness of the principles of hygiene and balanced diet — exposes the infant, as it exposed its mother, to severe stresses of infection (Fig. 11/2). The size of the infant at birth is closely related to its level of motor competence (Cravioto *et al.*, 1969). Equally, the size of the infant at birth is related to the height and weight of its mother, which is in turn dependent on the level of housing and sanitation which governs her health and nutritional status.

A malnourished infant becomes apathetic and does not respond to affection and stimulus from its mother; she consequently loses interest and pays less attention to it, producing further apathy. In many rural areas, the mother has to resume work in the field, and cannot devote sufficient time to the care of her child. Children separated from their families in hospitals or orphanages also become apathetic, although their diets may be adequate. However, children recovering from marasmus and kwashiorkor regain curiosity in the surrounding world, while electrical activity of the brain, which has been abnormal during protein malnutrition, is restored during recovery to a normal condition (Eichenwald and Crooke-Fry, 1969). It is therefore considered unlikely that emotional disturbance can be seriously implicated for the apathy of malnourished children.

Physiological evidence, while not conclusive, provides more significant information. The period of rapid brain growth in the human commences in the uterus, reaches a peak near birth, continuing during the first year of life. The production of brain DNA is two-thirds complete by birth, and ceases around 5 to 6 months after birth. Children who suffer from severe malnutrition during the first eight months of life show evidence of cerebellar damage at 4 and 5 years (Chase, Lindsley and O'Brien, 1969). In rats, the effect of under-nutrition can be interpreted as less protein and smaller cells in the cerebrum, without diminution of cell number. The cerebellum is apparently more severely affected than the cerebrum. Where pregnant rats are chronically malnourished, the foetuses are smaller and remain smaller, even if subsequently given normal nourishment. Their organs, including the brain, contain fewer cells. Placentae are reduced in weight, protein and DNA content, and show an increase in RNA content. In a pilot study with humans, 50 per cent of human placentae from a low socio-economic group show biochemical abnormalities similar to, although less marked than those seen in placentae from infants with intra-uterine growth failure (Winick, 1969a).

The stage of malnutrition governs its long-term effect. Early malnutrition in rats impedes brain division, and the animal does not recover. Malnutrition at a later stage results in reduction of cell size, from which the animal, if given an improved diet, can recover (Winick and Noble, 1966).

The critical period in the human brain as far as cell division is concerned is from birth to six months; severe under-nutrition during this period will curtail cell division in all organs, including the brain. Tissues from children who died of malnutrition during the first year of life showed a marked reduction in the number of cells, two having 40 per cent less than the normal (Winick, 1968). Little cell division occurs after 5 months of age; further growth is achieved by increase in protein, RNA and perhaps the lipid content of cells (Winick, 1968). The weight of the brain increases rapidly for the first two years of life, thereafter more slowly, reaching adult weight by adolescence (Winick, 1969b); 80 per cent of the adult weight is reached by 3 years of age. Protein-calorie malnutrition or marasmus in the first two years of life are likely to lead to permanent reduction in head circumference.

Cerebral metabolism alone accounts for 20 to 25

FIG. 11/2   Interrelation between biosocial factors and low weight gain in infants

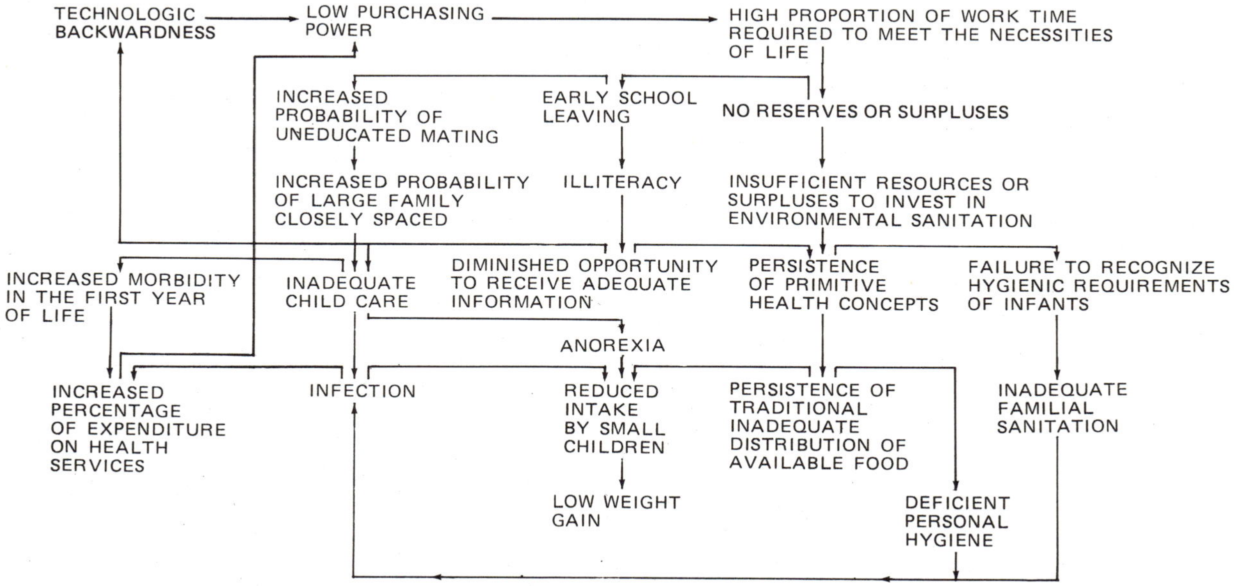

Source: Cravioto, Gaona and Birch, 1967

per cent of basal metabolism in human beings. In rats and swine, simple caloric restriction during lactation results in behavioural changes, but does not affect problem-solving ability; protein deprivation reduces also subsequent learning ability in these animals, and in their offspring (Eichenwald and Crooke-Fry, 1969). There is a reduction in certain cerebral enzymes and amino acids during a period of moderate protein deficiency in young and adult rats, with a relatively greater reduction in the younger animals. This condition is associated with diminished learning ability. In both children and animals who die from severe protein malnutrition, the electrical activity of the brain stops before that of the heart. This suggests that death is caused by a failure of the central nervous system, occurring primarily due to failure of brain function (Rajalakshmi, undated).

To what extent do these biochemical and physiological findings with animals and humans justify the conclusion that intellectual development is impaired by early malnutrition? To what extent can it be demonstrated that the capacity of the child and adolescent to acquire and use knowledge and experience depends upon an adequate level of protein intake during the critical period of brain formation?

Cravioto and his associates (Cravioto, Birch, de Licardie, Rosales and Vega, 1969) find that infants with low birth weights born to small mothers recover initially impaired motor competence during the first month of life: those with the lowest weight increase by 30 days do not. (Motor development and intelligence levels are not correlated). Mentally retarded American school-children, irrespective of socio-cultural factors, invariably have lower birth weights than children with an IQ of above 110 (Churchill, Neff and Caldwell, 1966). Severe motor and mental retardation has been noted among Peruvian children who have in all other respects completely recovered from a period of marasmus. These findings confirm those of Cravioto on children who have recovered from kwashiorkor, and demonstrate the similarity of the long-term effects of both marasmus and kwashiorkor (Cravioto, Piñero, Arroyo and Alcade, 1969). (See also Monckeberg (1971); Fig. 11/3.)

Early malnutrition causes neuro-integrative inadequacy, leading to impaired ability in reading and writing, school failure, and subsequent subnormal adaptive functioning (Cravioto, de Licardie and Birch, 1966). Such children are less competent in their adaptive capacity and more prone to the negative effects of a highly inadequate environment. They show less

social adjustment; this will ultimately lead to their raising their own children at a level certain to give rise to a new generation of malnourished infants (Cravioto *et al.*, 1969). In the Lebanon, a group of children under-nourished before 18 months had significantly lower IQ than a control group at the age of 4 to 5; there had been no evidence for an original difference in IQ (Botha-Antoun, Babayan and Harfouche, 1968). In India, each of a group of children in Andhra Pradesh who had recovered from kwashiorkor seven to eight years earlier was tested with three normal children, matched for age, sex, religion, caste, socio-economic status, family size, birth order and parental background. There was a clear difference in both intelligence and intersensory organization, with much more pronounced retardation with regard to perceptual and abstract abilities. However, the effect of emotional disturbance and loss of learning time involved in long hospitalization and low level of parental intelligence and resourcefulness also have to be taken into account (Srikantia, 1969).

Indonesian children aged between 6 and 7 years who had suffered from malnutrition five years earlier, and who, at 6 and 7 years of age, were 95 per cent of the average Indonesian height, were equally divided. The shorter group scored 12 points less than the taller group in the Goodenough IQ test. A significantly greater number of children weighing over 95 per cent of the standard weight for their age scored 90 and

FIG. 11/3 Frequency of mental deficiency among pre-school children in relation to intake of animal protein

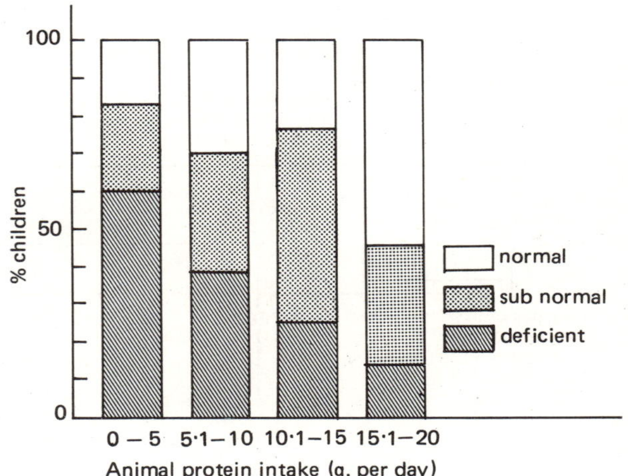

Source: Monckeberg, 1971

above in the IQ test. Among these same children five years previously, one-third weighed 100 per cent of the standard weight, and had an average IQ of 14 points higher than those who weighed less; most of these with an IQ of above 90 were among the heavier group. A significant observation of Indonesian workers is that children who have suffered from malnutrition and vitamin A deficiency combined five years previously have a significantly lower score; not only than children who had previously been healthy, but also than those who had been malnourished but without vitamin A deficiency (Liang, Hie, Jan and Giok, 1967).

In the Philippines, on the basis of a non-verbal intelligence test designed for rural areas, a correlation was found between head circumference and intelligence only in the 11 to 14 years age group, but a correlation between height and intelligence existed at all ages (Guthrie, Guthrie and Tayag, 1969). A correlation between head circumference, as well as between height and weight, and intelligence, has been noted by various workers in Latin America (Scrimshaw, 1969).

Even where children, both those who have recovered from early malnutrition and those without a history of ill-health, have been carefully matched for ethnic, socio-cultural and economic factors, it is difficult to eliminate entirely the differences which must exist between the care an infant receives from a relatively healthy mother and from a chronically malnourished mother. Such differences will occur in the same village, and the children continue to live, throughout studies such as those described above, in the same home atmosphere. Nonetheless, most of those conducting research in this field conclude that there is little doubt that delayed neuro-integrative development occurs with children on a low plane of nutrition who have not grown well.

Cravioto and his associates have pointed out that malnutrition may affect mental development both directly and indirectly; indirectly because a malnourished child cannot concentrate and does not learn while it is suffering from malnutrition; and it is frequently

sick. There may thus be interference with learning during periods of critical development, since it is believed that there is a correlation of opportunity with a given stage of development; if missed, such development does not take place. Equally, malnutrition causes changes in motivation. Apathy leads to diminished adult responsiveness to the child, resulting in diminished stimulation, learning, maturation and interpersonal relations, ending in significant backwardness in performance on later, more complex learning tasks. In addition to these effects, there is a likelihood that malnutrition may affect the development of intersensory organization directly, by modifying the growth and biochemical maturation of the brain, as has already been discussed.

Further long-term projects are in progress in Latin America, in which an attempt is made to eliminate socio-economic and cultural variables, and to clarify further the ultimate effect of early malnutrition on subsequent development. It is still not known what degree and nature of malnutrition are most destructive, how permanent are its effects, and up to what age. It is suggested that protein-calorie malnutrition occurring after the first year of life may not have irreversible effects, but it must be remembered that for such damage to be rectified, the child requires a balanced diet. In most of the rural areas of Asia, a reasonably adequate diet is not achieved until the age of 6 or 7 years, if then.

It is known that severe malnutrition in young infants will produce significant brain damage (Winick, 1969c). It is suspected that malnutrition during childhood impairs subsequent mental development in a number of ways. Since, therefore, improved nutrition will, directly or indirectly, help rectify all the factors which have been implicated in impaired mental development, it is obviously essential in the face of this menace, and without waiting for further proof, to plan the allocation of national food resources, and to organize rural extension and health services in such a way as to stress the importance of balanced nutrition of the vulnerable groups.

12 Food for Rural Asians

TWO WORLDS

THOSE who formulate the objectives of nutritional policy for rural peoples in Monsoon Asia base their recommendations upon a framework of world economy which is at variance with the requirements of the greater proportion of those who inhabit it. It is assumed that there must continue to be two worlds, 'us' and 'them', the one having access through purchasing power, geography or sheer luck of the draw, to a diversified, well-balanced diet in which much of the protein, and frequently more protein than is actually needed, comes from animal sources; the other, desiring and urgently needing at least some degree of improvement of the poor diets which are the basis of rural nutrition in Asia, about half the world's population.

The 'two world' philosophy reaches its apotheosis in the idea that the developed countries should retire a certain proportion of their land from food production. Such land should then be redeveloped so as to provide recreation and essential exercise for urban dwellers. To scientific workers in Asia, it must seem amazing that the reduction of milk production in western Europe and Great Britain, for example, can be seen as morally defensible when the embarrassing surpluses could be of such inestimable value in the nutrition of Asian children. In the words of Lyndon B. Johnson: 'It is almost criminal to have the capacity to produce that we have, and not to know how to distribute this and get it to the people that need it'.

At the 1972 meeting of the 24-nation Intergovernmental Committee of the UN/FAO World Food Program, it was stated that in 1971 about one million tons of highly-subsidized skim milk and dried skim milk had been used to feed livestock in the European Economic Community. In the Federal Republic of Germany alone, supplies to the value of U.S.$300 million, subsidized to the extent of U.S.$100 million, were used to feed calves and pigs. At the same time the world market price for a ton of dried skim milk increased from U.S.$300 at the beginning of 1971 to U.S.$750 at the beginning of 1972. Members of the E.E.C. acknowledge that agricultural production in the industrialized world must be restructured for a more equitable allocation of essential foods.

Particularly on the global scale, it has not been customary to promote maximum production of an agricultural commodity in an environment to which it is best adapted, beyond the needs of the country, including what may profitably be sold for export. For the economic security and profit of their members, the marketing boards and farmer producer groups of the developed nations, the first world, supported by international foundations and other bodies, take effective action to apply the principles of organized scarcity. These are, of course, a complete denial of the applications of ecology. The maximum productive capacity of the favourable environments is, therefore, not to be fully realized. A global increase of food production is held back just as much by these economic but non-ecological practices as by any lack of practical and administrative effort in developing countries, or by the so-called apathy of cultivators, produced by under-nutrition and malnutrition in the more difficult equatorial and monsoonal environments.

Therefore, it is argued, it is unrealistic to suggest that it would be sociologically wise and morally correct to create conditions in which agricultural producers everywhere would continue to grow the maximum amount of food of which their particular environment is capable, probably far above the present level of production, while maintaining present standards of incentive and profitability to producers. The economic and political delegates to United Nations Conferences on Trade and Development and other international bodies have been unable to evolve some method of getting that food to the people who need it. At the same time there is a public unawareness in the advanced world of the great dangers of maintaining present conditions of chronic under-nutrition and malnutrition among rapidly increasing populations, and of the pressures that are being built up within Asia, which in due course will affect the whole world.

The Asian food production scientist and field adviser and the nutrition specialist must realize that, in working for the improvement of rural diets, they are more or less on their own. They have to rely on the production of Asian foods from the Asian land. They must review all the food crops that are at present being grown in the region, discover how their yield may be increased and their quality improved, and try to ensure that what little is available of quality foods is used correctly in diets that approach some degree of balance, especially for the vulnerable groups. Certainly, the higher income groups and tourist centres will be able to afford the quality foods, and especially the proteins, fats and vitamins which may be produced expensively in Asia and will come increasingly from the advanced countries in the Asian-Pacific grouping. But the great mass of the Asian population has a poverty index level at which it is difficult to obtain even caloric requirements, let alone balanced proteins. The main concern of research and extension must therefore be how to maintain and improve existing diets, based as they are on cereals with generally ineffective quantities of legume protein and other nutrients (Table 12/1).

Table 12/1 has the usual defects of the statistics provided to and used by FAO for analysis. There is no distinction between urban and rural, nor between socio-economic groups within these major countries. There is no distinction between wheat-eating West Pakistan (Pakistan) and rice-eating, more populous and poorer East Pakistan (Bangla Desh), nor between the minority of wheat eaters and the majority of rice and millet eaters in India. The figures for percentage of protein from animal sources are suspect and therefore highly misleading.

COLLABORATION BETWEEN AGRONOMISTS AND NUTRITIONISTS

Matters relating to the production, consumption and composition of foods offer an excellent field for profitable collaboration between crop agronomists, animal production specialists, biochemists and specialists in rural nutrition. The problems to be faced concern the production, as efficiently and cheaply as possible, and within Asia itself, of all the crops that provide food for direct human consumption or indirectly through the domestic animal. These foods are:

(a) the sources of energy (foodgrains, starchy roots and tubers, sago, and, to a lesser extent, sugars and syrups, fats and oils);

(b) the crops that provide most vegetable protein (foodgrains, grain legumes, nuts and seeds);

(c) the sources of vitamins, fats, oils and minerals from plants; and

(d) all the many wild and cultivated plants which

TABLE 12/1

Degree to which some Asian countries obtain calories from wheat

Country	Wheat used per caput per day (gm.)	Percentage of total calories from wheat	Wheat calories as percentage of calories from all cereals and starchy foods	Percentage of total calories from all cereals and starchy foods	Percentage of protein from animal sources
Pakistan[1]	120	20	28	73	21
India	73	13	19	68	12
Japan	71	10	15	68	24
Taiwan	61	9	13	75	26
Ceylon	52	9	14	65	18
Philippines	25	5	7	71	33

[1] including East Pakistan, now Bangla Desh.

Source: Aykroyd and Doughty, 1970

are convertible by grazing or stall-fed livestock into products rich in protein of high biological value, as well as in vitamins, fats and minerals.

The production of these foods for direct or indirect human consumption is the field of the crop agronomist and animal husbandman. But their plans for food crop and livestock improvement must be worked out in association with the biochemist. By using careful methods of analysis that ensure accuracy and comparability of results, the biochemist has to assess the quality of foods and diets. If he and the nutrition specialist then state what foods should be produced to meet nutritional requirements, ethnic preferences and purchasing power of particular rural communities, it will then be the job of the land science specialists to say whether that type of production is ecologically, agronomically and economically feasible on a long-term basis in that area.

Something like the approach in Rajalakshmi's Table 43 (1969) is needed, giving land area required to produce specified amounts of different foodstuffs, and their cost according to diets for different age groups in the lower, middle and upper income classes (Table 9/5); or the calculations of Whyte and Mathur (1968), designed to express litres per day through-put of a milk plant in terms of the total number of hectares of cultivated land needed to produce the feeds and fodders needed to produce that milk from efficient bovines. *Times of India* of 9 August 1970 reports that a comprehensive scheme for studying the cost of cultivation of principal crops is to be undertaken by the Union Ministry of Food and Agriculture in association with non-official agencies like agricultural universities in thirteen States.

In 1958, an FAO/CCTA Technical Meeting on Legumes in Agriculture and Human Nutrition in Africa was convened at Bukavu, then the Belgian Congo (Chairman, A. Angladette; Technical Secretary, T.R.G. Moir (FAO,1959). Aykroyd and Doughty (1964) state that this meeting was remarkable in giving experts in both agriculture and human nutrition an opportunity to discuss the grain legumes from their respective standpoints and to pool their ideas. 'The Bukavu approach was at least a move in the right direction.' Until then the agricultural research centres in Africa had not given enough attention to the cultivation, improvement of yield and extension of a number of legumes which nutritional studies had shown to be of potential value in the African diet (Aykroyd and Doughty, op. cit.). There is a suggestion that this failing on the part of the crop people is due to lack of resources for research and extension — it may, however, be due equally to the opinion of the crop specialists that many of these grain legumes just would not make good economic crops for cultivation on a large scale, or even in village gardens.

The agriculturists and the nutritionists attending the Bukavu meeting applied different criteria in the classification of the grain legumes of central Africa. The agriculturists grouped fifty-three legumes into four categories:

(1) species the agronomic interest of which is not in question for all regions in Africa south of the Sahara, or at least for one of them,

(3) species without any present or future agronomic interest,

(2a; 2b) species intermediate between (1) and (3).

The criteria of the nutritionists in defining their three categories were:

(1) legumes, the food products of which are widely used and accepted for human consumption and for which there is satisfactory evidence that the products as eaten have good or high nutritive value;

(2) legumes yielding foodstuffs less well-known than those in category (1), and the nutritive value of which is not so well characterized; this category is divided into:

(a) those about which there is sufficient knowledge to justify study and possible subsequent upgrading to category (1);

(b) those of doubtful nutritional value or about which little is known, but which might nevertheless merit further study; and

(3) legumes which are rarely used as human food or only in small amounts, or which, on present knowledge of digestibility, toxicity and acceptability, cannot be recommended as human food.

Unfortunately there is not much evidence of further collaboration along the lines of the Bukavu meeting, and certainly not in Asia. One rarely finds that working parties and specialist panels in crop and livestock production contain practical nutritionists to provide the complete picture. The FAO/WHO or WHO study groups dealing with various nutrients of crop or animal origin for human nutrition do not enrol the assistance of at least one crop and one livestock specialist to tell them which of their idealistic nutritional objectives is feasible in the field or the farmyard and under what ecological conditions. The same may be said of the Protein Advisory Group of FAO, WHO and UNICEF. All these bodies which discuss and decide upon the optimal nutrition of rural Asians should also contain a trained anthropologist who would inform them of the possible degree of acceptability of new foods among different ethnic groups, and the method of introduction of change most likely to meet with success.

Some basic publications are equally unbalanced, since they deal only with specific aspects of what should be a closely co-ordinated subject. The FAO Agricultural Study, *Legumes in Agriculture* (Whyte, Nilsson-Leissner and Trumble, 1953) deals almost exclusively with those legumes which may be used for feeding domestic livestock, hardly at all with the agronomy and improvement of grain legumes for direct human consumption. The FAO Nutritional Study, *Legumes in Human Nutrition* (Aykroyd and Doughty, 1964) on the other hand, lacks the authenticity of agronomic and livestock presentation that could have been provided by the collaboration of a tropical agronomist with field experience.

The standard work, *Human Nutrition and Dietetics* (Davidson and Passmore, 1966) could be improved by the collaboration of qualified crop and livestock specialists with tropical experience. For example, the agronomists and animal husbandry specialists do not consider that the nutrition specialists are told what they should know about the land and its productivity in terms of food for direct or indirect human consumption. The major food crop of Asia, rice, is dismissed in a few words: 'Rice is the cereal of choice for most damp tropical climates. It grows best in the deltas of the great rivers of the tropics, since it is essentially a mud plant requiring an abundant water supply.' There should also be discussion, in this book and in *Legumes in Human Nutrition,* of the pasture, fodder and feed crops which, when fed through efficient animal converters, may contribute effectively and economically to the production of animal protein for human diets; also of the relative efficiency of grain and fodder legumes when expressed as the production of amounts of protein of specific biological value per unit area of land, the ultimate criterion for joint agricultural and nutritional planning.

Nutritionists sometimes state, in support of the increased use of grain legumes in farming systems, that the fertility of the soil is improved when legumes are grown in rotation with the usual cereals and cash crops of a particular region. It is, however, unlikely that the common grain legumes, with their relatively small root systems, have any effect on soil fertility, apart from a possible after-effect from any fertilizers which were applied to the legumes but not fully utilized. When

legumes are grown through to seed maturity, this represents a considerable withdrawal of minerals from the soil. In addition, many rural peoples harvest their grain legumes by pulling everything out of the ground, roots and all. It is generally accepted that the cultivation of groundnuts greatly increases the erodibility of the soil. Arguments regarding the beneficial effects of legumes on soil fertility may safely be raised only in respect of the pasture and fodder legumes.

QUALITY IN ASIAN FOODS

The relative quality of foods for human consumption may be expressed in a number of ways, for example, carbohydrate content, percentage of digestible crude protein, biological value of protein, content of and balance between essential amino acids in proteins, content of the different vitamins and minerals. A short list of common Asian foods and their content and biological value of their proteins is given in Table 12/2, bringing together data from several different sources. FAO (1969b) has summarized, with an annotated bibliography, national and international food composition tables, giving the proportion of food analysed, the nutrients included, the type of presentation of data and grouping of foods. This publication includes three international and seventeen regional tables, as well as 135 national tables for sixty-five countries. Analytical values for some 850 items of Indian foods are given by Aykroyd, Gopalan and Balasubramanian (1966). WHO (1969) has prepared a list of the nutrient composition of common foods used in countries of the Western Pacific Region, while individual countries have made their own analyses.

Other relevant studies include Cresta, Périssé and Autret (1969) on correlations between biological and chemical measurements of food quality; Cresta (1968) and FAO (1970a) on international tables of amino-acid content and protein quality of foods; Ramasastri and Mohan (1969) on the vitamin and amino-acid contents of Indian foods; and Autret, Périssé, Sizaret and Cresta (1968) discussing the protein value of different types of diets in the world, with wheat, maize and rice as the main source of protein, with or without a contribution from animal protein.

It would appear desirable to know more about the agronomic and ecological origin of samples of food selected for biochemical and nutritional analyses, especially soil fertility and deficiencies, use of fertilizers, availability and use of irrigation water, agroclimate and seasonal factors in relation to the growth cycle of the crop; varietal particulars, especially whether the crop has been improved by breeding or selection, or recently screened for protein and amino-acid composition; also interval between harvest and analysis, so as to relate chemical composition, for example of thiamine, to duration of storage.

Where data are available, the full range found in content of protein or other nutrients should be given in quality tables, to indicate the variability likely to be found, and hence the potentiality for varietal selection to the higher levels. Rajalakshmi and her associates (1969) have analysed the chemical composition of· different varieties of bajra from different sources; a range was found in the percentage of protein, carbohydrate, calcium, phosphorus, iron, thiamine and niacin, and a lesser variation in fat and riboflavine. A range in the calorie, carbohydrate, protein and fat value of buffalo milk has been found by the same workers. The Indian Agricultural Research Institute is finding variation in protein contents of grains from rice varieties collected from the hills of Assam, a supposed centre of origin and high variability of this crop. The International Rice Research Institute (IRRI, 1972), has evolved a plot technique and sampling procedure that can adequately measure protein content in varietal tests, in spite of the influence of environmental factors, such as time and rate of nitrogen application, plant spacing, time of harvest, crop season, and location. Variations in protein and amino-acid contents in genetic stocks of rice have also been studied in Taiwan (Tong, Chu and Li, 1970).

FOODGRAINS

The current emphasis is on the relative success in limited areas of Asia of the high-yielding varieties of cereals which their protagonists say are suited to wide areas of the tropics and subtropics. They offer promising opportunity for a break-through in agriculture and for the rapid transformation of the food and nutritional situation in developing countries (FAO, 1968).

In some areas these varieties, when used in suitable combinations with other inputs, have more than doubled yields per hectare and have dramatically increased the profitability of farming.

The full yield potential of these new varieties can be realized only when associated with adequate quantities of fertilizers, plant protection chemicals, and assured and controlled water supply and changes in traditional methods of cultivation. This will require investments in improving irrigation, drainage and flood protection, in the provision of massive quantities of fertilizers and pesticides needed, and the expansion and improvement of transport, distribution and storage facilities for the inputs and the resultant output. Other supporting services such as credit and extension will also have to be expanded and the quality of personnel improved; and modifications to the land tenure system may also be required in some countries....

Cereals occupy the major portion of the cultivated land in many countries, and generally represent the main staple of the diet. If the basic cereal requirements could be met from a smaller proportion of the gross cropped area as a result of increased yields, opportunity would be created for diverting land and water resources to other types of crop and livestock production. A more diversified and prosperous agriculture and an improved dietary pattern could then emerge. This argument for according first priority to cereals among basic food crops is reinforced by the break-through in developing high-yielding varieties of most major cereals, whereas similar progress has not yet been made with other key commodities (FAO, 1968).

The term 'green revolution' has been introduced into the popular and farming literature in Asia to describe the effects of the introduction into agriculture of these new, high-yielding 'miracle' varieties or cultivars, and their cultivation under optimal conditions of soil fertility and agronomic management. The new wheats of India, based on the Rockefeller Mexican dwarf cultivars which were themselves bred from dwarf strains from East Asia (Japan, Korea, China), the series of IR cultivars of rice produced at the International Rice Research Institute in the Philippines, the Japanese and the Taiwan rice cultivars such as Taichung, have all greatly changed the Asian foodgrain picture. The imports and plantings of high-yielding varieties of wheat and rice in the less developed nations have been tabulated by the Foreign Economic Development Service of the U.S. Department of Agriculture in co-operation with USAID (Dalrymple, 1971).

The application of fertilizers, particularly nitrogenous, is an essential component of the new agronomic technology. The grain yield per hectare of most high-yielding varieties of rice is doubled with applications of 200 — 250 kg. nitrogenous fertilizer per hectare. At this same level, protein content of the grain increases in different varieties in varying degree, by 25 per cent in IR—8 to nearly 70 per cent in C—6725. Cultivars IET 712 and C—6725 are most responsive to the application of fertilizers in both grain yield and protein content; the increased protein content appears to be in protein nitrogen (Indian Nat. Inst. Nutrition, 1970).

TABLE 12/2

The protein content and quality of protein in foods

	Protein percentage in edible portion		Protein content gm./100 calories	Biological value[2]	
Ideal protein				100	
Egg (hen)	12.4	13 to 13.5	7.5	96	100
Egg (duck)	13.0	16.5			
Meat (muscle)		20.6		80	
Beef (lean)	17.5		9.6		80
Pork	12.0	16.65			84
Fish, fatty sea	20.0[1]		11.4		83
” tilapia	17.5				
” medium cured fatty	40.0		15.3		
Milk, (cow, fresh)	3.5	3.31	5.4		75
” (cow, skimmed)	36.0		10.0		
” (powdered whole)	26.0				
” (sweetened condensed)	8.1	8.8			
” (unsweetened condensed)		35.6			
” (evaporated whole)	7.0				
Milk (buffalo)	5.8				
Soybean (grain)	38.5	39.85	11.3	75	
Soybean (fresh in pod)		19.5			
Soybean (sprouted)	6.2	11.5			
Other grain legumes	20 to 30	20 to 30	6.4	40 to 50	47
Rice (home-pounded)	7.1		2.0		
Rice (highly milled)	6.7				
Cooked rice		3.38		70	67
Congee (rice gruel)		0.81			
Wheat (grain or wholemeal)	10.5	12.4			
Wheat (flour)	8.6	10.8	3.3		52
Kaoliang	10.1	9.5 to 11			
Millet (*Setaria italica*)		9.59			
Millet (unspecified)		2.9 to 3.4			56
Maize (wholemeal)	9.5	7.7 to 9.2	2.6	55	56
Taro (*Colocasia*)	1.9	1.10	1.7		
Sweet Potato	0.6 to 1.3	1.08	1.1		

Sources: Column 1, World Health Organization, 1969
     ”   2, Ch'en and Li, n.d.[3]
     ”   3, Brock and Autret, 1952; Davidson and Passmore, 1966
     ”   4, Food and Agriculture Organization, 1965
     ”   5, Davidson and Passmore, 1966[3]

[1] There is wide variation in per cent edible portion and protein content among different species of fish.

[2] *Biological value* = the proportion of absorbed nitrogen that is retained in the body for maintenance and/or growth.

[3] See also: F.A.O. (1949); F.A.O. (1954); U.S. Department of Agriculture (1952); Her Majesty's Stationery Office (1962); Ang (1960); F.A.O. (1969a).

Parallel success has not yet been achieved with the dry-land crops, such as the millets, nor with upland rice, which covers a far greater area in Asia than paddy rice. But Asian scientists such as the Director of the Indian Agricultural Research Institute are issuing warnings, particularly about the use of fertilizers. The soils of the Indian subcontinent are old and tired; they have received little in the way of plant nutrients or organic manure for centuries. Perhaps they are not up to the new pressures to which they are now being exposed by the new technology. Excessive use of inorganic fertilizers may destroy the water-retentive properties of the soil. Greater emphasis on fertility-restoring rotations and the use of more organic fertilizers and green manures are necessary. But there is little doubt that plateaux of production are being reached on that 10 per cent of the cultivated land of Asia to which the high-yielding varieties are adapted.

Concern has been expressed about the ultimate effects of the reduction of the cereal varieties of Asia from *the many* of restricted ecological adaptation to *the very few,* high-yielding types of wide ecological adaptation. If a new fungous or virus disease, or insect pest, were to arise and the new varieties did not carry the necessary resistance, vast areas of cropland might well be affected before the plant breeders could evolve a new, resistant type. If it is possible to provide the cultivators on irrigated land with new cultivars each year, as is claimed by India, perhaps the danger may be averted. The risk applies especially to the dry-land settled and swidden cultivators who do not have ready access to plant protection facilities. Breeders will have to think twice before they breed new dry-land cereals in particular, of such wide ecological adaptation that they would eliminate the present low-yielding but more resistant indigenous types.

CROP IMPROVEMENT BY GENETIC METHODS

Apart from the emphasis on increased yields from high-yielding varieties grown under optimal conditions, great interest has developed on the variability found within existing cereal varieties in respect of protein content and the amino-acid proportions in the protein. This has led to a renewed screening of varietal collections on this basis, for example, in the joint project of the Indian Council of Medical Research Nutrition Research Laboratories and the Indian Agricultural Research Institute. Although the highly complex biochemical data obtained may at first sight appear rather irrelevant to village level workers in remote rural communities, they must be considered because of their important place in international and national nutrition policies.

The cereals provide 75 per cent or more of the calories, and from 40 to 70 per cent of the proteins in the diets of developing countries, with higher percentages in rural diets. The planners must therefore know whether the proteins of cereals can be improved to desirable levels by screening, breeding, selection or radiation genetics, or whether they will still require artificial supplementation. The collaboration that is called for between plant breeders, biochemists and food technologists can be achieved only at a relatively few centres which have the trained staff and the equipment for the refined techniques of analysis that are necessary.

Rice

The Indian Council of Medical Research and the Indian Council for Agricultural Research have been concerned with the nutrient composition and the essential amino-acid composition of the protein of ten of the *indica, japonica* and *indica* x *japonica* varieties, some of which have already been released for cultivation on a large scale. In most of these high-yielding varieties, the protein content is higher than average (6.4 to 11.3 per cent), but there is a negative correlation between protein and lysine content (Srinivasa Rao and Ramasastri, 1969). The new varieties have higher thiamine and calcium contents than the standard. However, in July 1970, the Union Minister of Food and Agriculture stated that, although the production of wheat in India had increased by 50 per cent in the preceding four years, and was expected to double again within the next six years, no remarkable results had yet been obtained with rice, India's most important foodgrain. High-yielding varieties have been developed, but they are not sufficiently resistant to pests and virus and fungous diseases, nor are they suitable for the waterlogged conditions of the wet-monsoon months. Research in these directions has to be intensified, more credit provided to the cultivators by the States, and the construction and maintenance of irrigation channels and the standards of water management on cropland greatly improved.

The cereal chemists at the International Rice Research Institute in the Philippines (Chandler, 1969) have analysed the grain from 8,000 varieties, and found a few that maintained a high-protein content during three successive generations. Unfortunately, none of these had a favourable plant type, and all were low in yield and relatively unresponsive to nitrogen. It seems to be clear that high (as well as low) protein content is an inherent character which can be incorporated into the germ plasm of the high-yielding varieties. Rice contains about 7.5 per cent protein, but only half that amount after milling and cooking. Under good management, some of the new varieties such as IR8 may contain 8 per cent. It is hoped to produce new varieties combining high yield with a protein content about 10 per cent, while still maintaining lysine at the normal level of about 4 per cent of the protein. It now appears that protein content can be increased 20 to 25 per cent without any reduction in grain yield (IRRI, 1972).

Protein content is strongly influenced by environment. In order to reduce variability due to environment, all pedigree rows and yield trial plots at IRRI which are to be evaluated for protein status are transplanted at 20 x 20 cm. spacing, and all nitrogen fertilizer is applied basally. The closer plant spacing and early nitrogen applications result in lower protein content and reduced variability (IRRI, 1972).

At IRRI, some 10,500 entries in the world rice collection have been screened for lysine content. There is a change in the slope of the regression curve above 10 per cent protein. The lower slope at high protein levels reflects the lower constant lysine content of brown-rice protein above 10 per cent protein. Milling reduces the proportion of lysine in protein, since the protein fraction with the higher lysine content, albumin, is more concentrated in the bran layers. IRRI conclude that, since lysine is not the first limiting amino acid in rice diets (see p. 152), 'improving the lysine content of rice protein is less important than improving the protein level without sacrificing lysine content in a breeding program to improve the nutritional value of rice' (IRRI, 1972).

Three of every four hectares of rice in Asia grow under rainfed conditions; confining bunds impound natural rainfall. A three- to five-year project on rainfed and upland rice began in Balacan and Nueva Ecija in 1971, involving co-operation between IRRI and the Philippines Agricultural Productivity Commission. The first year's results indicate the great potential for increasing yields under rainfed conditions. Average yields of between four and five tons per hectare have been obtained from experimental rainfed padis receiving adequate fertilizers, and treatment for weeds, insects and diseases. In that year of serious drought, combined with an outbreak of tungro virus, yields on farmers' fields were less than 0.5 tons per ha., because

of their general poverty and limited technology (IRRI, 1972).

Wheat

According to FAO (Aykroyd and Doughty, 1970), the Government of India hoped that by 1971 over 12 million hectares of land, correctly fertilized, with assured rainfall or irrigated, would be sown to new varieties of wheat, rice and other crops, resulting in an increase of 25 million tons in the total annual production of grains. In August 1970, M.S. Swaminathan forecast a production of 25 million tonnes by 1972/3, provided harvesting, threshing, storage and marketing were improved to supplement work on high-yielding varieties, on the breeding of cultivars adapted to different ecological conditions and on the dry-farming programme. Production in 1969/70 was estimated at 20 million tonnes.

But, as Michael Lipton notes in his review of Mellor, Weaver, Lele and Simon (1968), of some 95 million tons of foodgrains produced in 1967/8, the contribution of high-yielding varieties is estimated to range from 4 to 7 million tons. The small, credit-hungry farmers on the remaining dry-land areas represent 85 to 90 per cent of the cultivated area, to which the existing high-fertility-demanding, high-yielding varieties are not adapted. It was to assist these that Government of India initiated its dry-land farming project (Chapter 14).

In the U.S.A., it has been found (Schweitzer and Ries, 1969) that wheat seed that contains more protein following field applications of nitrogenous fertilizer develops into larger seedlings. Thus the content of protein in the seed is correlated with subsequent growth and yield, indicating that the amount of endogenous protein or of a proteinaceous moiety which is controllable may be an important factor in agronomy. There have, however, been reports from Asia that higher protein content in both wheat and rice is inversely correlated with lysine content (Deosthale, Suryanarayana Rao and Mohan, 1969).

Screening of fifty lines of wheat in India has shown protein content of from 8.6 to 16.9 per cent (a new variety is claimed to reach 15 to 30 per cent protein), but the variation in lysine content of the protein is small. This relative constancy of the amino acid may be useful in evolving varieties with high protein contents without detriment to the nutritional quality of the protein. If, however, the 1,000 grain weight of the new high-protein varieties remains the same as in the unimproved varieties, it is difficult to see how the proportion of some other component may not be reduced.

Barley

An increase in the protein and lysine contents would be important where this cereal is the staple, or is used in the feeding of non-ruminant livestock such as swine and poultry. One variety is known to have amounts of protein and lysine 20 to 30 per cent higher than the common ones; controlling factors are simply inherited and may be transferred to other varieties. Studies are in progress at Beltsville, Maryland, on the amino-acid composition of the protein induced by the changes in lysine and possibly also methionine. Biologic assays are being made to measure the results of changes in amino acid composition of barley proteins in diets of humans and non-ruminant livestock.

Maize

The discovery of the existence of major differences in nutrient composition associated with the genetic mutants, Opaque-2 and Floury-2 has led to extensive investigation. The original high hopes for the use of the opaque gene in human nutrition have not been realized, because of susceptibility to ear-rot, lower yield and unattractive appearance. In addition to the agronomic requirements of satisfactory yield, there are specific problems of protein levels, relative content of lysine and tryptophan, and grain appearance for acceptance by producers and consumers. By recombining certain genetic modifying factors, types with much harder endosperms are being obtained which retain the high levels of lysine and tryptophan characteristic of the Opaque-2 maize (CIMMYT, 1970-1).

The success achieved with high-lysine maize in north and south America should be important for that relatively small proportion of rural Asians who use this cereal as a subsistence staple. Already, high-lysine maize flour has been incorporated into a weaning food, Duryea, which can be used both as a bottle-feeding formula and as a gruel. A single serving of about 0.25 litre in the latter form provides about 6.8 gm. good quality protein, about 180 calories, and adequate vitamins and minerals. The higher lysine levels ensure more efficient use of the total protein. Germ plasm material with considerable variability is available, adapted to low, intermediate and high altitudes in the tropics. As in rice, however, the new varieties call for high agronomic efficiency on the best soils.

A protein content of 13 to 15 per cent is now a practical objective in maize breeding in the Americas.

The Indian workers find protein values range from 8.5 to 13.6 per cent (Ramasastri and Mohan, 1969). The lysine content of the protein varies from 1.70 to 2.69 per cent, with a possible trend towards a lower lysine content with a higher protein content. There is a significant negative correlation between higher protein content and methionine content. The leucine content of the protein (2.3 to 3.5 per cent) is lower than reported for American varieties, the lysine comparatively higher. Indian workers suggest that, in Opaque-2 maize, there is an inverse relation between lysine and leucine (the amino acid associated with incidence of pellagra); this is confirmed with some composite varieties.

Grain Legumes/Pulse Crops

Those species of the plant Order Leguminosae, which are grown for their grain for direct human consumption, are often said to be used widely in the vegetarian diets of Asia. Certainly, large areas of land are devoted to their cultivation —the species of *Cicer*, *Phaseolus* and other genera in the west of the region, and the soybean in the east. However, in view of the demand from the enormous human populations, the amounts of legume protein available per head are small, probably too small to provide a minimum effective intake for adults, much less for children. These crops deserve much more attention in agricultural research and extension. In spite of the low biological value of their protein, they would theoretically represent an important balance to the cereals, since some of the grain legumes contain important amino acids, especially lysine, which are deficient in cereal protein. Certain legume/cereal combinations may be regarded as a balanced diet for non-vulnerable groups without need for recourse to animal protein; other combinations do not represent a balanced diet (Aykroyd and Doughty, 1964); see p. 97.

Even if rural peoples could afford to grow or to purchase the large amounts of legume protein needed for their own diets, plus export to the urban areas, where is the land to be found? A vast acreage would be required, and could be provided only by the somewhat unlikely transfer of land now under cereals or cash crops (including foodgrains for export — a modern status symbol in Asia). The situation in this respect in India and China is discussed in Chapters 14 and 15.

In spite of the evolutionary diversity of the pulses (Hutchinson, 1970), high-yielding varieties of most grain legumes have not yet been developed. Again, FAO policy in this respect is quoted:

These fall into second place in our list of priorities because of their importance to a balanced diet, the need for diversification of production and the improvement of crop rotations. It is considered that the main strategy for FAO should therefore be to gather available information on these crops and to foster research in developing high-yielding varieties. This action should be initiated immediately in FAO, since there is a number of countries already advanced in cereal production, where there is an urgent need to lay a sound foundation for diversification. Already some countries (e.g. India, Iran and Mexico) are prepared to consider intensive effort in the development of grain legumes and oilseed crops and have taken the initial steps towards breeding varieties (FAO, 1968).

The traditional emphasis on breeding soybeans, for example, has been on increased oil content. It is now being found that the new varieties which have been evolved, combining higher grain yield with protein levels up to 15 per cent above standard varieties, have lower resistance to diseases and pests. The U.S. Department of Agriculture is also trying to produce late-flowering genotypes, to permit the growing of two crops per year in tropical latitudes. Workers in India appear to see considerable promise in this crop, but its acceptability in the Indian diet in preference to gram and other long-established pulses has yet to be proved. The Indian Agricultural Research Institute hopes to replace the present cultivated varieties of khesari *(Lathyrus sativus)* with new varieties low in the neurotoxin associated with lathyrism, a crippling disease of the nervous system caused by excessive consumption of khesari over long periods of drought and famine when other foods are unavailable.

LAND SOURCES OF ANIMAL PROTEIN

Some specialists in the advanced countries consider that it is quite unrealistic to contemplate even the maintenance of the existing forms of animal husbandry in most of the countries of Asia, and that to talk of expanding them is mere wishful thinking by biased enthusiasts. This is rather an over-simplification of the situation. Here we are concerned primarily with the rural people, who do not have the purchasing power required to obtain animal protein from elsewhere. They must either grow it themselves, or it must be available free or cheaply near at hand. The food habits, preferences and taboos and the appreciation of the need for a balanced diet are related to the

ethnic traditions and state of technological development of the rural people.

It is probably correct to say that the food situation in Asia, and particularly the deficiency of plant and animal protein, are such that every actual and potential source of cheap food, including cheap protein, must be exploited to the full. Nutritionists will probably recommend the maximum use of animal protein, provided it can be made available cheaply and without reducing the production of food grains (for calories) and cash crops (providing funds for the purchase of food and other essential commodities). Nutritionists may also agree that a satisfactory diet composed of a little animal protein of high biological value and a minimum effective content of important vitamins and fats might be easier to achieve than the large amounts of vegetable protein of half the biological value that would have to be provided from grain legumes to achieve the same result in terms of human nutrition.

Some authorities believe that for millenia the rural Asians have known how to design a balanced diet from plant sources only, by a judicious blending of the important cereals, grain legumes and vegetables, and therefore why all the fuss now about ensuring some animal protein in their diet? This again is incorrect. Until the relatively recent and rapid increase in human population, the rural people were in reasonable balance with the land resources. Scattered among the areas of shifting cultivation and adjacent to the more settled communities, there were areas of climax or secondary tree vegetation in which the people could obtain daily hors d'oeuvres of animal proteins from the forest fauna, from larger quadrupeds and birds down to insects. Increasing pressure of human population on the land has progressively eliminated this valuable and free source of food of high biological value. Even if shifting cultivation is practised correctly, with a sufficient period to permit the optimal regeneration of vegetative cover, this period will not be sufficient for progression in terms of animal ecology to permit the return of the forest fauna. To this degree and in these environments, the nutrition of the peoples has sadly deteriorated since the days of this wider symbiosis in a relatively balanced ecosystem.

A great contribution to rural diets is or could be made by the livestock kept under systems which may be grouped under the term of scavenger animal husbandry. Again the types of animals kept depend upon the geographical and ethnic traditions. Among scavenging animals around the village, one would consider primarily the pig, the hen and the duck. This is a form of animal production of an intermediate type that deserves much more attention on the part of the animal husbandmen and breeders. These would know how to create and maintain groups of intermediate-level animals on an average but not by any means ideal plane of nutrition, while the veterinarians would try to give greater protection against the diseases that are so characteristic of this type of husbandry.

In addition to those types of livestock that can obtain most of their food around the village and in the nearby fields, there are the free-ranging sheep and goats that also obtain their feed largely free of charge on the arid and semi-arid ranges. But apart from their occasional use for sacrifice, these do not generally represent a major source of animal protein for the rural peoples, who rather tend to maintain them and to sell their produce to the urban areas. These forms of animal husbandry do have the merit of not being dependent on feeds and fodders produced on cultivated land. They can therefore be developed to the extent that the environment and the natural plant cover will permit, without coming into competition with arable food and cash crops.

If increased investment and industrial development are going to raise the average gross domestic product per head per year, this will affect urban diets and greatly increase the demand, first, for the superior food grains, and then for foods of animal origin. It then becomes correct economic policy to provide the more expensive forms of animal protein at a price acceptable to the higher and middle brackets of urban purchasing power. This will divert that purchasing power from the food grains, and by reducing the demand, to some extent prevent an increase in their price, which would make them too costly for the lower income groups in both the urban and rural areas. The increased supplies of foods of animal origin that would then be required may be produced in the rural areas within marketing access of centres of population (administrative, industrial, tourist), to the financial benefit of the peoples in those rural areas. Or these foods of animal origin may be increasingly imported from countries with advanced forms of animal husbandry in the better adapted environments around the Asian-Pacific oceanic fringe.

There may be a period of increased shortage of animal protein in the food procurement areas around urban centres; if this period can be overcome or passed without excessive rural malnutrition, the ultimate higher economic level of the farmers may, it is to be hoped, gradually induce them to hold back some of the superior foods they produce, for home consumption. India is still mostly in the first stage, while some parts of Japan may have achieved the second stage, where increased sale of foods of animal origin to urban areas no longer adversely affects dietary standards in the rural areas.

It can be seen, therefore, that animal husbandry should, on grounds of both good economics and improved rural and urban nutrition, remain an important facet of land use planning in the region. Such planning requires greater regard to ethnology, the ecology of livestock production and to the establishment not only of intensive, but also of intermediate forms of animal husbandry, for local consumption especially in those rural areas far from urban markets.

NUTRIENTS FROM FISH

With its long coasts and seas that are calm for much of the year, salt-water fish are an important item of the diet in Asia, although their significance is sometimes exaggerated when daily intakes are considered. (see Appendix). Fish may be obtained from the sea, or from fresh waters of rivers and lakes, or may be cultivated as a 'crop' in paddy fields and ponds. The production of fish such as tilapia may be important in an intensive farming symbiosis, with the energy food provided by paddy, the protein by fish grown in the paddies, and by ducks which also manure the paddy and promote more insect growth to feed the fish.

Fish may be taken fresh, salted, dried or as fermented fish sauce, or may be processed in other ways. The depth of penetration of sea fish into country markets depends, in the absence of refrigerated rail cars, upon the way in which it is used. Dried fish can be sold far from the coast if acceptable, whereas fresh fish cannot be transported far inland, especially in humid tropical conditions. Thiamine is rapidly destroyed in fish and shellfish; there is none in dried fish (Postmus and van Veen, 1949). Some peoples, such as the Malays (Dean, 1961), consider freshwater fish to be a second-rate food. Others, for example the Cambodians, dislike salt fish (Delvert, 1961).

Fish can make a marked contribution to the diet as a source of animal protein, vitamins, minerals and fat. Small fish eaten whole are an excellent source of calcium in a rice diet particularly deficient in that mineral. It is frequently said that fish represents a major contribution to the Asian diet, and that its use makes it unnecessary to provide anything other than a little vegetable protein, such as soybean, as a relish

TABLE 12/3

Indonesia: Java and Madura:
Consumption of fisheries products per head by household expenditure classes, 1964
(kg. per head per year)

Fish product	*Up to Rp. 6,000*	*6,001– 10,000*	*10,001– 16,000*	*16,001– 30,000*	*Over 30,000*	*All households*
		Household expenditure per week (rupiahs)				
Fresh	1·2	1·8	2·9	4·7	7·4	3·4
Dried and salted	1·6	2·8	4·2	5·3	7·0	4·1
Shrimps etc.	0·2	0·2	0·3	0·7	0·7	0·4

Note: No conversion into dollar equivalent is offered because of the continued inflation during 1964 and the varying rate of exchange

Source: Krishnandhi, 1969

TABLE 12/4

Indonesia: consumption of fisheries products
per head by regions, 1964
(kg. per head per year)

Fish product	*Java and Madura*	*Outer Islands*
Fresh	2·6	16·1
Dried and salted	3·1	5·2

Source: Krishnandhi, 1969

TABLE 12/5

Indonesia: fish production by regions, 1965-7

	Production ('000 tons)	*Production per head (kg.)*
Sumatra	274	15·3
Java	140	1·9
Kalimantan	87	18·7
Sulawesi (Celebes)	123	15·3
Rest of Indonesia	49	6·1
All Indonesia	673	6·1

Source: Krishnandhi, 1969

in the eating of rice. It would be difficult to calculate the consumption of fish protein per head per day or per week, even in communities within reasonable access to a source of supply, but such figures as are available are not high. The benefit to be derived from regular consumption of even small amounts of fish protein has been noted in a coastal village of Trengganu, West Malaysia. Biochemical tests revealed uniformly satisfactory levels of serum protein in all examined. Measurement of skinfold thickness and mid-arm circumference demonstrated large muscle mass, also indicating satisfactory protein status (Wilson, 1970a). In Indonesia, fish consumption in kg. per head per year was (1940) 8.4; (1964) 9.1 and (1966) 11.4 (Krishnandhi, 1969). It is not clear how the figure for 1966 is related to per caput production (Table 12/5). Considerable differences between geographical regions and socio-economic groups are concealed by these figures for average consumption (see Tables 12/3, 12/4, 12/5).

MANUFACTURED AND FORTIFIED FOODS

There is throughout the world an increasing interest in unconventional foods derived either from existing plant or animal sources, or manufactured synthetically. The objective is to produce nutritious foods or supplements to existing low-quality foods, particularly for the developing world. If these manufactured and synthetic foods were to be generally acceptable in urban and rural diets, their costs would have to be kept within the range of low-purchasing powers by methods of mass production. However, results comparable to those achieved with complex, multiple fortification of diets have been achieved with simple, protein-rich foods based on locally available and familiar crops (Doraiswamy, Daniel, Rajalakshmi, Swaminathan and Parpia, 1971).

The Central Food Technological Research Institute, Mysore, India, has for many years been conducting research on manufactured foods and has evolved products based on balanced vegetable protein suitable for the nutrition of the vulnerable groups. Difficulties are experienced in introducing these foods on a large scale because of consumer resistance and lack of purchasing power. Studies on balanced foods of vegetable origin suitable for infants and toddlers have been made in Taiwan (Huang and Tung, 1968), and on coconut as a source of protein in the Philippines (Abdon, 1969). A high protein, pre-cooked weaning food containing 25 per cent protein is composed of rice flour, mung bean flour, fish protein concentrate, coconut skim milk solids with added vitamins. Limiting amino acids are methionine, threonine and isoleucine. The product may be safely stored for six months at room temperature (Payumo, Legaspi and Apolinario, 1972).

The FAO/WHO/UNICEF Protein Advisory Group finds (1970b) that there is ample evidence from animal studies and from observations on humans under controlled conditions in hospitals, schools and orphanages that improvement in nitrogen retention or growth occurs when either simple experimental diets or mixed diets typical of food intake patterns in certain regions are supplemented with the limiting amino acid or acids. The Group sees this as particularly apparent in infants and children who have been malnourished or are fed at low protein intakes. At higher protein intakes, cereal-based diets can usually provide sufficient protein for healthy adults, but this is often not true for adults suffering from acute and chronic infections, or for lactating women. So far, effects of supplementation have been observed mainly with lysine or methionine, although with no cereal-based diet are these the first limiting amino acids. Any decision as to the fortification of staple foods with amino acids must be made on a country basis.

The relevance of this work on unconventional foods to rural Asia may be questioned under four heads:

(a) cost of production — price to consumer; (b) acceptability by consumer; (c) logistics of distribution, especially in rural areas; (d) advisability of adding one ingredient to a diet of overall deficiency.

(a) Cost of Production

Most manufactured and synthetic foods and supplements are intended to increase the percentage of vitamins and/or protein, or to improve the balance of amino acids in the protein. Most are intended for direct human consumption, although the protein produced from the treatment of hydrocarbons of petroleum with yeast is being tested in western Europe and Japan primarily for animal feed, and thus for the production of animal protein for human consumption. Trials of these foods have shown that they are directly beneficial to nutritional status and are therefore of great potential value. In most cases, however, the economics of their application have not been fully worked out. Even if it were possible to take these foods into the bazaars of the villages in the rural areas and the initial resistance could be overcome, even a fractional increase in price above that of the common dietary ingredients would greatly affect their acceptability.

(b) Acceptability

The rural Asian, like the rest of us, is a very conservative person in regard to the foods which he accepts. Change in food habits is acceptable only where a food has become familiar and is known to be of value — for prestige, palatability, and only rarely because its nutritional advantages are understood. Reactions will vary widely from one ethnic group or sub-group to another. Even slight changes in the taste, appearance or behaviour during cooking of familiar staples may lead to their refusal or abandonment. Possibly one of the most acceptable techniques would be the fortification of existing foodgrains with lysine, because this does not affect taste or appearance; it is also potentially one of the cheapest methods of raising protein quality by creating a better amino-acid balance. The fermentation of starchy tubers of crops such as cassava with fungal organisms such as *Rhizopus* can result in a higher protein content (Stanton and Wallbridge, 1969). However, the acceptability and the economics of this process have also yet to be proved. Even less will rural people accept a commodity totally unknown to them, either as a food in itself or as something to be added to their staple food at an appropriate stage of cooking.

(c) Logistics

Enthusiasts for the supplementation of existing low-quality foods, particularly those deficient in proteins, may concern themselves with the ingredients and vehicles of fortification. Reference is rarely made to the great problems involved in bringing fortified foods to the rural areas, or the precise control of

attempts at fortification in the rural areas, though experience with vitamin fortification of rice in the Philippines may have served as a reminder of the difficulties involved.

At the Calcutta meeting of the Indian Association of Food Technologists in February, 1969, on the protein fortification of foods, the delegates were concerned with two major aspects of protein fortification; (a) the ingredients — cottonseed, fish protein concentrate, soybean, single-cell protein, groundnuts (especially isolates), amino acids; and (b) the vehicles of fortification — rice, milk, tea, salt, wheat flour and bread. It is apparent that even the ubiquitous rice is not a vehicle for fortification with a potentiality for wide distribution. In India only 10 per cent of the total rice consumed is milled where fortification can be applied. The rest is either home-pounded (50 per cent of the total) or treated on small, hand-operated mills in rural areas inaccessible to fortification. The situation in other rice-eating areas of Asia is similar. Vegetable isolates with a higher biological value than unprocessed grain legumes appear to be promising, until cost is considered; but where is there enough cultivated land to produce the extra amounts required? In India, isolates might be used instead of imported skim milk for supplementing toned milk (in which the fat content is reduced to 3 or 1.5 per cent). As with the fortification of salt, and even more, bread, the cost of the product would take it beyond the reach of the purchasing power of the rural and poorer urban peoples for whom it is most needed. Wheat flour seems slightly more promising as a vehicle, since the mills are more accessible to the fortification process. Although tea may be fortified with lysine with no apparent effect on taste, it is customary to drink tea between meals rather than together with meals. Thus the whole object of achieving better balance between amino acids would not be reached. The green tea consumed in much of Asia is not susceptible of fortification. Most of the cereal grains throughout Asia are subsistence crops, and thus totally inaccessible to fortification; an improved protein content or amino acid balance would have to be bred into the farmers' varieties.

Any discussion of the fortification of diets of the rural peoples must be largely academic. This is not to discount the value of fortification *per se,* whether with protein isolates from vegetable sources or with selected amino acids, to enhance the more diversified diets of middle-income city people which are still susceptible of considerable improvement. Most of the rural people, however, are living in subsistence economies, many adopting swidden and other dry-land forms of extensive cultivation and with diets largely deficient in terms of major nutrients. Apart from the limited availability of lysine and the even lower availability of methionine and its high cost, it is hard to visualize how one can contemplate the logistics of fortification of rural diets on any impressive scale. And even if it were possible to fortify the proteins, much or most of that protein would still be used primarily for energy under current conditions of calorie deficiency.

(d) Advisability

In reviewing the tendency to propose the addition of one component to the diet of rural Asians, it is necessary to refer to the biochemistry of balance and imbalance between all the components of the diet. The Report of the Joint FAO/WHO Expert Group on Protein Requirements (FAO, 1965) states with regard to amino acids in particular:

The possible effect of amino acid imbalance must be taken into account in any evaluation of the essential amino acid patterns of foods and in planning supplementation. One type of amino acid imbalance arises when the addition of a single amino acid or mixture of amino acids to a diet reduces the utilization of the dietary protein. Even a small increase in the concentration of certain amino acids can increase the needs for others when the total protein intake is low. Utilization of one dietary amino acid may also be depressed by addition in the diet of another structurally related to it. The two best-known examples are the interference by an excess of leucine with the utilization of isoleucine and valine, and the interference of lysine with the utilization of arginine. Large amounts of single amino acids added to experimental diets may induce various toxic reactions, including depression of growth. The most toxic amino acids are methionine, tyrosine and histidine, and their effect is most serious when the diet is low in protein. Not enough is yet known about the practical bearing these observations might have in relation to human diets, but they must be taken into account in studies of the biological effectiveness of essential amino acid patterns and in the amino acid supplementation of specific foods.

A paper submitted to the WHO Expert Committee on the Biochemistry of Mental Disorders (Rajalakshmi, undated) says: 'A deficiency or excess of individual amino acids is also found to affect central nervous system functions. . . . A deficit in learning performance has been found with an excess of phenylalanine.'

Even if it were possible to induce a moderate improvement in the biological value of a protein by fortification with lysine, this may well cause a growth spurt in children and adolescents, thus creating a sudden increased demand not only for more protein, but also for vitamin A, calcium, iron, and indeed all the nutrients essential for growth, so many of which are deficient in Asian diets. Night blindness was found in Javanese children who were showing such a growth spurt (Blankhart, 1967): 'probably induced by extra rations of milk powder containing about 400 i.u. of vitamin A daily: In these cases even the additional vitamin A apparently failed to satisfy the increased demand during the accelerated growth.'

Where food grains are the principal source of protein, and even if lysine is raised to the level of a reference protein, other amino acids, both 'essential' and 'non-essential', will become limiting before this level is reached, and the biological value may thus not be greatly enhanced; i.e. the usefulness of adding lysine in any amount may be questioned where diets are otherwise unbalanced.

The National Institute of Nutrition of India has studied the amino-acid composition of wheat, rice and mixed-cereal diets of pre-school children in different regions. In no case is lysine the first limiting amino acid. On wheat-based diets, isoleucine, valine and threonine are equally limiting, followed by the sulphur amino acids and then by tryptophan. With rice diets, tryptophan is the first, the sulphur amino acids the second and isoleucine and threonine the third limiting amino acids. In mixed-cereal diets, tryptophan is the first limiting amino acid, followed by isoleucine and then the sulphur amino acids. In adult diets in Gujarat, Maharashtra, Punjab, Tamil Nadu, Uttar Pradesh and West Bengal, isoleucine is the first limiting amino acid and valine the second (Indian Nat. Inst. Nutrition; 1970).

In south India, diets based on ragi *(Eleusine coracana)* supplemented with lysine caused significant increases in height, weight, nutritional status and nitrogen retention in school children (Doraiswamy, Rao,

Swaminathan and Parpia, 1968). Nonetheless, when the effect of lysine supplementation was compared with supplementation with leaf protein (Doraiswamy, Singh and Daniel, 1969), it was found that leaf protein produced a better response. This was because the amount of protein in the diet had thus been significantly increased.

Lysine supplementation of bread for children in Shikoku, Japan, has significantly increased height, weight, grip strength and standing broad jump over the controls (Niki, 1968). It may be assumed, however, that these Japanese children differ from those in south India in the higher purchasing power of their parents and an environment which permits greater diversity and balance in the diet, even before the introduction of supplementation in the diet (see also Chapter 10).

CONCLUSION

It is obvious that the rural people of Asia will continue to depend almost entirely upon their staple foodgrains as the principal source of nutrients. The research which has been discussed on the increase of yield and the improvement of quality of the foodgrains is therefore of great significance to the whole region.

There is a limited potential for increased production of animal foods from the land and the sea. This will never be enough to meet the protein requirements of the Asian diet, or even those of the vulnerable groups. Above all, it seems to be economically inevitable that the marketed animal product will remain beyond the purchasing power of the great mass of the population.

Fortification and supplementation of basic dietary items with manufactured and synthetic products may be technically possible, although perhaps not economically feasible. However, insuperable problems seem to arise in the logistics of supplying these fortified foods to the rural areas on anything approaching an adequate scale.

Part IV

NATIONAL AND INTERNATIONAL ACTIVITIES

13 Surveys, Policies and Programmes

INTERNATIONAL AGENCIES

SEVERAL Specialized Agencies of the United Nations are concerned with food and nutrition in Asia. The World Health Organization advises governments on health and nutrition, assists progress in the prevention of epidemic and endemic diseases, and assesses nutritional status. In association with the Food and Agriculture Organization, WHO regularly reviews human nutritional requirements in relation to current research and knowledge. WHO collaborates with FAO and UNICEF in the Applied Nutrition Program, which aims at providing balance in the diets of a certain percentage of the vulnerable groups, in the hope that the diets of others will gradually be influenced and improved. Education in food use and nutrition is included in the FAO Rural Youth Program. FAO, WHO and UNICEF collaborate in the work of the Protein Advisory Group, which is responsible for investigation and advice on high-protein foods, protein concentrates and protein mixtures, their production, nutritional evaluation, safety, acceptability, tolerance and marketing. The PAG has asked a Panel of Experts to formulate an international strategy to cope with the protein crisis in developing countries.

UNICEF announced (February 1971) that it proposes to extend its aid programme in South-East Asia to support health services, family and child welfare and education, in the following countries:

Malaysia: increase production and consumption of protein-rich and protective foods; assistance during 1971-6 to strengthen the community services programme

Philippines: youth activities among over four million school-leavers

Indonesia: community action for children and youths in rural areas; training of village-level social workers

Hongkong: improvement of day-care facilities for children of working mothers

South Vietnam: training of personnel and provision of equipment for care of orphans

Taiwan:
South Korea: improvement of health services
Laos: for children and youths
Thailand:

From its headquarters in Bangkok, the United Nations Economic Commission for Asia and the Far East (ECAFE) promotes those actions on a regional and national basis within Asia which may provide the economic background for an overall improvement of standards of living and hence of health and nutrition. The Asian Development Bank and the World Bank provide financial support for projects which receive technical approval and counsel from other United Nations agencies. Finally, the major responsibility for increasing the production or the provision of all types of foods rests with FAO, to the extent that its objectives, policies and budgets are acceptable to its member countries.

There are in addition numerous bilateral programmes and projects carried out by foundations from all over the world. The beginnings of regional or subregional collaboration between Asian countries themselves are reflected in the creation and activities of ASEAN, ASPAC and other groupings.

An indication of the views of WHO and FAO on current problems and future developments within Asia can be gained from addresses given by the Directors-General of these two organizations to the UNESCO Intergovernmental Conference of Experts on the Scientific Bases for Rational Use and Conservation of the Resources of the Biosphere, held in Paris from 1 to 13 September 1968.

The paper presented by WHO was entitled: 'Man's health in relation to the biosphere and its resources'. The ecologist conceives the term 'conservation' as the wise management and utilization of natural resources for the greatest good of the largest number. One may debate the position of man in such a universe, but only as to what level of hierarchy he may allocate himself. Man is not only dependent upon the resources of this earth; he himself is one of its most valuable resources. Man's history justifies the claim that he is also 'an endangered species'. The record of human disease makes clear that this danger is neither new nor predicted only for the future. More knowledge is needed about the relations between human populations and their potentials and those of the natural environment. The development of a comprehensive ecological knowledge is a necessary ingredient for planning a better world.

Diseases, for which the means of control was discovered over one hundred years ago, still challenge the biologist, the physician and engineer. Smallpox still rages through much of the world, and cholera in a new form has spread from its historic foci in Asia to the portals of Europe. Malaria, schistosomiasis, the enteric diseases, tuberculosis, leprosy, measles and cerebro-spinal meningitis are still well-established causes of morbidity and mortality. Other less known diseases like viral hepatitis and haemorrhagic fevers are arousing increasing concern. In many regions the health scene is dominated by the presence of malnutrition, kwashiorkor, nutritional marasmus, and other forms of protein-calorie deficiencies which affect millions of children.

In the impoverished, developing countries, the infant mortality rate, a sensitive indicator of public health, fluctuates between 200 and 300 per thousand births. Man dies early of the communicable diseases, and his life expectancy is less than 45 years. He is the easy victim of his debilitated internal and external environment. By contrast, in the developed world, man suffers least from the communicable diseases and has a life expectancy of some 70 years, with an infant mortality rate of 20 per thousand or even less. With some exceptions, he is well-fed, lives long, and hence encounters the penalties of the ageing process, particularly cancer and cardio-vascular diseases.

Man's health is influenced by environment, but much research still needs to be done on the ecology and natural history of disease. Any real change for the better in health for the 'third' world is contingent upon economic developments in agriculture and industry, upon the creation of skilled manpower and organization of health activity, and upon the provision of such environmental necessities as safe water and sanitation. Some will say that by reducing disease, society is subject to even greater hazards because of great population increases and shortages of food — six billion people in the year 2,000. One might choose the fatalistic road laid out many years ago by Malthus and take refuge in despair. We have not disposed of the problem, however, by choosing that debilitating route, because it leaves unsettled what is to be done with the billions of people already alive.

Better health is correlated with changes from wasteful patterns of high mortality and high natality to more productive patterns of low mortality, with a natality regulated as desired — whether this involves an increase or a decrease over previous levels. Family planning is being considered as an important feature of medical practice in the care of mothers and children and in the promotion of family health, in addition to whatever role it may play in relation to possible demographic problems.

In the FAO statement, a basic distinction was drawn between the prospects for the developed and developing countries — the 'two-world' hypothesis already introduced in Chapter 12. The most serious danger in the coming decades is seen to be almost certainly over-production in the developed world. There will be one feature in common in the developed world, namely, the retirement of surplus agricultural land for non-agricultural purposes. A highly mechanized urban society eats just as much as before, but takes less and less physical exercise. Thus, more land might be diverted from food production to recreation for urban populations, so as to provide that increased activity which would compensate for the decrease in energy expenditure during working hours.

The food situation in the developing areas is profoundly different. The demand for food is rising, and will probably continue to rise, at a historically unprecedented rate, probably at something between 3 and 4 per cent per annum for the foreseeable future. At least two-thirds of this will be due to increase of population. FAO has no statistical evidence to suggest that the world is proving incapable of feeding a rising population. For the developing areas as a whole, food production has just about kept pace with population increases in recent years, except for the serious setback in 1965 and 1966, due to extensive droughts in India, Pakistan and parts of Africa.

Critical excess and deficit of rainfall occurred again throughout the Asian region in 1972. The Director-General of FAO told an Asian Regional Meeting in New Delhi in 1972 that, during the preceding two years, the growth rate in food production had declined, and early hopes generated by the introduction of the high-yielding varieties were fading.

The outlook becomes even more uncertain when one takes into account the further increases in food demand resulting from rising incomes, as well as from urbanization. Meeting this additional demand offers the only real solution to the problem of nutritional deficiencies, seen in the chronically inadequate diets of millions of people, especially of children, and particularly lack of protein. The most effective remedy is to make people better off through general economic progress, and at the same time to ensure that food is available for them to buy with their extra money. Only by satisfying the additional demand for food associated with rising incomes, particularly from the poorer strata of society, can one hope in the long run to achieve a world that is free from hunger and malnutrition.

In recent years, the farmers of the developing countries have not succeeded in meeting this additional demand. Food aid has covered part of the gap. Scarce foreign exchange has had to be diverted to food imports. In many cases, rising food prices have created hardship for the poorest sections of the population.

Unless this performance can be dramatically improved upon, the world food problem will continue to give major cause for concern. What are the chances? Can the developing countries actually achieve an increase in food production over an extended period at the rate of 3 to 4 per cent per annum? FAO does not believe that a direct and unqualified answer is possible at present.

However, it is extremely doubtful whether real success can be achieved without a radical change in the demographic outlook. FAO is convinced that the developing countries *can* achieve an agricultural growth rate exceeding the rate of population increase, but this will not be accompanied by increases in employment. Furthermore, success in solving the food problem can probably be attained only at the cost of diverting investment capital and human resources from other areas, by some sacrifice of progress in the non-agricultural sectors of the economy. Rural as well as urban unemployment and under-employment are already at alarming levels, and no relief is in sight. Current demographic trends seem destined to lead to the inexorable growth of what has been called 'marginal population'. FAO believes that this is the gravest problem facing the world of today and tomorrow.

FAO INDICATIVE WORLD PLAN

This Plan, presented to the Second World Food Congress in June 1970, suggests to member governments in Asia that the bulk of investment expenditure on inputs, and allocation of human resources, should be concentrated on crop production (see Table 13/1). The four priorities are:

(a) A break-through in cereal production, the main staple of human nutrition, and the principal source of concentrates for livestock feed.

(b) An improvement in the nutritive value of the diet, through a greater contribution of cereals to the protein supply, and a more rapid rate of growth in the production of grain legumes, vegetable oils, fruits and vegetables.

(c) Increasing efficiency in production and processing of export crops, and reducing dependency on too narrow a range of crops by diversification.

(d) Creating additional income and employment by a more intensive use of physical resources and modern technology. The nutritional implications of this Plan have been presented by Autret and Périssé (1970).

The livestock production objectives (Table 13/2) indicate greater emphasis on pigs and poultry in which

TABLE 13/1

Asia and the Far East (excluding China);
FAO Indicative World Plan.
Proportion of daily nutritional supply
per caput from different plant sources
1962 and 1985

	1962		
	Calories	*Proteins*	*Fats*
Cereals	65·9	59·9	18·2
Pulses, nuts and seeds	9·4	20·0	15·7
Vegetable oils	4·1	—	32·4
Other food crops	14·3	6·7	2·7
Total plant products	93·7	86·6	69·0
	1985		
Cereals	61·0	57·5	14·4
Pulses, nuts and seeds	9·7	21·4	14·7
Vegetable oils	6·0	—	41·9
Other food crops	17·3	7·3	3·6
Total plant products	94·0	86·2	74·6

TABLE 13/2

Asia and the Far East (excluding China): FAO Indicative World Plan.
Calculations for livestock products, 1962, 1975 and 1985

	Meat			*Milk*			*Eggs*		
	1962	*1975*	*1985*	*1962*	*1975*	*1985*	*1962*	*1975*	*1985*
Production of livestock products (in thousand metric tons)	2,523	3,754	5,521	29,943	39,901	56,542	385	756	1,434
	Production	*Demand*		*Production*	*Demand*		*Production*	*Demand*	
Growth rates 1962-85, per cent per annum	3·5	5·6		2·8	5·4		5·9	6·4	
Production of meat (kg. per head of total population) and milk (kg. per cow in milk)	Estimated 1962	Proposed 1985		Estimated 1962	Proposed 1985				
	1·7	2·5		501	625				
Concentrate feed use (in thousand metric tons, in terms of 90 per cent dry matter)	1962	1985		Growth in feed used (per cent per annum) Quantity	Value		Growth in total annual production		
	8,242	27,978		5·4	3·6		3·3		

the rate of reproduction is much faster. High growth rates for milk and meat production call for an increase in herds, difficult to achieve in the face of a rising demand for meat. The key to dairy development is likely to be the rapid rise in urban demand for milk, even where people have not been regular milk users in the past. When the dairy industry has a very small base and where the environment is suitable, rapid growth may be achieved by the importation of alien cattle. The Plan envisages future growth not as a general expansion of the dairy industry, but as the development of planned production projects centred around consumption (urban) areas.

It is hoped that the national Asian studies, when completed, will be less urban-oriented, to part of that 10 to 20 per cent of the total populations who are already relatively privileged in respect of nutrient status. Or is it assumed that, by extending the two-world philosophy, there should continue to be two worlds also within a state; the 80 to 85 per cent rural population producing, with such strength and enthusiasm as may be provided by an all-plant diet, the expensive forms of animal protein for the urban areas?

If so, the Plan should show this now, and relate its suggestions to social status, occupation and relative purchasing power.

The Plan should also look more critically at the basic data of production provided by prestige-conscious governments and national planning authorities, particularly of those crops and products not included on schedules regularly reported to statistical authorities. This applies partly to grain legumes in India, certainly to the area under cultivated fodder crops, the production of concentrates, and the areas of good, poor and useless grazing land. The real availability of milk per head of population per day in India is probably about 0.01 litre; most rural people never taste milk. Allan McArdle estimates that egg production in India divided by total population works out at 12 eggs per year (the same in China; 250 per person per year in Great Britain); but the rural Indian or Chinese rarely has part of an egg with his meals.

It is when one considers the conclusions of the Plan in the Asian field in relation to actual conditions in the Indian village, Malay kampong or Philippine barrio, that one becomes very uneasy about its whole statistical bases and recommendations. The livestock recommendations that emphasis should be given to pigs and poultry are correct in relation to rates of reproduction and efficiency of conversion of feeds and fodders. However, feeds for these livestock must be produced largely from cultivated land in competition with or as a by-product of the food and cash crops. It seems a little unrealistic to ignore the vast areas of semi-arid and humid tropical grasslands or the areas lying semi-derelict after shifting cultivation for the production of sheep and goat meat or beef. The availability of these more costly types of meat for the upper-income groups would take the buying pressure off pig and poultry products, so keeping their cost down to reasonable levels. Even in the congested areas of China, there is still room for a specialized form of cattle husbandry (Whyte, 1972a).

REGIONAL CO-OPERATION

The South-East Asian Ministers of Education Organization has a programme of regional co-ordination in tropical medicine and public health. A programme of health and medical research and training is being carried out by seven national centres. These consist of a Central Co-ordinating Board at the Faculty of Tropical Medicine, Mahidol University, Bangkok, and national Tropical and Public Health Centres, each assigned responsibility for certain subjects: Indonesia (nutrition and radioisotopes); Laos (public health and helminthology); Malaysia (applied parasitology and entomology and medical and health laboratory technology); Philippines (rural health and rural medicine); Singapore (urban health and medicine and family planning); Vietnam (plague, enteric infection and communicable diseases); Thailand (general and clinical tropical medicine and hygiene and tropical paediatrics). Each national centre will offer formal teaching in at least one subject. A post-graduate course for a Diploma in Tropical Medicine and Hygiene is given in Bangkok; a course for Master of Public Health and Master of Science in Hygiene is offered in Manila; a Post-Graduate Course for Diploma in Applied Parasitology and Entomology in Kuala Lumpur; a Post-Graduate Course for Diploma in Applied Nutrition in Djakarta; a Training Course in Practical Nursing and Assistant Laboratory Technology in Laos.

A first Asian Congress of Nutrition was held at Hyderabad, India, in January/February 1971, under the auspices of the International Union of Nutrition Scientists, sponsored by the Nutrition Society of India and the Indian National Science Academy, and supported by regional governmental and commercial organizations, by UNICEF and USAID. It is hoped to hold Asian Congresses of Nutrition at regular intervals, the second was held in the Philippines in 1973.

The Central Treaty Organization (members: Iran, Pakistan, Turkey, United Kingdom and the U.S.A.) held a Conference on Combating Malnutrition in Pre-school Children, in Islamabad, Pakistan, from March 18 to 22,1968. Problems, plans and activities in Iran, Pakistan and Turkey were discussed and recommendations made regarding protection of autonomy of institutions of nutrition research and training; inter-country exchange of information; post-graduate training; further CENTO conference, National working conferences and meetings of national food manufacturing and research organizations; co-ordination of media for publicity and education; and support of voluntary organizations. It was recognized that while malnutrition was most critical among the pre-school age group, many of the above recommendations were applicable to older groups, and measures should also be applied to those as far as possible.

NATIONAL ACTIVITIES

Nutrition surveys and research have been carried on to different degrees in the countries of Asia for some decades. Some countries now appreciate the importance of nation-wide investigation of diets in order to bring about improvements; others are drawing up national nutrition plans; the government of one country has adopted a national nutrition plan aimed specifically at improving the diet of pre-school children.

Detailed analyses should be presented for all Asian countries with populations over 100 million. Insufficient information is available from Pakistan and Indonesia; India and China are dealt with in Chapters 14 and 15 respectively.

Pakistan

In 1962, a nutrition survey of East Pakistan (now Bangla Desh) was commenced, under the joint sponsorship of the Directorate of Nutrition and Research, Ministry of Health of Government of Pakistan, the United States National Institutes of Health, and the Department of Biochemistry and Nutrition, University of Dacca (1966). These studies were designed to determine nutritional status so that action might be taken to improve health. Rural locations in each of East Pakistan's (Bangla Desh) seventeen districts and five urban locations were selected for study. Dietary evaluation, clinical examination and biochemical study were carried out. An examination of seasonal variations was begun in 1964 at the completion of the general study. Deficiencies of vitamins A and C depend on seasonal availability of fruits and vegetables. The general conclusion was that malnutrition affects the health and well-being of at least half the population of East Pakistan (Bangla Desh), and especially the vulnerable groups (Marks, Reiner and Ahmad, 1965).

The first phase of a nutrition survey has been completed (Rahman, 1968b), and re-survey is proceeding on a limited scale to determine the siting of pilot projects for the improvement of nutritional status of vulnerable groups. Studies are in progress to establish norms of growth rates for children. The Nutrition Research Laboratory is conducting analyses of common foods, and laboratory evaluation of diets. A pilot project in public health and nutrition to reduce malnutrition among infants, children and mothers has been initiated (Rahman, 1968b). The Government plans to establish a National Nutrition Institute, to conduct systematic and specialized studies on malnutrition, to develop supplementary foods, and to start feeding programmes for vulnerable groups. Programmes of nu-

TABLE 13/3

Pakistan: production of major food crops in West Pakistan
and East Pakistan (now Bangla Desh), 1960-7

(in million tons)

Year and Province		Rice (cleaned)	Wheat	Other cereals	Sugar-cane (raw sugar)
1960–61[1]	E. Pak.	9·52	0·03	0·07	0·40
	W. Pak.	1·01	3·75	1·67	1·15
1961–62[1]	E. Pak.	9·47	0·04	0·07	0·44
	W. Pak.	1·11	3·96	1·80	1·41
1962–63[1]	E. Pak.	8·73	0·05	0·06	0·48
	W. Pak.	1·08	4·10	1·94	1·82
1963–64[1]	E. Pak.	10·46	0·03	0·04	0·54
	W. Pak.	1·17	4·10	1·82	1·59
1964–65[1]	E. Pak.	10·34	0·03	0·05	0·62
	W. Pak.	1·33	4·52	2·03	1·84
1965–66[1]	E. Pak.	10·33	0·04	0·05	0·76
	W. Pak.	1·30	3·87	1·77	2·23
1966–67[2]	E. Pak.	10·50	0·04	0·06	0·77
	W. Pak.	1·30	4·20	1·85	2·05
1969–70[3] Planned	E. Pak.	12·73	0·06	0·07	0·70
Targets	W. Pak.	1·72	5·40	2·22	2·13

Source: [1] Government of Pakistan, Central Statistical Office, *Statistical Yearbook 1965 and 1966*, op. cit., Table 42, pp. 76-9
[2] Government of Pakistan, Ministry of Finance, *Pakistan Economic Survey 1966-7*, op. cit., Statistical Appendix, Table 6, p. 12
[3] Government of Pakistan, Planning Commission, *The Third Five Year Plan 1965-70*, (Karachi: June 1965), Table 2, p. 398

Note: Other Cereals include Maize, Millet, Sorghum, Barley and Gram

Source: Khan, 1969

trition education will be developed, and a cadre of workers trained.

The Jinnah Postgraduate Medical Centre, Karachi, the Council of Scientific and Industrial Research Laboratories, Lahore, the Agricultural University, Lyallpur, and the Model Child Welfare Centre, Lahore are conducting nutrition programmes.

Maternity and Child Welfare Centres and Rural Health Centres distribute skimmed milk, dietary supplements and vitamin tablets supplied by UNICEF and CARE (420,000 persons annually). Two hundred Lady Health Visitors are trained annually for 734 Maternity and Child Welfare Centres.

An Inter-Departmental Committee on Nutrition, with representatives from the Ministries of Food, Agriculture, Education, Commerce and Information has been established by the Ministry of Health. The Committee proposes an increase in fish production and the development of duck farms, the poultry industry, and cattle and goat breeding. Increased production of grain legumes is proposed. The production of materials for teaching nutrition and hygiene in the Teachers' Training curriculum is recommended, with school garden programmes in rural areas, cookery classes and model kitchens in girls' schools. Industrialists are urged to provide subsidized meals to workers, and Municipal Boards should have an expert dietitian as a member of staff (Rahman, 1968b).

In a study of food consumption and its long-term perspectives, 1961–86, Hasan Khan (1969) considered the relative income levels and consumer preferences of West and East Pakistan separately, and, correctly, broke down his estimates of food consumption, 1961–86, further into rural and urban.

Khan's conclusions are:

(a) If agricultural programming, negligible at present, is to be useful, analysis of demand for food must become an integral part of the development exercise.

(b) If people are to be provided with a better diet, well within their means, an assessment of the dietary needs of the socio-economic groups must be made through nutritional surveys.

(c) The so-called 'crash programmes' for achieving self-sufficiency in foodgrains are ill-conceived. Targets for wheat and rice in particular will have to be raised (Table 13/3). Khan would not agree with Hodson (1969) that the 'green revolution' has made it possible to strike an overall balance between food supply and population 'though this is not necessarily true of particular regions, nor is it necessarily permanent'. There is an immediate need to allocate ad-

ditional resources to the sectors of livestock, fisheries, fruits and vegetables, to provide a better balanced diet. Failure to act will add to the gravity of an already alarming situation, thus generating new frustrations for all involved in the task of economic development (Khan, op. cit.).

Nepal

Since information on food consumption and nutritional status is limited, FAO, at the request of the Government, has made recommendations: a nutrition survey should be conducted by the Ministry of Food and Agriculture, acting through the Food Research Laboratories and in close co-operation with the other Ministries and agents concerned. The research programme in the laboratories would include the establishment of a small plant for processing soybeans and for the production of a high-protein infant food based on this grain legume.

Ceylon (now Sri Lanka)

Research in nutrition has been carried out for over thirty years at the Medical Research Institute, with further studies at the University of Ceylon, and clinical observations by medical workers. A high incidence of under-nutrition and malnutrition among lower socio-economic levels seriously affects the vulnerable groups in particular (de Silva, 1956; Bibile *et al.*, 1949; Cullumbine, 1951).

In 1961, the National Ceylon Committee of the Freedom from Hunger Campaign, wishing to focus national attention on the importance of nutrition, sponsored an Applied Nutrition Project. The plan was accepted by Government, and in 1966 a nutritionist from FAO began work, planning and carrying out training and education in nutrition. The Applied Nutrition Project is sponsored by the Ministries of Health, Agriculture and Education, the Department of Fisheries, the Ministry of Home Affairs and various voluntary organizations. The first phase involved selection and training of staff, and of villages and schools, and collection of base-line data. During the second phase, this staff carried out nutrition and agricultural extension in the selected villages, aimed at introducing new practices in food production and changes in meal patterns.

Strengthening of the nutrition element in the training of para-medical workers has begun, and the Agriculture Department is undertaking a major revision of the training of extension workers. A great gap still exists in the training and employment of women workers in home management and social welfare in rural areas. A major step towards filling the need for technical skills, including home science, has been taken with the introduction of a new, diversified curriculum for secondary schools.

It has been recommended that a National Food and Nutrition Board be set up, composed of members from the departments and other bodies concerned with food production, import and marketing, health, education and social welfare, nutrition and medical research. This Board would consider all planning for food production and distribution, and prepare a national food policy based on the country's nutritional needs. It was hoped that practical training in nutrition might be incorporated into the field training of all para-medical workers, agriculture extension officers, rural development and colonization officers and school teachers (MacIntosh, 1968).

Malaysia

Nutrition, particularly of the vulnerable groups, has been a primary concern of the Nutrition Division of the Institute of Medical Research, since its inception nearly fifty years ago. The Government of Malaysia has formulated Rural Development Plans to raise the standard of living of rural peoples. An important component of the national plans was the Rural Health Plan, involving a network of rural health units, each comprising a main centre, four sub-centres and twenty midwife stations, each unit to serve 50,000 people. In 1960, there were eight main health centres, in 1968, there were thirty-nine, with 148 sub-centres and 760 midwife stations. These centres are staffed by public health personnel, nurses and midwives; advice on nutrition is part of their activities. Training in applied nutrition is given by the Institute of Medical Research to senior government officials concerned with food production, health, welfare and education. Rural health workers are trained by the Medical and Health Office.

The assistance of FAO was sought to advise on the training of teachers of home economics at primary, secondary and specialist levels (Aleid, 1960). In 1957, the Department of Agriculture appointed a Lady Junior Agricultural Assistant, to find out whether a woman would be more successful in persuading women land owners and farmers to adopt changes to promote increased food production. The experiment was so successful that it has been expanded. The Community Development Office, the Ministry of Agriculture and the Institute of Medical Research send travel-

ling exhibits to kampongs, explaining the importance of quality in the diet of vulnerable groups, and giving demonstrations of the production and use of local fruits, vegetables, chickens and eggs.

Singapore

In the present situation of rapid urban development throughout the island, it is becoming increasingly unrealistic to talk of rural communities. Those areas which might still be included in the rural category are so exposed to urban influence in one form or another that they are not comparable with rural areas discussed elsewhere in this book.

The Maternal and Child Health Department of the Public Health Division operates centres for rural families, but to which the residents of nearby housing development for city workers may also come. Women who cannot afford suitable baby foods are given 450 gm. full-cream powdered milk per week or per fortnight for their infants. Infant cereal foods and Marmite are also given when available. Mothers and children are given free vitamin pills and tonics. Demonstrations in some clinics show how weaning diets may be prepared from inexpensive local foods including porridge, cooked with fish and vegetables, and mashed banana or papaya rich in vitamin A. The foods are then fed to their infants by the mothers attending the demonstration.

The School Health Service covers both rural and urban schools, and includes routine medical examination, the treatment of minor ailments and nutritional defects, the supervision of supplementary feeding and the issue of non-fat milk to needy children. Defective health is more common among new entrants than others, and anaemia more common among children from rural areas, where hookworm infestation is prevalent.

Two types of school-feeding schemes are in operation. Slightly undernourished children are supplied during recess with free skim milk flavoured with Milo. The second scheme serves children belonging to less privileged families. A fortnightly ration per child consists of 450 gm. full-cream powdered milk, 225 gm. vitaminized skim milk, 112 gm. Ovaltine for flavouring, 112 gm. fresh butter, six fresh hen eggs and six oranges.

Thailand

As a first stage of a national nutrition policy, the Government in 1960 planned a pilot project in applied nutrition, involving the Ministries of Public Health,

Agriculture, Education and Interior. The province of Ubol was selected because of the known presence of nutritional deficiency diseases and the high concentration of population of low socio-economic status. Assistance was requested from FAO, WHO and UNICEF. The ultimate aim is to develop and strengthen a central organization capable of defining and implementing a national food and nutrition policy, and to gain initial experience from the project at Ubol.

Action at the pilot project was planned in three main phases: orientation of key personnel and training of personnel selected from the pilot area; collection of basic data; establishment of a co-ordinated field service to operate through health service, schools, agricultural service and the Community Development Programme. The first two phases began with the inception of the project in 1960; in the third phase, experience gained was extended to villagers. This has involved training courses for farmers, housewives, midwives, village committee members, sanitarians, teachers, student health workers, police students. A school lunch programme presents problems of staffing and finance (Thomsen, 1966).

The Department of Agriculture has increased extension services in the north to stimulate the production of legumes, vegetables, fruit trees, cash crops and the use of compost. Agricultural extension is carried on by youth clubs, aimed at young people between the ages of 10 and 20, and stressing legumes, poultry and pigs. Clubs for women are organized by the Departments of Community Development and Health. The Applied Nutrition Project, with these Departments, has drawn up a programme of activities involving instruction in food demonstration, food preservation (mainly pickling), health, and sanitation (Nielsen, 1965).

FAO has advised the Government on the curriculum in nutrition at the College of Education, on nutrition training courses for teachers, and the composition of cheap, high-protein lunches for secondary schools (Eastwood, 1971).

Indonesia

A blueprint for a food policy and applied nutrition programme was established at a workshop convened jointly by the Indonesian Institute of Sciences (LIPI), and the National Academy of Sciences, U.S.A., held in Djakarta in May 1968. It is not known whether this food and nutrition programme has yet received government approval in full or in part, whether it has been established by law, or whether the necessary budgetary provisions have been made.

Assessment of food supply and allowances (recommended by the Workshop). Food Balance Sheets should be compiled, on a national and regional basis, taking the 1963 figures for available foodstuffs as estimates of the food supply in 1968 (Table 13/4), and subject to the difficulties of collecting reliable information from remote communities and outer islands. Special attention should be given to the production not only of the main food crops, but also to the increased availability of protein-rich foods. Results should be checked through regional and group surveys, nutritional surveys or food consumption surveys.

An attempt should be made to solve the widespread problems of vitamin A deficiency, which cause much blindness and increased susceptibility to infection. Any of the following methods would be nutritionally acceptable; improved utilization of sources of plant carotene, especially green, leafy vegetables, yellow fruits and red sweet potatoes, along with increased fat intake to improve the efficiency of carotene absorption; development of sources and utilization of red palm oil and/or shark liver oil; and purchase of concentrated vitamin A preparations for oral dosage.

Tables of dietary allowances and of protein and calorie requirements should be drawn up and adjusted periodically; national average requirements per day should be taken as 2,100 calories and 55 grammes of protein.

Family Planning. The population growth rate is estimated to be 2.6 per cent. A family planning programme should be given priority in the Five-Year Development Plan, designed to cover the whole country, but more especially Java, Bali and Madura.

Food Policy and Nutrition Programmes. A food and nutrition policy should be established by law under a Central Scientific Advisory body, preferably through LIPI.

An FAO consultant (van Veen, 1970) analysed food production targets of the Five Year Plan in relation to the Workshop's nutritional targets. If production targets are achieved, calorie needs may be met, though unequal distribution may result in under-nutrition among lower socio-economic groups. There will still be a serious shortage of protein. The consultant drew up a programme of work for the Food and Nutrition Unit. His proposal for the establishment of an Advisory Committee on Food and Nutrition was ac-

TABLE 13/4

Indonesia: food available per person per day, expressed as calories[1]

	1951	1952	1953	1954	1955	1956	1957	1958	1959
Rice	832	902	911	940	867	931	896	927	929
Maize	159	182	200	293	207	203	188	261	203
Cassava	262	284	327	338	314	316	340	378	402
Sweet potatoes	45	77	71	68	60	81	80	89	83
Soya	28	28	28	37	31	31	29	36	36
Peanuts	25	27	28	36	31	33	33	33	36
	1351	1500	1565	1712	1510	1595	1566	1724	1689
Other foods[2]	97	194	189	203	226	204	207	219	211
	1448	1694	1754	1915	1736	1799	1773	1943	1900

	1960	1961	1962	1963	1964	1965[3]	1966[3]	1967[3]
Rice	995	895	923	805	888	879	837	839
Maize	233	211	295	209	314	192	248	243
Cassava	354	342	346	339	330	292	370	349
Sweet potatoes	75	68	99	81	102	69	56	52
Soya	36	34	30	26	29	25	24	24
Peanuts	36	31	34	30	33	24	36	28
	1729	1581	1727	1490	1696	1481	1571	1535
Other foods[2]	217	210	247	211	179	205	200	195
	1946	1791	1974	1701	1875	1686	1771	1730

[1] *Source*: Statistical Pocket Book, Central Bureau of Statistics, Indonesia
[2] Wheat, sugar, coconut, fat, palm oil, fish, meat
[3] Preliminary figures

Source: Indonesian Institute of Sciences, 1968

cepted by the Government, and he drew up a framework to guide the Committee's policy.

On the basis of a UNICEF report stressing the low economic level of the people and the limited resources of Government, the Protein Advisory Group considers that measures for improved nutrition in Java must be unsophisticated and applicable at the local level. Declining production of soybeans and groundnuts and limited supplies of animal protein are causing concern. The Protein Advisory Group believes that UN Agencies should give particularly high priority to a feasible source of protein for the vulnerable groups.

Hong Kong

Hong Kong is highly urbanized, and only a relative-ly small proportion of the total population of about four million can be regarded as truly rural.

The Medical and Health Department of the Hong Kong Government distributes free milk powder (skim milk, half-cream and full-cream) to infants and young children through Maternal and Child Health Clinics. The skim milk powder has been received free of charge from UNICEF in gradually diminishing amounts. In 1970, only 31,500 kg. were received.

A voluntary organization, the Children's Meal Society, receives an annual Government subvention of HK$150,000 for the supply of at least one balanced meal a day to children in certain schools in Kowloon and the New Territories. In 1971 7,000 to 8,000 meals were served daily, at a cost of HK 20 cents per meal. The organization aims at serving 14,500 meals a day.

TABLE 13/5

Hong Kong: history of public assistance

Form of assistance	Commencing from	Ending on	
Cooked meals	1948	6th January 1969	
Dry rations	about 1951	7th March 1971	
Rice	1962	7th March 1971	3·5 kg. per adult per week
Cash	June 1967	to certain categories of recipients	
Cash	January 1971	to all approved applicants	

The Social Welfare Department of the Hong Kong Government provides public assistance to rural communities. This programme has changed over the years from the provision of cooked meals, dry rations and rice, to the provision of cash assistance (Table 13/5).

Approved applicants were given cooked meals if they lived within half a mile of a distribution centre or kitchen, and dry rations if they lived further away. Residents in rural communities were normally given rice, unless they suffered from specific illnesses or disabilities. It was assumed that they could obtain their own animal protein (poultry) and vegetable requirements. The ingredients of the dry rations and cooked meals are shown in Tables 13/6 and 13/7.

Before 1971, cash assistance up to the maximum of H.K. $33 per adult per month was given in lieu of food to the chronically ill or seriously disabled who had difficulty in collecting rations or attending de-

TABLE 13/6

Hong Kong: public assistance: scale of dry rations

Unit: 1 Share (2 Diets a Day) Per Week

Item	Quantity
Rice	[1] 3·15 kg.
Tinned fish or	850 gm.
Luncheon meat or	340 gm.
Corned beef	340 gm.
Vegetable	1·57 kg.
Peanut oil	90 gm.
Tea	14 gm.

[1] 2·36 kg of rice per share per week for recipients of two shares and above

TABLE 13/7

Hong Kong: public assistance: scale of cooked meals

Unit: 1 Share (2 Diets a Day) Per Day

Item	Quantity
Rice	340 gm.
Meat or	55 gm.
Tinned fish or	112 gm.
Nam Yu (salt cakes made of Chinese yam)	112 gm.
Vegetable	225 gm.
Peanut oil	14 gm.
Salt	5 gm.
Tea	2·5 gm.

TABLE 13/8

Hong Kong: number of recipients of public assistance and expenditure in August 1970

	Total no. of cases receiving assistance in Hong Kong, Kowloon & New Territories	*Total expenditure in August 1970* *H.K.$*	*Total no. of cases receiving assistance in rural communities*	*Total expenditure in August 1970* *H.K.$*
Rice	984	31,853.35	984	31,853.35
Dry ration	2,046	166,500.00	331	20,158.00
Cash	3,984	210,245.58	190	8,351.65
Total	7,014	293,359.93	1,505	60,363.00

partmental kitchens for cooked meals, to those who were certified by medical practitioners as requiring special diets because of illness, and those who could not for various reasons collect dry rations.

The limit of $33 a month for cash payments was fixed in April 1967 on the basis of the cost of rations purchased in bulk by the Government at that time, and intended to provide 1,500 calories a day. The Director of Social Welfare increased cash assistance per month up to a maximum of $60 when a special diet was required for medical reasons.

A new public assistance scheme was put into effect in 1971. From January onwards, the figure of $33 per month was raised to $40, and the conversion of all public assistance into cash was begun. From April 1971, the criteria governing eligibility for assistance were widened. An eligible single person living alone without any income may receive up to $70 per month with an additional amount for rent. Each of the first three eligible members in a family may get up to $50 per month, while the next three receive up to $40 each a month, and the remainder $30 each, with additional amounts for rent, school expenses and any essential travelling expenses. The level of income is expected to be sufficient to maintain an adequate diet.

Families who have lived in Hong Kong for at least one year with a per caput income below the amounts in the preceding paragraph may be eligible for assistance, while children are regarded as adults for assessment purposes. Additional needs, such as the provi-

sion of special diets, may be covered. Those aged between 15 and 55 in good health are eligible only if they have to remain at home to look after young children or sick and disabled family members, or if they are receiving education or vocational training.

The Philippines

The Four-Year Socio-Economic Plan gives prominence to increased food production and intensified work in human nutrition. Surveys show the presence of widespread malnutrition and low intakes of protective foods (see case studies in Appendix).

It has been established that malnutrition is a serious public health problem, as the result of extremely rapid population growth, low crop yields, inadequate exploitation of agricultural potential, linked with need for agrarian reform, deficient food distribution and processing, and widespread ignorance of the essentials of a nutritious diet. The diet consists mainly of rice and fish (Aguillon and Valdecañas, 1969).

Eight surveys covering different regions show that, while cereal intake is adequate, total calories are only three-quarters of recommended levels. Protein, although one-third of animal origin, is 14 per cent below recommended levels; fat intake is very low. Calcium and riboflavine meet only one-third, vitamin A one-half, thiamine less than two-thirds of recommended levels (Quiogue, Villavieja, Ramos, Alejo, Roxas, Salamat, Kuizon, Bayan, Matawaran and Gervasio, 1969). These conclusions require some modification in view of the 1970 revision of nutrient requirements (Intengan and FNRC, 1970). Requirements for some items, particularly protein, have been reduced considerably (see Table 9/12, p. 108).

A high incidence of communicable diseases may be traced to poor nutrition, especially the leading causes of death in the Philippines — pneumonia, gastro-enteritis and bronchitis. The fatality rate from measles and the mortality rate of the 1 to 4 age group are respectively about 29 and 11 times higher than in the United States, further indicators of precarious health and nutrition status.

Workers have stated that full co-ordination and co-operation of all government and private agencies will be necessary, with active steps to bridge the gap between research and its application. It has been recommended that technical leadership be provided by Government, with financial support and use of multilateral or bilateral assistance where necessary. The following order of priorities would be adopted: (a) infants and pre-school children; (b) pregnant and nursing mothers; (c) other children, especially adolescents; (d) the aged, and (e) other adults.

A National Nutrition Programme is to be set up under three components: food research; nutrition research, and applied nutrition.

Priorities under the Food Research Programme are:

(1) to develop new products from indigenous food resources for eventual use in mothercraft feeding centres as replacement for donations; strengthen local food technology institutions so that quality control of their products can be assured, and market possibilities studied;

(2) to improve methods of food preservation, processing and fortification for better utilization of local food resources and for assuring round-the-year supply; and

(3) to set up standards for food products and food additives.

Priorities under the Nutrition Research Programme are:

(1) expansion of local institutional capability to undertake clinical and biochemical studies, animal experimentation and feeding tests, with emphasis on new local food products developed for the alleviation of malnutrition in young children; and

(2) collection of data needed for the establishment of Filipino standards for the evaluation of nutritional status.

Priorities under the Applied Nutrition Programme are:

(1) alleviation of malnutrition in pre-school children and pregnant and lactating mothers through the operation of barrio mothercraft centres, focusing activities on those in the lower socio-economic levels;

(2) improving nutritional status of the population as a whole, and of mothers and children in particular, through widespread nutrition education activities directed to key members of the community, leading to increased production and consumption of local foods; and

(3) enhancing the competence and number of qualified personnel.

The Food and Nutrition Research Center (FNRC) has four Divisions: Medical and Applied Nutrition; Nutrition Surveys; Nutrition Research Laboratory; Food Research Laboratory. A National Co-ordinating Committee on Food and Nutrition established by FNRC in 1960 was expanded in 1966 to become the National Co-ordinating Council on Food and Nutrition (NCCFN), with the Director of FNRC as ex-officio Chairman, and three committees: Nutrition Research, Food Research, Applied Nutrition. The Chairman has specified the activities which should be undertaken by the member agencies of the NCCFN (Pascual, 1971).

Taiwan

A statement on Taiwan, prepared for the WHO Seminar on Methods to Improve Nutritional Standards at the Village Level, held in Manila in January 1964, was published subsequently in the *Chinese Medical Journal* (Hsu, 1964).

Important problems are:

(1) lack of specific content for nutrition education which people could readily accept within their means;

(2) lack on market of ready-made cheap protein food for children;

(3) periodic stratified random nutritional surveys necessary to supplement dietary surveys already made are required, as a basis for national economic and nutritional policies;

(4) cheap methods for reducing helminthiasis, particularly intestinal parasites;

(5) extension of family planning (birth rate fell from 36.3 per 1,000 in 1963 to 28.5 in 1967; natural increase from 3.0 to 2.3 per cent); and

(6) establishment of an organization for food technology and control.

Malnutrition at the village level is shown by disturbance in growth of babies during and after weaning; severe clinical malnutrition is rare, but riboflavine deficiency is frequently seen. Internal parasites aggravate unbalanced diet, due to low availability of animal protein, insufficient content of B-complex vitamins, and low level of available iron. Average calorie intake per caput of rural people in 1962 was 2,278 per day, 123 calories less than in the 1961 balance sheet (due perhaps to a better balanced diet, with increased intakes of animal protein, fat and thiamine).

Since the land is already used intensively and to the full, and every farmer has his pigs and poultry, a village food production campaign can produce only limited results. Policy is directed towards increased unit production and number of crops per year, shift from crops of low to high cash value, utilization of marginal and tidal lands, use of more efficient, faster growing animals, extension of sea fisheries, introduction of new fruits and vegetables, better animal feeds. The number of persons supported per hectare of cultivated land increased from 7.32 in 1946 to 14.73 in 1967.

In 1961, the Medical Co-ordination Committee of the Ministry of the Interior established a Sub-Committee on Nutrition, to co-ordinate the nutritional work of all governmental and voluntary organizations, and to advise the government on nutrition policies and programmes. Out of 324 farmers' associations, 189 had in 1962 a home economics worker to advise housewives on nutritional practices. Farmers' associations in Hualien, Ilan and Hsinchu counties had established six pilot soybean milk processing cottage plants, to process farmers' soybeans into milk for home consumption. The Medical College of National Taiwan University has conducted feeding trials with infants, comparing whole soybean meal with cow's milk and spray-dried soybean milk powder (soybean milk is about one-fourth the cost of cow milk powder).

More than 800 primary schools have constructed standard latrines, and 280 have been supplied with piped water (Taiwan, JCRR, 1968a). A school lunch programme undertaken in indigent areas has provided 250,000 pupils with wheat, milk powder and edible oil contributed by the U.S. Government. Some 5,000 primary school children aged 6 to 12 years take part in a cheese feeding programme, a study of the physical growth and development of children fed supplemental high-protein food, compared with those on an ordinary diet. The processed milk cheese and milk biscuits are donated by the New Zealand Dairy Production and Marketing Board.

South Korea

Up to 1967, nutrition and dietary surveys had not been made, apart from small-scale surveys for particular areas. Chai (1967) began to analyse the everyday foods, to survey the kinds of foods that are eaten, and to record the nutrient intake, conducting also blood and urine analyses and clinical examinations. The technique of the International Committee of Nutrition for National Defense was adopted. A three-month survey was carried out of 27,417 individuals in urban areas, mining and industrial areas, and in agriculture, fishery and forestry. A two-month survey followed, of 6,054 individuals in 33 districts of the country. Biochemical, clinical and dietary studies were carried out in a farming village of Kyung-Gi Province.

Rice represents 55 per cent of total food intakes, with barley and other grains. Intake of animal foods is only 3.5 per cent of total food; in the forestry and mining areas people receive only one-fourth to one-fifth, and in farming areas, only one-half that of urban areas.

Protein deficiency is widespread, particularly among pregnant and lactating women. Calcium intake is low. Sources of riboflavine and vitamin A are limited, and intakes suboptimal. While intakes of thiamine, niacin and vitamin C appeared adequate, clinical examination revealed signs of deficiency. The main deficiencies in the Korean diet are, however, animal protein, fat, calcium, riboflavine and vitamin A. Chai (op. cit.) considers an intensive programme of nutrition education to be essential, concentrating especially on maternal and child nutrition.

At the request of Government, an FAO consultant advised on nutrition education in primary schools (Yang, 1966). An Applied Nutrition Project was planned, through the Office of Rural Development, Ministry of Agriculture and Forestry. The same consultant (Yang, 1970) set up pilot projects on the production and preparation of high protein foods, methods of preservation, provision of sanitary water, and training in education. It was recommended that food consumption targets should be defined as a basis for planning and increased production of cheap, protein-rich foods.

The formation of a Food and Nutrition Council has been agreed by Government, to formulate policy and co-ordinate major programmes. A plan of operations for a school nutrition education project has been prepared. School feeding started in 1953, with skim milk provided by UNICEF, and has subsequently been continued by CARE; by 1965, 38 per cent of all children attending primary schools were included. Fifteen meals a month (out of twenty-four school days) are provided, composed in rural areas of 60 gm. cornmeal and 30 gm. skim milk powder. This allocation is not considered enough, and the addition of hot soup made of local vegetables, soybean and dried fish would be desirable.

Japan

The Nutrition Section of the Health and Welfare Ministry is responsible for surveying the state of urban and rural nutrition and for setting nutritional standards (see Table 9/13). Within this Ministry, there is a Research Group on Essential Amino Acids, staffed by leading academic nutritionists, and a Sub-Committee on Amino Acid Supplementation.

The Health and Welfare Ministry conducts annual surveys to assess current nutritional standards. A review (Insull, Oiso and Tsuchiya, 1968), describing diets and nutritional status together with changes over the preceding twenty years, reported that the national diet was still low in total fat, cholesterol, animal protein and sugar, high in total carbohydrate, adequate in total protein and high in salt. As more foods of vegetable origin were consumed than in western countries, dietary fat was rich in linoleic acid. Nutritional status was good, without evidence of any gross nutritional deficiency. Mature adult stature had been increasing annually since World War II. Dietary changes showed lower intake of carbohydrate with higher proportion of simple sugars, and increased proportions of fat and animal protein. In 1963, cereals provided 67.0 per cent of total calories. Rice provided 31.7 per cent and fish 23.1 per cent of total protein (Insull *et al.*, op. cit.).

The 1968 survey by the Health and Welfare Ministry (*Japan Times*, 1970b), was carried out during five days in 16,500 households in 346 districts. The average daily intake was 2,214 calories, 74.9 gm. protein, 44.6 gm. fat, 375 gm. carbohydrates and 529 mg. calcium. Fat consumption has increased by 91 per cent, and animal protein intake by 35 per cent since 1958. In 1968, 3.5 times more fruit, and 2.7 times more meat were eaten than in 1958, while rice consumption dropped by 13 per cent over the decade. The targets set by the Health and Welfare Ministry for intake of calories, protein, vitamin C and fat in 1975 had already been reached in 1968, while intakes of vitamin A, thiamine and riboflavine are still below the targets.

There is a considerable gap between well-fed and ill-fed families. About 15 per cent of Japanese households had less than 2,000 calories per head per day,

500 calories below the recommended level. However, 20 per cent of families received more than 3,000 calories per head per day. Rural households eat considerably less fruit, meat and milk than urban families (see also Chapter 7, pp. 76-8).

The Health and Welfare Ministry has undertaken a revision of standards for height, weight and rates of growth, in view of these improved intakes. It is expected that there will be a slow but steady increase in stature, and a gradual disappearance of the present distinction between rural and urban diets. This is due to rapid industrialization and the development in rural areas of side-line occupations. Thus a progressive improvement in child physique is anticipated.

Heights and weights of those in the 0 to 20 years age group in 1970 are 3 years above the 1967 standards; i.e. in 1970 a child of 9 years of age has the height and weight of a child of 12 in 1967.

In 1970 the average weight of an adult man of 25 years is 58.9 kg., and of a woman, 49.7 kg; the same man is 165.5 cm. in height, and the woman 153.8 cm. Standards for all age groups have been worked out (Japan, Health and Welfare Ministry, 1969).

The Health and Welfare Ministry has revised recommended protein intakes, in view of the improved quality of protein in the diet, more of which now comes from animal sources. Recommendations for protein intake for different age groups are given in Table 9/13. A distinction should be made between bottle-fed and breast-fed infants, since research in Japan has shown that both total serum protein and serum albumin are lower in the former. Special recommendations for bottle-fed infants are therefore given (op. cit.). After weaning, it is recommended that at least 5 per cent of total protein should come from animal sources, especially egg and fish, to supplement miso (soybean paste).

Conclusion

In this chapter, the activities of most of the countries of the region in the fields of nutrition research, education and planning have been discussed.

Emphasis throughout this book has been given to the importance of understanding the land ecosystems of Asian countries before nutrition science can be applied, and plans for greater food production made. It is on this broader basis that the specific problems of the two largest countries of the world, India and China, are discussed in the following chapters.

14 India

INDIA is one of the leading countries of Asia in appreciating the magnitude of the food/population situation, and in taking steps designed to cope with the enormous problems that face the nation. Only information which is new and supplementary to that presented elsewhere in this book and by Whyte (1968a) is given here.

Government of India for its 1961 Census adopted the following criteria for definition of urban and rural peoples. Areas deemed to be urban:

(a) municipalities and notified areas;
(b) military cantonments;
(c) places satisfying the following three conditions:
(i) population exceeds 5,000;
(ii) at least three-fourths of the working population depends upon non-agricultural pursuits, and
(iii) density of population exceeds 1,000 per square mile.

(d) localities, though not in themselves local bodies, which are contiguous to a city or town and have urban characteristics as (ii) and (iii) above.

The figures for population in 1951, 1961, 1971 and 1976 adopted by the Reserve Bank of India are given in Table 14/1 (Madalgi, 1967).

TABLE 14/1

India: estimates of population
by Reserve Bank of India

Population (millions)	1951	1961	1971	1976
Total	361	439	560	630
Urban	62	79	105	123

Source: Madalgi, 1967

DEMAND FOR FOODGRAINS

The Reserve Bank of India has examined the demand for foodgrains to be expected by the year, 1975/6, calculated separately for rural and urban areas, as a guide to the scale of the necessary production effort (Madalgi, 1967).

The Nutrition Advisory Committee of the Indian Council of Medical Research defines the Indian reference man as an adult of 20 to 30 years of age, weighing 55 kg. On each working day he is employed for eight hours in an occupation which is not sedentary, but does not involve more than occasional periods of hard physical labour. The average requirements for Indian reference man and woman respectively are 2,780 and 2,080 calories per day, or an average of 2,100 calories per day. Allowing for losses between the retail level (the level at which food intake is actually measured) and the physiological level on account of losses due to spoilage and storage, food requirements at the retail level are estimated at about 2,250 calories per day. These calories come from the entire diet of foodgrains, sugar, fruit, vegetables, meat, fish, eggs, milk, oil and fats, to the extent to which these items are consumed. The urban population will need foodgrains (cereals and grain legumes) enough to provide 66 per cent (grain legumes being about 10 per cent) or 1,500 calories per caput per day; the corresponding figures for the rural people will be 80 per cent or 1,800 calories.

On this nutritional basis, Madalgi (op.cit.) calculates the consumption demand for foodgrains from rural and urban areas by two alternative methods. The demand will be about 130 million tonnes, on the assumption that the distribution of projected national income in 1975/6 will be the same as during the period 1953/4 to 1956/7, and that the level of foodgrain consumption of different expenditure classes will broadly conform to that observed in 1959/60.

It will be 130 million tonnes on the assumption that the aggregate private consumption (at 1960/61 prices) will increase at the rate assumed by the Perspective Planning Division of the Bank, and that expenditure elasticity of demand for foodgrains will remain at 0.6 and 0.3 for rural and urban areas respectively. On strictly nutritional grounds, the demand will be 114 million tonnes.

Therefore, 22 to 23 million tonnes is a fairly reliable estimate of urban demand, and 106 to 107 million tonnes for rural demand. As the agricultural sector has to meet a demand of about 19 million tonnes from the non-agricultural classes in the rural areas, the marketable surplus is about 39 to 40 million tonnes. Of this, some 4 million tonnes is expected to be produced in the urban area, giving a net availability of 3.5 million tonnes for consumption (0.5 million tonnes for seed and feed). Thus the rural sector will have to generate a marketable surplus of about 36 million tonnes. This is possible only if total gross production is about 150 million tonnes, which calls for an assured annual compound growth rate of about 5 per cent.

INCREASING FOOD PRODUCTION

For some years, Government of India, operating independently or in association with Ford Foundation, has been conducting over 100 Intensive Agricultural Projects throughout the country. Into these selected areas have been introduced the ingredients of the new technology — improved high-yielding varieties, greater availability and correct use of fertilizers, increased availability of irrigation water and better water management, and crop protection, supplemented by ample credit, advisory services and marketing arrangements. The areas selected were, correctly from an economic point of view, situated on the more promising soils where irrigation was already available for much of the land. In view of limitation of funds, technical staff and other needs, it was undoubtedly wise to concentrate on areas where a reasonably good return could be expected on the inputs.

Inevitably, the yields of crops and so the economic status of the more prosperous farmers on the good land have improved. The gap between those farmers and the far greater proportion of smallholders with little irrigation facilities and poor financial resources has become much wider. This is an essential fact of agrarian life on the variable soils of any country, but it could not be accepted as part of the land policy of the Congress Party of Mrs. Indira Gandhi. The President of the New Congress, Mr. Jagjivan Ram, has said that:

the beneficiaries of the so-called breakthrough in agriculture are not those who are living on a pittance of a few rupees per month, but the privileged minority of substantial farmers and middle cultivators. With 47 per cent of farm families owning only one acre of land (usually dry) and 22 per cent having no land at all, with only 3 or 4 per cent of the big cultivators enjoying all power, wielding all influence and appropriating to themselves all the skill, resources and expertise that Government agencies have to offer, the poor villagers have little to thank anybody for.

This is the political basis for a new agricultural policy involving far greater attention to the dry-land farmers of India, announced by President Giri, at the Indian Agricultural Research Institute in February 1970. The President again referred to the imbalance between the prosperous and poor farmers, and also to the fact that progress had been achieved in increasing the yields of certain foodgrains, but not of others (those grown on dry-land). The different rates of economic progress between irrigated and unirrigated farms posed another imbalance which had 'serious social implications'. Dry-land farmers in low-rainfall areas — 49 million hectares — had yet another handicap; the relative proportion of landless labour was high. The President accompanied his address with the release of a new publication entitled *A New Technology for Dryland Farming* (IARI, 1970). A Co-ordinated Research Project has been undertaken under the auspices of the Indian Council of Agricultural Research, involving the establishment of fifteen main centres and eight sub-centres in moisture-deficit regions, to undertake research in soil management, harvesting of water, new crop varieties and agronomic practices.

Dry farming areas are defined as those which receive an average annual rainfall of 750 to 1,125 mm., spread over ninety-one districts in eight States. Assistance is being provided by the Government of Canada (Can. $1.5 million) on a grant basis, in the form of agricultural machinery, laboratory equipment and fellowships for the training of Indian scientists at dry-land research centres in Canada. Related to this contribution is another grant ($0.7 million) for a ground-water hydrological survey of the hard rock areas of Andhra Pradesh, to obtain quantitative data capable of extrapolation to other parts of the Deccan.

Two other developments relate to the dry-land programme: (a) an Irrigation Commission to study future development; and (b) a computer study by Government of India Meteorological Office at Poona.

The return on the vast inputs involved in a programme over such a large proportion of the cultivated land of India cannot possibly compare with that obtained from earlier investment on the best and intermediate types of land. The dry-land development programme is not an economic investment; it is a necessary social and a shrewd political investment. The plans are vast and complex. They must be linked with a survey of the further irrigation potential in the dry-land tracts, and with a study of drought expectancy in all the ecological regions. The latter will provide a basis for planning cropping programmes and particularly the accumulation and location of adequate buffer stocks of foodgrains for the inevitable periods of crisis. Can these plans be carried out quickly enough to have any marked impact within a reasonable time?

A comprehensive survey of all aspects of land use, agriculture, animal husbandry and forestry in India was made in the first decade of this century by the Royal Commission on Agriculture in India, presided over by Lord Linlithgow (Government of India, 1928). The report of this Commission provided the basis for agricultural development for many years thereafter. The Government of India announced (September 1970) the formation of a National Commission on Agriculture, under the chairmanship of C. Subramaniam, to make the first overall review since the Royal Commission.

The Indian Council of Agricultural Research maintains through its Research Institutes and supported projects research on increased food production and better and more intensive use of the land. In his address at the 1970 Convocation of the Indian Agricultural Research Institute, the Director (Dr. M.S. Swaminathan)[1] described projects relating to food production. These include studies on soil micro-nutrients that are becoming limiting factors in areas of intensive cropping; effect of excess of inorganic fertilizers on water-retention of soils; better crop rotations; breeding of improved cultivars of sorghum, bajra (*Pennisetum typhoides*), maize, grain legumes, wheat, barley and the minor millets — all important contributors to the dry-land project. The minor millets may be high in lysine but low in digestibility. The dwarf basmati rice cultivars may introduce a 'rice revolution', but reports of high susceptibility to disease are made from Uttar Pradesh. Farmers are having difficulty with the

---

[1] Now Director-General, Indian Council of Agricultural Research.

IR8 and Taichung Native No. 1 cultivars of rice — the straw is difficult to cut, and the coarse grain does not bring a good price on the market.

NUTRITION RESEARCH AND TRAINING

The Indian Council of Medical Research investigates all aspects of human nutrition through the National Institute of Nutrition, Hyderabad (established 1919). The Central Food Technological Research Institute in Mysore is concerned with manufactured foods; products based on satisfactory balance of vegetable protein suitable for the nutrition of the vulnerable groups. Full-scale manufacture, distribution, and consumer acceptance were the subject of an international symposium, *New Foods for National Development,* held in Bangalore in 1967, and attended by members of the food industry, food technologists and food adminstrators (Indian Institute of Management, 1967).

Nutrition research is also carried on by centres of higher learning and hospitals throughout India, notably by the Department of Biochemistry, University of Baroda (Professor C.V. Ramakrishnan and Dr. R. Rajalakshmi), the Nutrition Research Unit of the Christian Medical College and Hospital, Vellore, and the Sri Avinashilingam Home Science College, Coimbatore (Principal, Dr. R.P. Devadas). A *Nutrition Research Profile,* covering different aspects of nutrition research throughout India, has been compiled by the Food Resources and Regional Development Division of the U.S. Agency for International Development, New Delhi (Kar, 1968).

The functions of the National Institute of Nutrition are:

To carry out research in the laboratory, hospital, and field, on dietary and nutritional problems with a view to elucidating the factors responsible, and to evolve appropriate methods of treatment and prevention; to train young scientists in research methods in nutrition and allied subjects; to train workers in public health and community development in nutrition to enable them effectively to participate in Nutrition Action Programmes; to advise Government and other organizations on problems of diet and nutrition; and to help in the spread of knowledge among the general public through popular publications and other educational media.

A special supplement of *The Indian Journal of Medical Research* (volume 57, no. 8, August 1969) contains articles dealing with research at Hyderabad, in honour of the fifty years of the Institute's existence.[1] Work at the Institute during the year 1968/9 (ICMR, 1969) includes: the systematic screening of germ plasm of various foodgrains for protein content and quality; toxic principle in the seeds of *Lathyrus sativus*; introduction of US-26 variety of groundnut, which combines good yield with better quality of oil and aflatoxin resistance; absorption of carotene from fruits and vegetables in a mixed diet; skin changes in kwashiorkor; conversion of carotene into vitamin A in malnourished children; status of the thyroid gland in kwashiorkor; altered mental status due to pellagra in relation to excess of dietary leucine; efficiency of absorption of iron during pregnancy; nutritional status of school children and pregnant women in relation to size of family; distribution of processed foods to rural children; prevention of vitamin A deficiency; fortification of wheat flour with lysine; nutritional osteomalacia.

The National Institute of Nutrition is conducting a field study on nutrition and infection at the Rural Health Research Project, Narangwal. Data on nutritional status and morbidity patterns have been collected from four groups of children: (1) those receiving medical care; (2) those receiving nutrient supplements; (3) those receiving both medical care and nutrient supplements; and (4) controls. It is planned to observe the children for two years in order to define any clear differences which arise in the various groups.

The work at Baroda has been presented in the textbook *Applied Nutrition* (Rajalakshmi, 1969). Parts I and II deal with basic principles of nutrition, Part III with diets (with suggestions for meal planning, nutritional care of particular groups, diseases of malnutrition), and Part IV with community nutrition (diet and nutrition surveys, including a checklist for interview as Appendix), nutrition and human development, and the production of food in relation to population. R. Rajalakshmi and C.V. Ramakrishnan have been concerned with the formulation and evaluation of low-cost balanced meals from locally available materials, and with observations of the effect of dietary protein on visual discrimination, learning and brain biochemistry in the albino rat.

The work of the Sri Avinashilingam Home Science College is presented in the monthly journal, *Journal of Nutrition and Dietetics,* of which the College Principal, Dr. R.P. Devadas, is Editor. They have concentrated on nutritional status of vulnerable groups in rural areas of Tamil Nadu State, and the effect on nutritional status of various dietary supplements.

DIETS FOR VULNERABLE GROUPS

The School Lunch Programme is carried on in most States, under the sponsorship of the School Health Committee of the Ministry of Health of Government of India (Radharukmani and Devadas, 1964), under the control of State Governments, and in collaboration with the Applied Nutrition Program, CARE and other agencies. The number of children covered in each State varies greatly, from those in one or two rural Districts, to a good distribution in the rural areas of the whole State. There is special emphasis on the children of low nutritional status in the cities of Bombay and Madras. In some cases skim milk and/or vegetable protein supplements are provided; in other areas, the entire meal including the staple.

THE CHILDREN'S CHARTER

In February, 1969, the National Nutrition Advisory Committee of Government of India accepted a plan to combat malnutrition, as a culmination of years of study and pressure by leading Indian specialists in nutrition, supported by bilateral aid organizations, especially USAID, and by the specialized agencies of the United Nations, WHO, UNICEF and FAO.

The Plan is based on a 7-point proposition:

(1) Well over two-thirds of the children of India are suffering from malnutrition, and from deficiency diseases such as beriberi, goitre, pellagra, anaemia and rickets.

(2) Malnutrition during childhood leads not only to physical retardation, but also to debilitating mental effects which are perhaps irreparable.

(3) The productive capacity of these persons, and therefore of the nation, will be seriously limited until successful efforts are made to combat malnutrition.

(4) The cost of combating malnutrition by raising the nutritional status of children would be far less than either the cost of the fall in productivity resulting from malnutrition, or the cost of treating a malnourished population.

(5) Combating malnutrition involves both increasing food production (to meet calorie deficiencies)

---

[1] Topics covered are: 'The Nutritive Value of Foods' (Ramasastri and Mohan, 1969); 'Studies on Nutrient Requirements of Indians' (Rao, 1969); 'Protein-Calorie Malnutrition in Indian Children' (Srikantia, 1969); 'Vitamin A Deficiency in Indian Children' (Reddy, 1969); 'Nutrition in Pregnancy and Lactation' (Belavady, 1969); 'Studies on the Pathogenesis of some Nutritional Deficiency States' (Gopalan, 1969b); 'Lathyrism' (Nagarajan, 1969) and 'Aflatoxicosis' (Tulpule, 1969).

and improving the quality of the food consumed (to meet nutrient deficiencies). Certain portions of the population are at present so deficient in calories that their deficiency in protein cannot also be considered. Government of India hoped, however, that the 'green revolution' might make it possible to overcome much of this calorie deficiency within the next few years, and that it might then be possible to tackle the problem of deficiencies of high-quality protein in the diets of the lower-income groups.

(6) Infant mortality in India is estimated to be 140 per thousand live births, plus an additional 200 deaths per thousand during the ensuing pre-school years. By overcoming protein and vitamin deficiencies of children, India could do more to reduce disease and infant mortality than by any other health measure.

(7) It is believed that the means are readily available to attack the problem of quality in foods, provided there are simultaneous efforts significantly to improve distribution to the vulnerable groups in the community, and at the same time — and above all — to limit population growth.

A linear programming exercise made on a computer by the Indian Institute of Public Opinion, under contract with USAID, was designed to determine the best way of reaching the 'target group' — those children between the ages of 1 to 6 years whose nutrient deficiencies are the greatest, within the shortest time and at the least cost.

Deficiencies in protein (including animal grade or high-quality protein), vitamin A and iron are the three nutrient deficiencies requiring the most urgent action. Dr. Kalyan Bagchi has estimated that some 25 million children may go blind because of prolonged vitamin A deficiency; at least as many again are threatened with impaired vision and the eye diseases resulting from less severe deficiency of this vitamin. These deficiencies are most severe among pre-school children, from 1 to 6 years, or 20 per cent of the population (now totalling 550 million) in the lower income groups, here defined as having a per caput expenditure per month of less than Rs. 25 (approximately U.S.$3.30; see Table 7/4). These groups represent 70 per cent of the population. The lower the income group, the lower will be the nutritional status of the child. A higher incidence of infection and intestinal infestation limits the absorption and utilization of food — therefore more protein per kg. body weight is required.

An increased interest in the improvement of nutrition is shown by the adoption of a National Nutrition Policy, the inclusion for the first time of a chapter on nutrition in the Fourth Five-Year Plan, the establishment of a formal Inter-Ministerial Policy Committee to overcome fragmentation of responsibility, the adoption of the principle of fortification (a seminar on the subject was held in Calcutta in February 1969) and the inauguration of a variety of specific projects under this general policy.

But the final objective of efforts was achieved in December 1969, when the Working Committee of Prime Minister Indira Gandhi's New Congress Party directed the Government to levy a national cess on all taxes, to provide funds for the improvement of nutrition of pre-school age children. The objective was to raise Rs. 350 crores per year (U.S. $476 million) to provide a balanced diet to 80 million children up to the age of 5, and also to nursing mothers. This is the so-called Children's Charter. A few days after the announcement of the Charter, the Old or Opposition Congress Party passed a similar resolution in its Convention at Ahmedabad, Gujarat: 'While India cannot ensure socialist equality to the people here and now, our earnestness has to be shown in what we do for our children. The Congress therefore attaches the highest priority to the provision of nourishment and particularly high-protein food, to all the children. . . .'

This scheme was to be implemented by the end of 1972, through a National Commission on Children's Welfare. The first stage is a programme of nutrition to cover two million children up to 3 years of age (1 million in tribal areas and one million in the slum areas of the great cities). The maternal and child health centres and family planning welfare centres in the rural areas are to be used for the child nutrition programme, and supplements to be distributed as follows:

Children up to one year	skim milk powder, providing 120 calories, and 12 gm. protein per day for 250 days a year.
Children from 1 to 2 years	one unit of skim milk powder and one unit of processed food, providing together 300 calories and 12 gm. protein per day.
Children from 2 to 3 years	one unit of processed food.

1.6 million children will be receiving vitamin A capsules in the first year.

The Children's Charter is regarded in India as one of the most constructive ideas to emanate from political quarters for many years. It certainly has a sentimental, vote-drawing appeal through its focus on children. An adequate source of funds for the purchase of ingredients within the country has been evolved. It is, however, highly doubtful whether the ingredients required for a nutritional policy to cover some 80 million children can be made available from the present or potential resources of Indian agriculture and animal husbandry (see following section). The Charter does not appear to take specific account of the nutritional requirements of the other members of the vulnerable groups of Indian society, namely, the pregnant and nursing mothers. Their nutrition is fundamental to the physical and mental health of the children who are subsequently to come within the scope of the Charter. India's high infant mortality is due above all to the defective nutrition of the mothers.

However, even if this ambitious and excellent programme is only partially successful, if it reduces the deaths of pre-school children from 340 per thousand to a more morally acceptable figure, and if the children of the future are sound in body and mind, India will inevitably be faced with a sudden population explosion of great magnitude. This will create even greater problems in terms of education, employment, housing, health, and — above all — food. The provisions of the Charter can be truly welcomed only if there is a parallel programme for population control on a more drastic and effective basis than any which has been attempted to date.

RESOURCES OF QUALITY FOODS

Quality foods considered by Government of India specialists and their advisers for the better feeding of children include:

(1) *High-protein cultivars of foodgrains.* So far, high protein content has been inversely correlated with yield. Recently, however, a variety of wheat has been produced in which it is claimed that a protein content of from 25 to 30 per cent corresponds with good yield. One must ask whether, if the grains of such a variety are of the usual size, what other ingredients have been lost in order to allow for the increased amount of protein nitrogen. Also it would be necessary to know whether the balance between amino acids has been affected in the production of such a high-protein grain.

(2) *Bal ahar.* This simple, processed children's food contains cereal grains, oilseed protein, milk or gram (chickpea), vitamins and minerals, all of which are commonly used in the Indian diet. Further, the area under grain legumes such as chickpea is tending to fall, and total production is being maintained only by achieving higher yields per unit area. A considerable increase in production of these components must therefore be obtained to meet the needs of 80 million children.

(3) *Toned milk.* High-fat buffalo milk reduced to 3.0 or 1.5 per cent fat by mixing with skim milk or protein isolate solution. The calculation made by the Ministry of Food and Agriculture regarding the potential availability of milk for toning is suspect. Total estimated milk production, and therefore availability of milk per head of population, are exaggerated. The initial stages of implementation of the Charter are being carried out with skim milk, partly supplied by CARE.

(4) *Oilseed flours and concentrates.* Only a small fraction of India's oilseed is used for human consumption once the oil has been extracted. Oilseed is, however, the basis of the concentrate ration for the dairy and poultry industries, which are already in direct competition for concentrates, and a certain proportion is exported to obtain foreign exchange. The product prepared for cattle feed is not sufficiently refined for human use, particularly because of aflatoxin content.

(5) *Amino-acid fortification.* Over 80 per cent of the protein consumed is derived from cereals, in which amino-acid composition is unbalanced, particularly in respect of lysine.

(6) *Vitamin and mineral fortification of staple foods.* This is relatively economic, although India does not yet produce enough vitamin A.

(7) *Fish Protein Concentrate.* India does not produce adequate fish for economic production, and there are additional difficulties on account of the strong taste of this supplement.

(8) *Meat and eggs.* These are produced in India in such statistically insignificant quantities, and at such high cost, that they cannot be regarded as a potential resource for meeting quality protein deficiencies.

(9) *Increased production of pulses, fruits and vegetables.*

(10) *Single cell protein.* This is grown as microorganisms on hydrocarbons to produce concentrates to fortify suitable foods. This technology is still in its early stages, and a product suitable for human use has yet to be found.

MILK PRODUCTION AND DISTRIBUTION

Problems relating to the production of milk have been discussed fully elsewhere, particularly in relation to the cattle problem (Whyte, 1968a). It is difficult to be optimistic about the outcome of the costly projects designed to achieve the Indian Council of Medical Research target of an average of 170 gm. milk per day per head of population, more for the vulnerable groups, less for mature people. The total number of productive bovines with different lactation yields required to achieve this national target, or to provide the through-put of individual milk processing plants, has been worked out as a basis for planning (Whyte and Mathur, 1968).

There are Intensive Cattle Development Projects distributed throughout the country. These are designed to lead to the improvement of dairy bovines, in so far as this is possible in the particular conditions of India (see Chapter 12 in Whyte, 1968a). But the dairy development programme of Government of India and the States, in association with U.N. agencies, is urban-oriented. Efficiency of extraction of milk from rural areas is the primary objective. Protagonists of this programme state that one-third of the now greater production in milk procurement areas remains in the villages. This is not confirmed by doctors and nutritionists, who find that over 90 per cent is taken to the collecting and chilling centres for transport to the urban milk plant. It is extremely difficult to visualize how this trend may be reversed, until the rural people reach the economic status at which they may be able to afford to resist the power of the market, and hold back some milk for their families.

The production of milk in the rural areas around the major cities of Delhi, Bombay, Calcutta and Madras is being increased by Operation Flood. This is designed to flood these cities with good, clean milk, and to force or induce the city milk producers to move out into the rural milk procurement areas, and so to become suppliers through the milk plant. The Agricultural Finance Corporation has promised Rs. 15 crores[1] for transport of livestock and grants and loans to help producers to become established in their new locations. The necessary ingredients for the reconstitution of the amounts of milk required are to be imported under the United Nations World Food Program.

THE STUDY OF RURAL CHANGE

Four Agro-Economic Research Centres were established in 1954 under the patronage of the Union Ministry of Food and Agriculture at Delhi, Poona, Santiniketan and Madras. Subsequently, others were

[1] crore is 10 million

established at Gwalior, Jorhat, Anand and Allahabad. One of the main objectives is continuous village survey, designed to gauge rural change by comparing two sets of data on the economy collected at two points of time, usually at five-year intervals. The selection of a village for study is therefore related to the presence of forces of change, e.g. a new irrigation project, urban impact, establishment of an industry nearby, community development project, *panchayat,* etc.

One example of the outcome of these studies is the report on the village of Dispur in Assam (Goswami, 1967). Changes affecting the life of the villagers which occurred between the first survey in 1955 and the second in 1961—2 were observed. During the intervening period the village had undergone rapid transformation. Prior to 1955 (or more accurately, before Independence), the village did not attract new settlers. It was then inhabited by two indigenous communities of Assam, the Kacharis and the Koches. Now with the growth of industrial activities and urbanization around Gauhati, and the increasing opportunities for employment, the importance of agriculture as a source of income has declined. Shrinkage of the area of cultivable land has also contributed to the decline of agriculture.

CONCLUSION

In spite of all these efforts, it is difficult to be optimistic about the nutritional status of the rural people of India (80 per cent of a total population of some 550 million) in the next two or three decades.

In considering the degree of imbalance between human population (which must continue to increase at its present rate over this period) and natural resources, it is essential to be clear about the true meaning of the term 'national self-sufficiency in food', as used in international circles. In terms of foodgrains alone, one has to distinguish between political self-sufficiency, which is at present stated to be about 130 million tons per year, and nutritional self-sufficiency. Most of the rural population is existing at a level which represents some fifty per cent of minimum required calorie intake. For the foods which provide quality and protection in the diet, the gap is even wider. Thus *nutritional* self-sufficiency demands a vast increase in the production of all foods.

The achievement of optimal nutritional targets has long been beyond the productive capacity of the Indian land and farming systems. Those responsible for agricultural policy are coming to realize that it is extremely difficult to achieve even the present political target of 130 million tons of foodgrains per year. It had been hoped that foodgrain production would reach 125·9 million tons by 1973-4, but production in current years has been: 1969-70 — 99.5; 1970-1 — 108.4; 1971-2 — 104.7; 1972-3 — 100 million tons.

Whatever limited success may be claimed for the green revolution has been achieved at the expense of increased production of the grain legumes which are so essential in diets devoid of animal protein. The nutritional status of the vulnerable groups in partic-ular remains intractable at its present level of misery: 200 to 250 per thousand children die before twelve months of age, 400-500 per thousand before five years of age.

There is also persistent and increasing imbalance between the major forms of land use. The National Forest Policy, designed to conserve the productive and protective role of the forest covers, is consis-tently disregarded. The result is ever-increasing damage to the cultivated lands and progressive desic-cation of the environment as a whole.

15 China

THE status of rural nutrition in China has been reviewed elsewhere (Whyte, 1972a). Therefore only the salient points are discussed in this Chapter.

CHINA IN MONSOON ASIA

Specialists in the production, distribution and utilization of food are profoundly interested in the nutrition of the urban and rural peoples of the Chinese People's Republic. It is impossible to define precisely the actual situation in China because the basic data are almost wholly lacking. Nor is it possible to be even approximately exact in estimating the degrees, if any, of under-nutrition and/or malnutrition in the absence of the essential dietary surveys and their associated clinical and biochemical examinations.

The isolation of China has tended to create the belief that China is somehow fundamentally different from the rest of the world, that the problems of land use, agriculture and human nutrition are in some way unique, and that greater production of food is not subject to the same natural laws and hazards that apply in the rest of Asia. The more densely populated and hence the most critical parts of China are, however, part of Monsoon Asia. The land systems or eco-systems, the soils, the climax and secondary forms of vegetation, crops and cropping systems, domestic livestock and types of animal husbandry, and the pests and diseases which affect production, are all those of that vast region of Asia that has a monsoonal eco-climate. Some authorities consider that 'greater Southeast Asia' extends up to the Tsinling Mountains in China (Lebar, Hickey and Musgrave, 1964).

It is possible, with long experience of monsoonal land use, agriculture and animal husbandry anywhere from Pakistan to Japan, and with the limited data which are available up to mid-1970, to discuss the problems and assess the potentialities of the Chinese land on the basis of comparable situations elsewhere. Bardhan's (1970) broad comparison of recent policy and performance in Chinese and Indian agriculture may serve to put things into perspective, as a sequel to earlier comparative studies (Ishikawa, 1967; Malenbaum, 1959; Raj, 1967). Bardhan refers to the fact that in both countries the availability and reliability of economic information are at their worst in respect to agriculture (non-availability, continuous changes in coverage and reporting systems, occasional deliberate mis-reporting, lack of impartiality). Nevertheless, it is possible to extract some comparative data from Bardhan's study, which relates to the period 1952/3 to 1964/5 (see below and Table 15/2).

The maximum biological productivity that can be achieved with full use of inputs, under dry-land conditions (100 per cent utilization or one crop per year), and the high levels that can theoretically be obtained with full and correct use of irrigation water (200 per cent utilization or two crops per year in the north with monsoonal summers and temperate winters, and 300 per cent or three crops per year in the monsoonal southern provinces) is governed by the environment in all its macro- and micro- manifestations — the cyclic and seasonal fluctuation between excess, adequacy and deficit in rainfall, combined with a range of maximum and minimum temperatures.

Where Chinese agriculture today differs from that of its neighbours in Monsoon Asia is in the form of political and administrative organization, the efficiency of extraction of food from the rural areas for the urban centres, industrial communities, those rural areas producing industrial crops such as cotton and soybean, and the military, to the detriment of standards of rural nutrition (as also happens with a market economy), and in the comparative incentives to work among the cultivators of a centrally directed regime.

The physiological characteristics and food habits of a people change only exceedingly slowly, even if new foods become available and accepted as part of the cropping pattern or of the diet. We have no reason to suppose that any new foods have become part of the regular diet of rural Chinese. There is an extensive literature on Chinese health, food habits and practices up to about twenty years ago. Much work has been done more recently on the present nutritional status and practices of the overseas Chinese. Thus it is possible to make a fairly accurate assessment of the nutritional requirements and responses of the rural people of mainland China.

In spite of the non-availability of scientific data or publications on rural nutrition in China today, it is nevertheless possible to show what facts have to be considered in an assessment of the situation. One may draw conclusions which, although necessarily tentative, are more closely related to the criteria of nutritional science than the assumptions which are based on actual or hypothetical figures of cereal production alone — on quantity, without due consideration of quality of foods. In the absence of any reliable data from China on production since 1959, it is necessary to consider the position from the opposite angle, that is, to express accepted nutritional targets per head of population per day or per year, in terms of the hectares of land or the numbers of livestock needed to produce these amounts of food. These may be equated against the estimates of production made by outside observers.

DEFINITION OF URBAN AND RURAL COMMUNITIES

A State Resolution of the Chinese People's Republic in 1955 defined urban and rural areas (Chen, 1966):

Urban areas (towns and cities) are those where a municipal people's council or a people's council of the *hsien* level or above is located, except for mobile administrative units in the pastoral areas. Urban areas are also those with 2,000 inhabitants or more, of whom at least half are engaged in pursuits other than agriculture. Places of 1,000 to 2,000 population may also be classified as urban, provided these are industrial, commercial, transport, educational or research centres, or are residential areas of workers, and provided at least 75 per cent of the population is non-agricultural. Finally, places with sanatorium facilities in which patients constitute more than half of the local permanent population may also be classified as urban. All other areas are considered rural. The same criteria are applied to city suburbs. They are rural if the majority of the population is engaged in agriculture.

It is appropriate in a study on China, with its special system for the procurement and distribution of foodgrains, to distinguish between (i) rural communities whose foodgrain allotment represents a share of what they themselves have produced, or is given in exchange for some commodity such as soybeans or cotton which they have produced; and (ii) urban communities, who grow no food for themselves, and who are entirely dependent on allocation from the State foodgrain pool.

ECOCLIMATE OR AGROCLIMATE

A climatic basis for a nutritional assessment in China may be obtained from a map of climatic regions and climatic types (Fig. 15/1). The chief climatic controls are those of the winter and summer monsoons. Most of the population of China lives in a monsoonal ecoclimate. Huang Ping-wei (1961) states that 46 per cent of the area of China is in the Eastern Monsoon Sector, 27.3 per cent is Mongolia-Sinkiang Highlands (part of the Eurasian steppe-desert zone) and 26.7 per cent is the Chinghai-Tibetan Highlands. The Eastern Monsoon Sector is broken down further into areas, sub-areas and zones. The Chinese ecoclimate is not a separate entity, but part of an Asian zone which is only now coming to be studied and interpreted as an ecological unit with great local diversity in terms of land use, crop and animal husbandry and standards of human nutrition. Much of China comes within the influence of the Bengal summer monsoons, and probably some 70 to 80 per cent of the population lives and farms in provinces affected thereby (C.S. Chen, 1970).

POPULATION

Neither Peking nor anyone else knows the size of the population of Communist China. Ironically, this lack of population data may be more frustrating to the non-Chinese analyst who is constantly searching for figures in order to construct economic indexes and to make political and social prognostications than to the Chinese themselves, who are well aware of the existing population pressures but are not overly concerned with the precision or timeliness of the statistics available to measure them (Orleans, 1969).

Data on total population in 1950, 1960 and 1965 are published in the U.N. *Demographic Yearbook,* the U.N. *Monthly Bulletin of Statistics* and U.N. *World Population Prospects.* The U.N. estimates for 1950 and 1960 appear to the FAO statisticians to have been based on available official data for China, and to have been considerably rounded to reflect uncertainties in them. Figures for the later years appear to

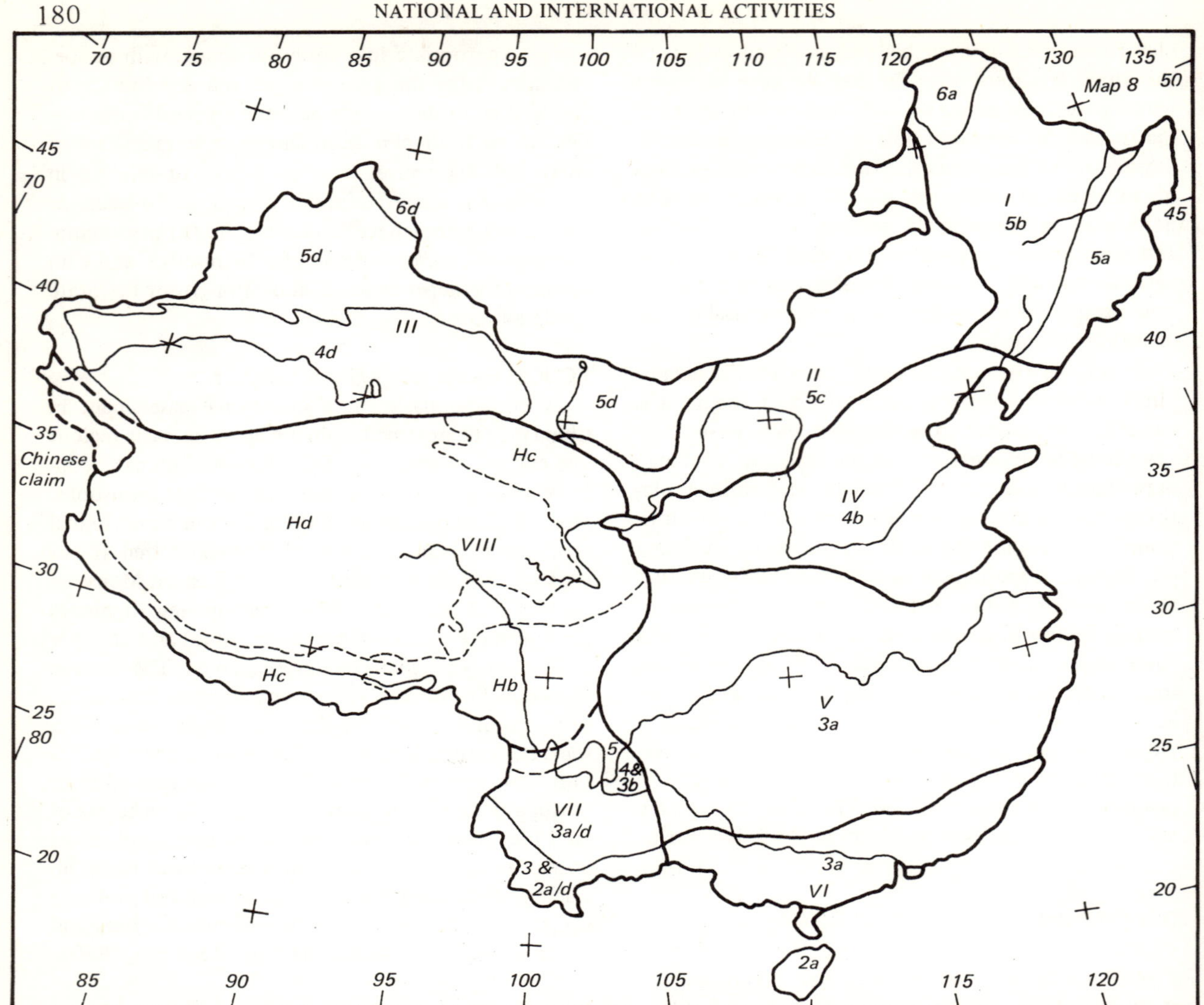

FIG. 15/1   China: climatic regions and climatic types

Primary Climatic Regions

Eight Primary Regions	*Climatic Types*[3]	*Warmth*[4]	*Dryness*[5]
I NORTHEAST	6a/–/–/–/–	Cold temperate	Wet
	5a/5b/–/–/–	Temperate	Wet/Semi-wet
II INNER MONGOLIA	–/–/5c/–/–	Temperate	Semi-dry
III KANSU-SINKIANG	–/–/–/6d/–	Cold temperate	Dry
	–/–/–/5d/–	Temperate	Dry
	–/–/–/4d/–	Warm temperate	Dry
IV NORTH CHINA	–/4b/–/–/–	Warm temperate	Semi-wet
V CENTRAL CHINA	3a/–/–/–/–	Subtropical	Wet

have been obtained by applying a constant annual increment of 10 million. This implies an annual rate of growth of around 1.5 per cent compound, which appears low as compared with the rate of growth indicated by the official Chinese estimates of total population and of birth and death rates available for 1952–7, and quoted in the U.N. *World Population Prospects.* No substantial reduction in the rate of growth has been assumed for recent years in view of the absence of any reports of success for family planning campaigns.

Various estimates of population are summarized in Table 15/1. For the calculation of food resources and requirements, it is appropriate to take the figure for 1970 of 800 million ±6 per cent; and further, to say that 80 per cent or 640 million, again ±6 per cent, are rural people (some authorities say 85 per cent).

Figures for annual rate of growth of population (column 2 of Table 15/1) are relevant to projections for agricultural planning, regulation of food exports and imports and a preliminary estimate of the sequence of events in a future crisis, should population outstrip actual and potential sources of food.

PRODUCTION AND DISTRIBUTION OF FOODGRAINS

The major objective of policy is the provision of foodgrains for the urban and rural people. Reference should be made to Donnithorne's study of output, procurement, transfers and trade (1970), and of the influence of factors such as transport difficulties and lack of storage facilities on the procurement programme. It appears that each province and the urban areas within each province are largely dependent upon the production of that province. Her conclusion in respect of foodgrains is, with a population of 750 million and a grain output of 190 million metric tons in 1967, output per head would have been 253 kg. per annum, 'marginal, perhaps just sufficient, if evenly spread. The same output with a higher population figure would give an overall deficiency in grain.' In translating these figures into consumption per head, allowance should be made for the amount of grain

---

VI SOUTH CHINA	3a/–/–/–/–	Subtropical	Wet
	29/–/–/–/–	Tropical	Wet
VII EASTERN TIBET [SIKANG]-YUNNAN	–/5b/–/–/–	Temperate	Semi-wet
	–/4b/–/–/–	Warm temperate	Semi-wet
	3a/3b/–/–/3a/d	Subtropical	Wet/Semi-wet
	–/–/–/–/2a/d	Tropical	Wet s., dry w.
VIII TSINGHAI-TIBET	–/Hb/Hc/Hd/–	Cool to cold	Semi-wet/semi-dry/dry

1) The division is that of a 1959 scheme prepared for the Committee on Delimitation of Natural Regions of the Chinese Academy of Science by Chang Pao-k'un, Chu Kang-k'un, et. al.

2) West-to-east divisions are based on indices of relative dryness; south-to-north divisions are based on temperature zones. The eight primary and 31 secondary regions (omitting the 32nd, the South China Sea) comprise 20 climatic types, most of which are shown on the map.

3) Combinations of warmth and dryness are shown by number-letter notation. Numbered zones, for China, are all monsoonal. Letter H, for Tsinghai-Tibet, indicates non-monsoonal, plateau-type climate.

4) Stated as the sum of daily mean temperatures (°C.) for duration of active growing season (≥10°C.) as follows:

1	Equatorial	about	9000°
2	Tropical		≥ 8000°
3	Subtropical	4500°	– 8000°
4	Warm temperate	3400°	– 4500°
5	Temperate	1600°	– 3400°
6	Cold temperate		< 1600°

5) Stated as the ratio of potential evaporation to precipitation. Authors postulate equilibrium (=1.0) for zone of Chinling Shan and Huai River.

	< 0.50	–*Very Wet*; water drains
a	0.50-0.99	–*Wet*; water drains
b	1.00-1.49	–*Semi-wet*; deficiency of water
c	1.50-4.00	–*Semi-dry*; irrigation is needed
d	> 4.00	–*Dry*
a/d		*Wet* in Summer, *Dry* in Winter

TABLE 15/1

China: population according to different estimates (in millions)

Source	Percentage annual increase, compound	1950	1953 Census Year	1955	1958	1960	1965	1970
China (official) (from Field, 1969)	1·6		575	602	647	667	700	780*
United Nations	1·6	560				650	700	760
FAO (1969)	2·0	547				686	764	845
U.S. Bureau of Census (Aird, 1968)			578/ 576	599/ 703	637/ 650	662/ 682	715/ 743	770/ 805*
Chou En-lai (Hou, 1968)	2·0 2·5					667	744	848*
Orleans (1969)	1·6	567	589	608	640	658	705	757
Chandrasekhar (1967)	2·2	552	588	614	662	690	769	858*
Frisen (Snyder, 1970)								760

* Figures for 1970 estimated on basis of earlier years and percentage annual increase

used for seed, livestock feed and export, for brewing and other industrial uses and for losses during transport and storage after harvest. The amount imported should be added to the gross production figure.

Donnithorne's conclusion about the increased contribution of vegetables, meat and eggs to a falling caloric intake is highly debatable:

On most outside estimates of China's grain output and population for the last few years, consumption per person must have declined since 1957, yet it is thought that in the areas from which information is available, the per capita calory intake of food is roughly the same as in 1957. This has come about as a result of the increase in output of vegetables, meat and eggs, thus representing an improvement in the quality of the diet. These subsidiary foodstuffs have been grown largely on the private plots which flourished in the 'Liuist' period of 1962–65 and which do not seem to have been seriously reduced, in most places, during the Cultural Revolution.

More ominous in terms of quality in the diet is her suggestion that the supply of grain from other parts of China for the great cities and for the deficit provinces might no longer be organized by administrative measures, but left to the influence of market forces:

The difficulties encountered by Peking in trying to extract grain from surplus provinces would not occur if both centre and provinces permitted the bulk of the harvest to be sold on the free market. At present while a fairly legitimate, no more than grey, free market exists for grain, only small quantities apparently seep through on to it. With a larger free market in grain, resources (private plots, labour, fertilizers, etc.) at present devoted to vegetable and livestock production might be switched to grain.

A comparison of Chinese and Indian agriculture has been made by Bardhan (1970) in respect of grain production, rates of growth in production and yields, soil nutrients, potential and effective irrigation, vulnerability to floods and droughts, economics, use of labour and the proportion of foodgrain production extracted from rural areas. It is to be hoped that someone with access to more recent data will bring Table 15/2 up to date. There have been considerable developments in both China and India since 1965–8. Bardhan's conclusions are:

For India one can, no doubt, expect that with the significant improvement in supplies of agricultural inputs and investment, Indian agricultural performance may be much better in the next decade than it has

TABLE 15/2

Comparison of Chinese and Indian agriculture over the period 1952/3 to 1967/8

	China		India	
	1955	*1965*	*1955*	*1965*
Gross sown acreage under all crops (million ha.)	151·1	156	144·1	157·9
Index of multiple cropping (gross sown acreage under all crops) (percentage)	137·2	143·1	112·8	114·8
	1952	*1965*	*1952*	*1965*
Yields per hectare in processed foodgrains (metric tons) *rice*	1·78	2·19	0·81	1·07
wheat	0·62	0·72	0·78	0·9
all foodgrains	1·11	1·3	0·59	0·75
Production of processed foodgrains (million metric tons)	124·9	161·8	61·67	89·0
Production of foodgrains in kg. per caput per annum	217·2	222·3	164·0	182·0
	1952 to 1967		*1952/3 to 1967/8*	
Annual (compound) rate of growth of output of foodgrains (percent)	2·7		3·0	
Linear regression analysis on bases of year-to-year output of data for growth rate (percent)	1·9		1·7	
	1955	*1965*	*1955/6*	*1964/5*
Consumption of chemical fertilizers per hectare of gross cropped area (N + P_2O_5 + K_2O in kg.)	1·7	10·2	0·9	4·9

Source: Adapted from Bardhan, 1970

been in the past. But a large part of her development effort will remain seriously constrained by her backward institutional framework and archaic administrative setup.

Whether or not the better potential for China will be effectively used will depend to a large degree on whether from time to time the Party does or does not avoid the temptation to force the pace of things in the face of technical feasibility, to go in for hastily conceived crash programs, or to bring about further reorganizations of land institutions without due consideration of peasant incentives.

No comparative study of two economies is complete without a consideration of the distribution patterns, but we have chosen not to discuss it here out of considerations of space as well as our belief that most people will hardly deny that the pattern of income and wealth is likely to be more egalitarian in China than in India. We may only note that the welfare effects of a more egalitarian distribution may be substantial in countries like India or China with millions of people at the near-subsistence level of consumption.

LAND RESOURCES

Elsewhere is presented (Whyte, 1972a) a discussion of the land types and farming systems, with the State emphasis on investments directed towards the 'areas of high and stable yield' equivalent to the intensive agricultural projects in India, of the state of the forest lands, and the possibility of developing a hill-land type of grassland/animal husbandry. The broad soil types and figures for fertilizer requirements and availability are given. Vast projects of water conservation should be evaluated in relation to the gains and losses of cultivated land.

It is necessary to consider a number of plateaux of production (see Chapter 16), in relation to environment and population density in so far as these govern the return from inputs of economic factors (water, fertilizers, plant protection, improved varieties) and seasonally available manpower. It would be an interesting study to express the potential regional maxima in China in the form of a block diagram (see Figure 16/1).

Did the land of China cease to be able to maintain the people on a reasonable plane of nutrition as long ago as 1750 to 1775, when the population was 250 million (Ho, 1959)? Since then, the state of equilibrium between the people and the land resources has deteriorated progressively (see Whyte, 1972a). It is one of the main objectives of the present Government to try to recover that equilibrium, by improved land use and farming practices and maximum reclamation of wasteland and extension of irrigation facilities, but with a human population over three times greater than that of 200 years ago. Recovery of equilibrium would be expressed primarily in the maintenance of good nutritional standards for non-rural peoples, while at the same time ensuring a great improvement in the standards of rural nutrition, particularly of the vulnerable groups.

Have yields of food crops per unit area reached a static level with the use of all available organic fertilizers? Hou Chi-ming (1968) refers to a continued low level of production in the post-1961 years, which has been variously ascribed to weather, the Great Leap Forward and the rural Communes. Hou considers rather that, during the most severe years of 1960—1, the food shortage in the rural areas might have been so serious as to inflict lasting damage to the health and physical strength of the peasants and to reduce the number of draft animals considerably. All this should have resulted in a shortage of farm labour, due partly to the substitution of human labour for animal power. However, Hou finds no evidence to suggest such a shortage since 1960. He proposes that the agricultural setback may not be really a temporary slump, but rather that it reflects the basic stagnant nature of Chinese agriculture:

The apparent inability to break through the 1959 level of production, despite considerable increase in labour force, strongly suggests that output ceiling may have been approached within the framework of traditional technology and inputs. Any significant increase in production may not be forthcoming unless modern inputs or new production functions are introduced.

Has China yet begun to use the high-yielding varieties? Dalrymple (1971) gives the American consensus of opinion, based upon radio and other reports:

On balance, it would seem very likely that the Chinese have imported at least small quantities of I.R.R.I. seed. But whether the seed has been imported in large quantities and/or has had any significant impact to date is not at all certain and may never be. The more important questions, however, concern the increased yield potential and area devoted to the new varieties, whatever tehir origin. And on these points we seem to have little solid information as yet.

The continued use of conventional improved cultivars is probably done on the advice of the plant breeders, who must be well aware of the dangers of the widespread introduction of high-yielding varieties into rural areas where soils are not sufficiently fertile, where water for irrigation is inadequate, and fertilizers and pesticides in short supply.

RURAL/URBAN RELATIONS

Attempts to achieve maximum productivity by better farming practices, use of fertilizers and irrigation water are designed to increase procurement from rural areas; the produce of the land, be it from the forests, the grasslands or the cultivated land, is intended for sale and consumption in urban and industrial areas, or for export to earn foreign exchange. In common with many Asian countries, China is stimulating maximum production by the great majority of the population for the benefit of a minority, and the more efficient the extraction of food from the rural areas, the less diversified is the rural diet.

Donnithorne (1970) gives a clear account of the history and development of the tax and procurement system in relation to foodgrains and other crops. Tax is levied in respect of crops of all kinds — grains, potatoes, vegetables and industrial crops. The tax, which seems to vary between 4 and 19 per cent, is based on the normal yield of all crops reckoned in terms of the main grain crop of the area. The grain taken by the State in agricultural tax and the compulsory deliveries (the so-called 'commodity grain' as distinct from grain grown for home consumption) seem to vary around 23 to 34 per cent of total output in any one year.

It would not, however, be correct to say that this represents the requisitioning of some 30 per cent of the crop for 15 per cent (the urban proportion) of the population. The State also needs grain to supply to the farmers otherwise engaged on the production of industrial crops, and for export (rice).

Presumably because of limited production, the extraction of livestock produce from the rural areas is even more intense and efficient, since the rural diet is almost entirely vegetarian. Some of the incentives applied to induce the rural people to part with their pig and other meats, eggs, etc. have been given by Myrdal (1966) (1961 data). Every goat delivered entitles one to coupons for 6 chi of cotton material or one sheepskin or goatskin. When pigs, goats or eggs are sold to the State, the household receives, as well as cash payment, permits to buy for:

one goat	six chi[1] of cotton material *or* one goatskin *or* sheepskin
one pig	one set of cotton underclothes *and* one pair of galoshes *and* one or two hand towels
one jin of eggs	half a jin of sugar

Prices paid by the State for animal products sold privately in 1962:

pigs per jin of liveweight	0.43 yuan[3]
goats per jin liveweight	0.43
eggs per jin[2]	0.795

Prices paid (per jin) by the grain office in Yenan hsien:

	Yuan
Wheat	0.10
Millet	0.06
Millet, 'sticky millet'	0.065
Maize	0.065
Black beans (*Vicia faba*)	0.08
Soya	0.08
Long beans (*Phaseolus vulgaris*)	0.075
Green beans (*Phaseolus mungo*)	0.10
Buckwheat	0.065
Kaoliang	0.065
Jute seeds	0.15

[1] chi: 10 chi = 1.333 oz.
[2] jin: 1 jin = 1.333 lb.
[3] yuan: 100 RMB = US$49.75

DIET IN RURAL AREAS

Maps of regional agroclimatic zones, of systems of land use and of the crops and domestic livestock indicate rural dietary patterns, particularly with regard to the staple foods. In China it is only in years of crisis caused by climatic fluctuations or other factors that food is brought in from elsewhere, as a temporary loan to be repaid in subsequent years. Food also has to be provided where the cultivators have to concentrate on the production of non-food crops. Change in dietary habits and status will occur only where marked change in farming techniques and crops takes place, for example, following the introduction of irrigation. 'The end result of the type of land utilization of a country is the standard of living it provides for its population' (Low, 1937).

It is assumed that China will ensure sufficient foodgrain consumption per caput from domestic and imported sources to meet calorie requirements. No attempt is made to give estimates of intake per caput of calories or nutrients, since there are no valid bases for such estimates. It is true that it has become fashionable for countries to take figures for total grain production, decide on availability per caput, and from this, with no knowledge whatsoever of intake of other essential foods, to calculate calorie, sometimes even certain nutrient intakes. This is no way an accurate indication of actual food intake per caput or of nutritional status.

It seems that diets deteriorated in quantity and quality during the period when the Communes were first set up, and improved following the re-introduction of the private plots.

The only study of rural nutrition on a country-wide basis in China ever made is the survey organized by J. Lossing-Buck in 1929–33, covering 22 provinces, 38,256 families in 186 localities. A review of his findings appears in Whyte (1972a), together with details of more recent information from scattered localities. (See also Case Studies Nos. 77, 78, 79, 102, 103, 104, 125, 131, 139.)

Today it is claimed that 5 per cent of the total cultivated area is regarded as private plots, the allocation to individual families varying according to numbers. Doubtless a similar range of crops is grown as was found by Buck and his team. Out of reach of the large towns, it is possible that the rural market for vegetables has diminished. Specialist horticulturists farm only near large urban markets; traditional rural vegetables, in season, are those of least nutritive value, the pumpkins, gourds, cucumbers, melons and

Chinese cabbage (Wolff, 1962). The question is whether as much of today's production from the private plots is sold as was sold 30 years ago (from 20 to over 50 per cent). If so, the diet must be quantitatively even more deficient in respect of quality foods.

Animals in China are reared for draft, to provide organic manure, and as a cash crop for urban areas and for export. Meat and fish are purchased in very small amounts for festivals. Eggs are rarely eaten on the farm. Efficiency of control and compulsory disposal to the State, together with illegal private transactions, probably ensure that extraction of livestock products from the rural areas is at least as effective as it was 30 years ago.

Two fundamental factors cannot have changed greatly — the pattern of production of the major crops, and the dietary habits and preferences of the population. Two major changes have, however, occurred. Local harvest crises are mitigated by foodgrain loans from the Central Government. Improved access has made possible greater efficiency of extraction of food for urban areas. This applies to foodgrains, and to foods of plant and animal origin rich in high quality protein, vitamins and minerals. It appears, however, that the State procurement plan meets with considerable resistance, especially during periods of political upheaval or local climatic crises. During the Cultural Revolution, some rural producers not only shared much of their crops among themselves, but even raided stores in which State buffer stocks were maintained.

It is no doubt national policy that the rural peoples should grow quality foods on their private plots to diversify their diets. However, the incentive for the farmer is not better nutrition for his family, but production of a marketable commodity. In the years before 1956, prices offered by the Marketing Co-operatives were so low that many subsidiary crops were abandoned. A free market was re-established in 1956 for vegetables, fish, poultry products, etc., a small, perhaps sub-standard proportion of which would be reserved for the home. During 1961–4, the commune system was largely abandoned, and the village once more became the administrative unit (Wenmohs, 1967). Each family was again given a private plot, its size depending on the number in the family. Private production of poultry for home use and for sale was encouraged. While the increase in grain output during this period was largely due to better weather, some credit must also be given to the increased energy and enthusiasm of the rural cultivators. After 1966, however, the private plots and subsidiary production came

into increasing political disfavour, being said by Peking to lead to 'spontaneous capitalism' (Wenmohs, op. cit.). By 1972, this phase had passed, the principle of the private plot had returned to favour, and the production of foods of animal origin was to receive particular emphasis.

Thus three factors — the reduction in size of the private plots; increased efficiency of extraction of all foods from rural areas; and the natural inclination of the Chinese farmer to sell produce for cash — are obstacles to the improvement of the rural diet with quality protein and vitamins. This is of particular significance in the correct nutrition of the vulnerable groups.

THE VULNERABLE GROUPS

It does not appear that China has evolved a nutritional policy directed primarily to the vulnerable groups, comparable to the Children's Charter in India. Yet the propositions associated with that Charter must apply with equal force to the children and other members of the vulnerable groups in China.

Chinese folk tradition, like that of most other Asian countries, makes a number of specific recommendations for the nutrition of the pregnant and nursing mother. Unlike the countries of South-East Asia and the Indian sub-continent, however, Chinese customs include a number of protein-rich foods of animal origin (Whyte, 1972a and Chapter 10). It is unlikely that family budgets in China today will permit the regular use of such luxuries, even when locally available, or that the mother alone would take enough of them.

In China, as elsewhere in Asia, weaning has traditionally been a gradual process, and denial of the breast may not take place until 3 years of age or later (Chapter 10). Small pieces of animal food may be boiled with the congee and removed before feeding. Vegetables are not usually given until later, when it is considered the child is able to digest them. The duration of breast-feeding — that is, how long the mother is able to carry her infant on her back while working — is crucial, since it is extremely unlikely that adequate animal protein (and consequently vitamins and minerals also) can be provided during her absence by the old woman who looks after the small village children during the day.

Adequate supplies of good quality protein, minerals and vitamins are necessary for growth from weaning throughout childhood, with increased requirements during adolescence. Again, there is no information on the composition of school meals on which to base an assessment of their adequacy. In view of the overall lack of animal protein and legume protein and of the low per caput availability of vegetables, it is, however, unlikely that children's needs throughout their growth are fully met.

Thus for the vulnerable groups as a whole there is a critical deficiency of proteins, vitamins and minerals. Deficiencies of these nutrients were reported in various sources some twenty years ago, and are found among Chinese communities today in South-East Asia whose diets do contain small amounts of animal protein. Both before and after World War II, there was evidence of vitamin A deficiency among children in China (Flowers, 1948), beriberi was common, and there are frequent references to rickets, confirming the severe dietary deficiency of calcium found by Maynard and Swen (1937). However, people throughout the world appear to subsist in good health on calcium intakes far below recommended levels; it is probably only the vulnerable groups who are likely to suffer. Some authorities consider that dietary deficiencies of calcium and vitamin D are likely to disappear when a child can walk and is exposed to sunlight, synthesizing vitamin D and thus mobilizing more of the calcium in the diet. Deficiencies of other vitamins were also noted (Jelliffe, 1968a; Whyte, 1972a). We have no evidence to show that the nutrient deficiencies have been remedied. The most severe of all is likely to be calorie/protein deficiency, especially in early childhood.

PRINCIPAL SOURCES OF CALORIES

In China, carbohydrates are again the principal source of calories. China's staples are shown in Fig. 15/2. A map of the distribution of crops is a direct

FIG. 15/2 China: principal land use and cropping regions

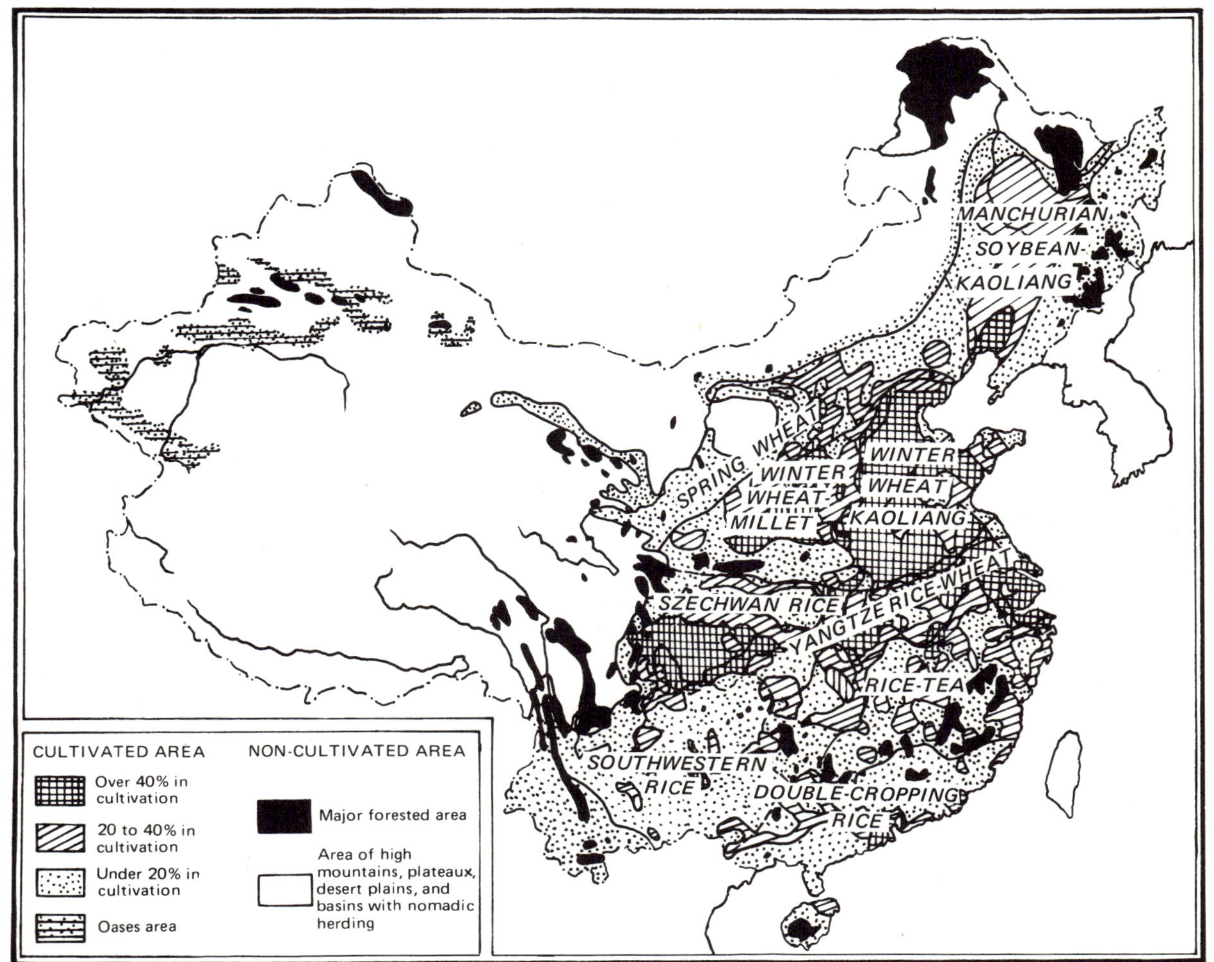

indication of the plant foods which are the basis of rural diets. Rice is the staple of over 70 per cent of the people, particularly in the southern monsoonal provinces. Wheat and kaoliang are the staples in the north. Maize is not popular, and is largely reserved for livestock feed. It is, however, eaten by the mountain-dwelling peoples (mostly non-Han), who also consume buckwheat, other cereals and roots and tubers, depending on environment. In China, as throughout the region, sweet potato is a low-prestige food; it is frequently denied that the rural peoples of the south are still obliged, as they were in the past, to supplement their rice supplies with this crop.

The first requirement of any policy designed to feed a population is the provision of calories. It is obvious that the Government of the Chinese People's Republic is fully aware of the overriding need to provide at least a minimum quantity of foodgrains for all the population, urban and rural. (See table 10 in Whyte (1972a) for calorie intakes.) Foodgrain supplies are ensured by procurement from the rural areas after the needs of the farming population have been considered, plus import of wheat, primarily for the great cities of the north. There is considerable discussion regarding the actual level of foodgrain harvests in recent years (see Table 11 in Whyte, 1972a, for grain areas, yields and production, as estimated by the U.S. Consulate, Hong Kong, for the years 1953 to 1968).

China exports fine rice to Cuba, Sri Lanka, Pakistan, Hong Kong, Malaysia, Singapore and Japan. Every ton of rice exported is roughly equivalent in cash value to two tons of wheat imported (Table 15/3). Any fall in rice exports may be due to increased demand from a larger population, increased rural resistance to procurement or lower production.

SOURCES OF PLANT PROTEIN

To ensure maximum production and availability of proteins from foodgrains, the following steps would have to be taken:

(a) Introduction of high-yielding varieties so that the total production and thus protein yield per hectare is increased. China had an earlier generation of improved varieties, but may now have begun to use China-bred or introduced IRRI types of the so-called high-yielding varieties of rice, which have been associated with the green revolution elsewhere in Asia.

(b) Screening of all existing varieties within China to assess protein content of the grain. Work elsewhere in Asia indicates that there is a large variation within the existing genetic material; for example, in wheat varieties, this ranges from 12 per cent in conventional varieties to a new one containing 25 to 30 per cent protein.

(c) In a diet relying almost entirely for its protein upon foodgrains, it is the amino-acid content and proportion which is the important factor. Therefore screening of existing varieties has to be undertaken also for amino-acid content. The technique of biochemical analysis has still to be perfected, being subject to considerable margin of error (FAO, 1970a). There is no reason to doubt that the breeders in China are fully aware of this approach.

(d) If protein needs cannot be met from conventional foodgrains eaten alone or in association with appropriate grain legumes, it has become customary to consider fortification (see Chapter 12). The considerable problems of fortification of a subsistence crop with synthetic amino acids would have to be overcome. Lysine fortification of rice diets in India has been shown to be inferior to fortification with leaf protein.

TABLE 15/3

China: imports and exports of foodgrains

(in 1,000 metric tons)

	1967	1968	1969	1970
Wheat imports	4,133	4,329	4,600	4,500

	1959	1963	1966	1967
Rice exports	1,700	513	1,150	1,000

Source: U.S. Consulate, Hong Kong, 1970

TABLE 15/4

China: soybeans as a source of plant protein: nutritional targets for total and rural populations at different levels of intake (gm.) per caput per day, expressed in terms of the land areas required to produce them

Population (million)	Soybean intakes at three levels (gm. per head per day)		Total amounts required per year (kg.)	Average yield per year (kg./ha.)[1]	Total approximate area of land required under edible varieties[2] (hectares)
800 (total)	(a)	30	8,760,000,000		12,500,000
	(b)	40	11,680,000,000	700	16,700,000
	(c)	50	14,600,000,000		21,000,000
640 (rural)	(a)	30	7,008,000,000		10,010,000[3]
	(b)	40	9,344,000,000	700	13,330,000[3]
	(c)	50	11,680,000,000		16,700,000[3]

(a) provides adequate protein in an adult diet

(b) and (c) are higher levels to allow for the special requirements of the vulnerable groups.

[1] (Nutrition Division, Plant Production and Protection Division, Economic Analysis Division, FAO, 1967)
[2] mostly to be grown on private plots
[3] existing area about 8.5 million hectares, mostly under industrial varieties

Diets based on foodgrain cereals plus grain legumes differ in terms of amino-acid balance. Nutritionists have shown that a diet based on a judicious mixture of plant proteins is equal in value to a diet containing animal protein. But probably nowhere in Asia are grain legumes available or consumed in quantities sufficient to ensure this desirable balance. In China, a satisfactory diet could theoretically be obtained by means of the soybean, by far the most valuable grain legume in protein content.

It is generally assumed that the rural people obtain soybean from their private plots. However, when one compares resources of soybean in relation to requirements, the situation is highly revealing (Table 15/4). If we are to provide an average of 40 to 50 gm. soybean per head per day for the total rural population of 640 million (this average takes into account the different requirements for soybean of different sections of the population), this would mean that the whole of the private plot area (assuming that they are and will remain at 5 per cent of the total effective cultivated area) would have to be sown to edible varieties of soybean, and that the yield per hectare would have to be *double* that obtained in the larger units where oil-producing varieties of soybean are grown for industrial purposes or for export. Yields on private plots are likely to be lower than on the large-scale units, because they are usually located on poorer soils and fertilizers are not allocated to their owners.

Certain factors reduce the value of protein from vegetable sources. One is the loss of protein which occurs in processing. The total content of protein in rice grain is ±8 per cent. Cooked polished rice contains only 3.38 per cent protein (Table 12/2). Mature soybeans containing nearly 40 per cent protein are available in the rural areas for only a limited period of the year. The protein content of the rest of the plant, consumed green throughout growth, is much lower (Table 12/2). The method of preparation of the mature grain legume greatly affects its value. When finely ground, as in soybean curd, absorption of protein during digestion is high. But the most common method of preparation in rural areas is boiling, and protein absorption is much lower. Intestinal diseases and infestation further reduce the amount of absorption of plant protein. Soybean sauce, that ubiquitous ingredient of the Chinese diet, is of insignificant value as a source of protein (FAO, Nutrition Division, 1966).

SOURCES OF ANIMAL PROTEIN

It is generally agreed that the rural people of China are virtually vegetarian. Most of the pigs produced are purchased for the use of the urban and industrial areas, for the military or for export (nearly 2 million pigs with average dressed weight of 50 kg. imported annually into Hong Kong). There is no uniform system for rationing of pig meat in Chinese cities. Supply is subject to seasonal factors. When pig meat is plentiful, it is freely sold, but in times of scarcity it may be rationed for periods of several months at a time. To achieve the levels of consumption in other Chinese Asian communities, Singapore, Taiwan and Hong Kong (11, 16 and 25 kg. pig meat per head per year respectively), China would need 340, 500 or 800 million pigs. The present pig population is probably about 160 million, giving 5 kg. pig meat per head per year if calculated on the basis of a human population of 800 million.

Poultry (hens and ducks) make an infinitesimal contribution to the animal protein composition of the diet, when calculated on the basis of products per head per year (Whyte, 1972a).

The use of beef and milk is insignificant in the rural diet. Goats are reared in the north, but mutton consumption is largely confined to the non-Han pastoralists of the grasslands of the north and west. Fish, fresh or dried, does not appear to play a regular part in the diet of the rural peoples other than those living near coasts, along important water-courses and on lakesides.

STATUS OF RURAL NUTRITION

While calorie requirements are ensured by State intervention, the rural cultivator in China is expected to obtain quality and diversity in the diet from his private plot. If these are actually 5 per cent of the total effective cultivated area, this means that the rural peoples have at their disposal 7.5 million hectares for the cultivation of their protective foods.

Animal protein in nutritionally effective amounts has long ago disappeared from the rural Chinese diet. It would appear that the amount of protein available from grain legumes, especially the soybean, is also completely inadequate. Vegetables of relatively low nutritive value are consumed in small amounts, and supply is subject to wide fluctuation in seasonal availability, with deficits in winter in the wheat zone, or in the dry monsoon period in the rice zone. Thus foodgrains are expected to provide not only the bulk of the calories, but also most of the protein, to the extent that their composition of essential amino acids permits, as well as some minerals and vitamins.

In attempting to assess the status of rural nutrition in China, and even after allowance has been made for adaptation to a lower plane of nutrition (Chapter 11), it is obvious that there are severe deficiencies in important foods and nutrients, and that the vulnerable groups of the population are most at risk. When the present and potential production and consumption of animal foods, grain legumes and vegetables are related to the ratio of cultivated land per head of population (nutrition density per unit area) it is difficult to see how the rural Chinese diet can be improved on the scale required.

It has been shown that the overall characteristics and crises of a monsoonal environment apply just as much to China as to the other countries of the region. Into this pan-Asian category come the epidemic and endemic diseases which must be tackled not by mere exhortation and incantation, but by the methods which have been adopted in Asian medical science. A scientific approach is required for the recognition and treatment of diseases which are the manifestations of, or are aggravated by, nutritional deficiencies.

Part V
CONCLUSION

16 Man and the Asian Environment

EQUILIBRIUM IN ECOSYSTEMS

THE ultimate utopia of the practising ecologist is a reasonable degree of equilibrium between the environment and the components of the ecosystems for which he is responsible, defining equilibrium as that illusory ecological condition, especially unattainable in Asia, in which none of the components of the economic ecosystem lacks food, water, light and optimal ambient temperature. An analysis of any economic ecosystem in Asia should first consider the adequacy or deficiency in quantity and quality of the foods and nutrients available for the crop plants, domestic animals and human beings. Plans for improvement of ecosystems, for the raising of man and the other economic components from one level to the one above, must be based upon such an analysis and on the ecological feasibility of the operation. This is the ecological basis of the pre-investment survey. But the survey and the subsequent development activities should be based not upon the highly suspect statistical data in central planning departments, but upon the analysis of ecosystems in a random statistical sample of villages, or other social unit, selected within a recognized land system or catchment basin.

An analysis of field studies by anthropologists, rural sociologists, historians, geographers and doctors reveals how widespread ecological regression has become in Asia. Thus we find deterioration in nutritional standards and health wherever population pressure on land is heavy, either because too many people are drawing on a static or dwindling food resource, or because of the spread of nutritionally inferior staples. Those who suffer most are the vulnerable groups, the infants, children and pregnant and nursing mothers, whose protein needs are not adequately met from predominantly vegetable sources. There is an increasing volume of medical literature to demonstrate that the mental and physical effects of defective nutrition in the early years are irreparable.

In analysing rural ecosystems, it is the human beings who should be given first priority. Applied plant ecology should be directed to those communities, wild genera and species and cultivated crops that provide food for man and feed for livestock. Applied animal ecology should concern itself primarily with those domesticated and wild animals that provide food for men, draft for their fields, and clothing for their backs.

In short, the study of Asian economic ecosystems should start with human ecology. This particular branch of ecological science as it relates to human nutrition has not yet been precisely defined, nor has a field methodology been developed. It is to be hoped that a handbook on field methods may be available soon, so that data may be collected by the specialists in all the relevant disciplines, working singly or in teams.

CONFIDENCE OR DOUBT?

That part of the developing world known as Monsoon Asia has an urgent need to attempt to bring the production and/or availability of food into equilibrium with its population. This region has been described as the golden fringe to a beggar's mantle, contrasting thereby the deceptive luxuriance of the tropical monsoonal and equatorial vegetation and crop plants with the bleak continental lands of extra-monsoonal Asia to the north. Too many people (about two-thirds of the world's population) have chosen these lands of Asia and contiguous areas in which to live and to multiply enormously. As a result, the region is faced with great economic and political problems, many closely related to standards of human nutrition now and in the coming decades. To combat these, the Vice-Chancellor of the Chinese University of Hong Kong, Dr. Li Choh-ming has said (July 1970) that Asians should seek more than a political association and a common market — they should seek a regional identity. No Asian country can afford to exist in isolation, whatever her affluence or productivity — they must look to the well-being of the whole region.

A tempered confidence in man's ability to feed himself has, for some, replaced the despondency of a decade ago. Typical of this view are the conclusions reached at the Symposium of the (British) Society of Chemical Industry in 1967, when it was agreed that there are no biological limitations to the problems of meeting the world's food needs by A.D. 2,000, that the technical knowledge to do so already exists, and that all the constraints are social, political and psychological. Adequacy of future food supplies is a problem of social persuasion and of the communal capacity of the species man, not of the biology of the plant and animal species which produce his food (Lucas, 1969). Hutchinson (1968) would agree that the technical difficulties have been overcome for the present, but that in the future the land/man ratio would become critical in the absence of control of human population. The planner and the agricultural scientist do not appear to accept that the technical success of a new field technique is far less than its biological and technical maximum potentialities. Even in the advanced countries, there is marked dilution of achievement between the research institute and the pioneer farmers on the one hand, and the average farming community on the other.

It is said by some that, by applying advanced techniques, there will be no insuperable problems in feeding Asia's hundreds of millions, provided the poverty and apathy of the average cultivator can be overcome, and the average purchasing power of all Asians, urban and rural, increased. Others feel that these obstacles cannot be overcome in time, that seeds of high-yielding varieties, fertilizers, pesticides, irrigation water and technical advice are not always available where needed, and that marketing and credit facilities are inadequate. The results of the much-vaunted green revolution apply only to a limited percentage of the total cultivated land, and will affect the nutrition of only a small proportion of the rural population. The further spread of the new technology may not be as rapid as early successes suggested (Wharton, 1969a), particularly in its extension from irrigated to dry-land agriculture (see Chapter 14). There is a great danger, according to the Rockefeller Foundation (report for

1969) in the reduction in the number of crop varieties which is a sequel to the introduction of one new high-yielding variety over large areas. If new races of fungus or virus diseases were to appear, for example a new rust, to which the high-yielding types of wheat do not carry resistance, much of the wheat crop could be eliminated very quickly. The heavy doses of chemical fertilizers that are needed may pollute the environment.

There are few countries in the world which can claim to be entirely free from under-nutrition and malnutrition among a certain proportion of their populations. But governments are unwilling to admit the existence of a degree of hunger and malnutrition that might be taken as a silent witness of the relative failure of their particular political and economic system. They frequently present figures for average food consumption or for the availability to all their people of, for example, sources of plant and animal protein and vitamins that do not bear close analysis at the rural level. And this applies also to the analyses of population. National figures, and hence the U.N. statistics based upon them, for total populations and percentage annual rates of increase are equally unreliable and represent under-estimates. As Hong Kong's former Commissioner for Census and Statistics has said: 'In many of these (Asian) countries, despite the World Population Census Programme, there had been no census, there was no registration of rural births and deaths, and even if these figures had been available, there was nowhere near enough know-how to deal with them' (Barnett, 1967).

It would be unprofitable to embark upon a discussion of the probable total, urban and rural populations of Asian countries. The present consensus regarding the 1970 population of China is presented in Chapter 15. It is possible to be reasonably accurate in respect of India (Chapter 14). Estimates for these and the other mammoth countries of Asia, Bangla Desh, Pakistan, Indonesia and Japan, may be found in the UN publications: *Demographic Yearbook, Monthly Bulletin of Statistics*, and *World Population Prospects*, and in the writings of many demographers.

RURAL NUTRITION

Under consideration is the nutritional ecology of 1,600 million people, that is, half the world's population. The prevention of widespread famine is ensured by State or international intervention. Animal protein in nutritionally effective amounts has long disappeared from the rural Asian diet. It would appear that the

TABLE 16/1

Levels of adequacy of calories and proteins in Asian diets

Nutrition grade	Calories	Animal protein	Legume and foodgrain protein
A	Adequate	Adequate	Present, but not essential as source of protein
B	Adequate	Becoming scarce	Become essential as source of protein
C	Adequate	Absent	Only sources of protein
D	Adequate	Absent	Grain legumes become inadequate, therefore balance in dietary protein deteriorates
C	Calories maintained at minimum requirement by government control or international aid	Absent	Grain legumes insignificant, dietary protein from foodgrains unbalanced
D	Calories always or seasonally inadequate	Absent	Foodgrain protein used as calories

amount of protein available from grain legumes is also completely inadequate. Vegetables may be consumed in small amounts; there is wide fluctuation in seasonal availability, with deficits, for example, in winter in the northern zones, or in the dry monsoon period in the rice zones. Thus foodgrains are expected to provide not only the bulk of the calories, but also most of the protein, to the extent that their composition of essential amino acids permits (Table 16/1).

Even after allowance has been made for Asian man's adaptation to a low plane of nutrition, it is obvious that there are severe deficiencies in important foods and nutrients, and that the vulnerable groups of the population are most at risk. When the present and potential production and consumption of animal foods, grain legumes and vegetables are related to the ratio of cultivated land per head of population (nutrition density per unit area), it is difficult to see how the rural diet can be improved on the scale required. If in future, efforts have to become concentrated on increasing production of foodgrains to feed an ever-increasing population, the rural people will continue in that nutritional half-life which is so characteristic of Monsoon Asia.

Nutrition and medical specialists can recognize evidence of malnutrition in general, and protein malnutrition in particular, especially among the vulnerable groups. This is reflected in high rates of infant and maternal mortality and deaths of children of pre-school age; low birth weights; low growth rates (weight, height, skeletal development) from 6 months, which may persist to maturity; high degree of susceptibility and low resistance to gastro-intestinal, respiratory and other diseases; impaired neuromotor development; limited life-span and premature senescence, particularly of women. Clinical and biochemical investigations reveal evidence of multiple deficiency of nutrients. The apathy, lethargy and lack of initiative for which the Asian worker is so often blamed are due in large part to malnutrition from early life.

FORECASTS AND TARGETS

In making long-term projections of food requirements on a national or local scale in the coming decades, it is necessary to have reasonably accurate figures of population and of their requirements, for foods of quantity and quality, broken down into mature and vulnerable age groups. This can be done only very approximately, since accurate data of present populations and annual rates of increment are lacking (Sukhatme, 1966).

It is also difficult, in view of wide variation between individual human beings, to determine a minimal effective intake of locally available foods or of essential nutrients. This is especially true of children, since growth and development take place at different ages under different conditions of environment and nutritional status. Nutritional recommendations therefore contain a margin of safety, designed to protect the majority of a population, and taking into account differences in weight and height and in efficiency of utilization and conversion of foods.

Recommendations must therefore be treated with caution when used as a yardstick to assess the adequacy of existing diets, when suggesting improvements in the diet, or when calculating food production targets to meet new dietary requirements. Some authorities have suggested diets to meet nutritional requirements based on locally acceptable and available foods (Chapter 9). These may form the basis for comparison with existing diets and for calculating food production and import targets. The average rural Asian, provided he is healthy and despite heavy intestinal infestation, may be able to subsist on a diet in which the protein, and also some minerals and vitamins, are considerably below recommended levels.

There are several ways of forecasting the future demand for food and of defining the production targets that have to be achieved. The numerical global and regional generalizations that are made for the benefit of the press and to shock the public into awareness cannot stand up to statistical analysis; 'cereals supply half the total of 80 million tons of protein available each year' or 'an increase in the protein content of cereals from 10 to 11 per cent would mean 5 million tons of protein more per year'.

The FAO Indicative World Plan is an attempt to be more precise. Its objective is to estimate what production will be needed by 1985 to meet the nutritional and other demands of the population at that date. The percentage increases above present levels are related to the policies of the member countries, not always synonymous with ideal nutritional objectives. But the calculations of food available per head are based on the very shaky foundation of government statistics, which Myrdal (1968) and many others have shown to be quite unreliable or non-existent. The colossal regional and national totals that are produced by the Indicative World Plan may be of some value to the planners in the national capitals, who talk the same language, but who are utterly remote from and unfamiliar with conditions at the village level.

Another method is to calculate what would be needed in terms of land area, crop land and numbers of livestock to meet minimum targets of human nutrition proposed by international or national authorities. This has been done for soybeans in China (Table 15/4), pigs in Taiwan (Whyte, 1972a) and milk in India (Whyte and Mathur, 1968). The daily inputs or through-puts of milk schemes (from 2,500 to 250,000 litres) are expressed as (a) total bovine population and bovines in milk with yields of from 250 to 2,500 litres per lactation, which will be needed to provide these daily levels of production, (b) amounts of concentrate feeds and green and dry fodders that these bovine populations will need if fed according to Indian standards, and (c) areas of crop and other land needed to produce these gross requirements. Fabulous yields of herbage may be obtained from the high-fertility-demanding African grasses grown with clean irrigation water plus heavy dressings of nitrogen and stable manure, or with cowshed wash, or with urban sewage which has been correctly treated (Whyte 1968a). Cooper (1970) compares an annual biological potential yield of over 20 tonnes dry matter per hectare in western Europe with a potential of over 40 tonnes per hectare in the tropics.

It is, however, again quite unrealistic to use these calculations in relation to the all-India nutritional targets of desirable milk intake per day proposed by the Indian Council of Medical Research and accepted by the Union Ministry of Food and Agriculture. Most people in India never taste milk. The daily production of milk is probably less than 10 per cent of the total needed to meet ICMR targets.

Thus the appendix to this book brings the discussion down to a more local level. Although the 140 case studies do not represent a random sample, they do contain sufficient information to show how unreliable and removed from reality government statistics and planning can be. The actual levels of average human nutrition in the rural areas are so low that even an increase of 10 or 20 per cent in the availability of food will not begin to provide the great majority of rural Asians with a satisfactory intake. The figures of 1, 2 or 3 per cent increase in world food production put forward by international agencies can have little relevance to hundreds of millions of rural Asians. In any case, the only real increases in Asian production are confined largely to those specially favoured areas where the new technology (including the high-yielding varieties) is biologically and economically applicable. Most rural Asians are farming land of which the productivity is actually decreasing. The increased production following the use of high-yielding varieties (in 1969, 22 million tons in Asia) has gone primarily to the urban areas or for export.

Would it not be more realistic to survey and plan from the particular to the general, to change from the present technique of planning primarily for the *urban* minorities, and to give more attention to the needs and potentialities of the *rural* areas? Could the statistician not design a study plan for rural production and dietary surveys, varying the number and scatter of sampling units according to topography, with obvious contrasts between the uniformity of the Gangetic Plain and the great diversity of mountain catchments in Indonesia or the Philippines? Could not the agronomist join forces with the nutritionist, and prepare simple checklists with agronomic criteria to parallel those given for health and nutrition by the World Health Organization (1969), and so provide data of greater value than the miscellaneous collection in the appendix, which is all that is available at present? Co-ordinated studies of this type would provide the realistic alternative to the daydreams and wishful thinking of New Delhi, Peking, Jakarta and the other capitals of Asia.

PLATEAUX OF PRODUCTION

Agricultural production over areas of cultivated land as vast as those of Asia does not progress by leaps and bounds. Claims for localized increases of 25 per cent or more cannot be extrapolated for application to whole regions. Having allowed for the marked fluctuations characteristic of the monsoonal ecoclimate, it is usually found that increases in crop and livestock yields per annum or per decade are small.

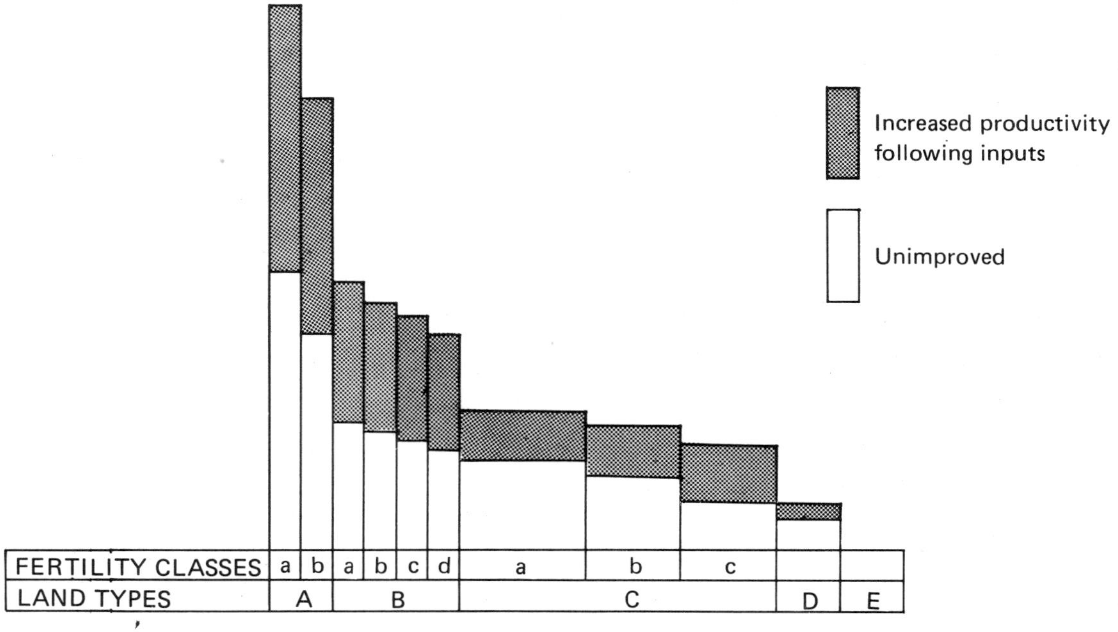

FIG. 16/1 Plateaux of production before and after introduction of maximum biologically effective and economically acceptable inputs in a theoretical catchment with the percentage of land types and cropping intensities shown below:

Percentage of area

A. with two fertility classes (a) (b) 10
cultivated land with year-round irrigation, = 200 to 300 per cent cropping

B. with four fertility classes (a), (b), (c), (d) 20
cultivated dry land with one reliable monsoon crop every year, but no source of irrigation water

C. with three fertility classes (a), (b), (c) 50
less good cultivated dry-land with three reliable crops in five years, but no source of irrigation water

D. shifting cultivation, with one good and one or two less good crops in fifteen years 10

E. secondary forest 10

They proceed by steps, following the use of improved agronomic practices, from one plateau to another, each successive step becoming more difficult and costly to achieve than the last. Each step has its own biological maximum, governed by environment, to which it may rise in relation to the economic inputs which are applied. On rain-fed land without supplementary irrigation, successive plateaux may be achieved, first with maximum use of organic manures, second with optimal economic use of inorganic fertilizers, in both cases with improved but not high-yielding varieties. On cropland depending upon rains in the wet monsoon season and irrigation in the dry, higher maxima may be achieved. On land with supplementary irrigation throughout the year, with fertile soils, optimal use of organic manures and inorganic fertilizers, plant protection and high-yielding varieties, the top and ultimate plateau of yield and production may be achieved. The higher one climbs, however, the better must be the technological efficiency of the cultivators. Intensive animal husbandry in the monsoonal environment also demands a higher standard of management, nutrition and disease control than is necessary in temperate countries.

It may be asked whether yields of food crops per unit area in China, for example, have reached the static level which would be achieved with maximum use of all available organic fertilizers, according to ancient Chinese custom, plus a limited amount of inorganic fertilizers on the best land. Hou Chi-ming (1968) states that: 'apparent inability to break through the 1959 level of production, despite considerable increase in labour force, strongly suggests that an output ceiling may have been approached within the framework of traditional technology and inputs. Any significant increase in production may not be forthcoming unless modern inputs or new production functions are introduced.'

The plateaux of production that may be recognized in all the ecological and economic ecosystems of Asia would appear to provide a good basis for series of block diagrams. These would indicate the various maxima which might be expected in each — the biological, the economic, and the real level related to human ecology and response (Meadows *et al.*, 1972).

ECONOMIC AND POLITICAL CONSIDERATIONS

Lester Pearson has said: 'Neither our ecology nor our morality can survive the contrasts that exist between half the world engulfed in misery, half careening towards the supposed joys of almost unlimited consumption.'

The present book has been an objective study of one aspect of applied ecology as it affects the rural population of Asia, which provides a good proportion of that first half of the world mentioned above. All people working within Asia or in other parts of the world for the good of Asia can evolve their own interpretation of the situation described here. They may agree or disagree with the fundamental premise that any form of economic determinism or political ideology can operate only within the limits imposed by the environment and by the degree to which that influence can be reduced or modified by modern technology. The problems still remain in all their variety and severity.

It would require a parallel study fully to present the economic and political counterpart to this ecological study. A basic assumption behind much economic and political discussion of Asian development is that the nutritional privileges of the advanced world shall be maintained. There is much talk of gaps between the developed and undeveloped nations in trade, in standards of living, in gross domestic product per head of population (Table 16/2), availability of foods

TABLE 16/2

Gross domestic product
per head of population, 1969

Country	U.S. dollars per annum
Hongkong	611
India	74
Indonesia	539
Japan	1,628
Korea	225
Malaysia	344
Pakistan	129
Philippines	206
Singapore	773
Taiwan	,334
Thailand	181
Australia	2,401
New Zealand	1,821

Note: There are some surprising discrepancies possibly due to different methods of calculation

Source: *New Nation*, Singapore, 6 March 1971

of quantity and quality, and other economic criteria. There is a theory that population growth is the only force powerful enough to compel rural communities to seek newer and more productive agricultural methods. The sequel is the belief that it is quite wrong to provide food aid; this has the effect of reducing their efforts to get themselves out of their predicament. Conversely, an Asian country already greatly helped by technical assistance and food aid has said that foreign aid is a new kind of slavery. Some consider that 'the day of the pessimists is over', because of the supposed success of the green revolution, and that we are moving into an era of surpluses of foodgrains (but with no purchasing power to buy them).

The rural Asian cultivator is a poor man. It is therefore a question how, on that percentage of the total cultivated and irrigable area that will respond to the new technology, the cultivators may be induced to retain some of their increased and perhaps more diversified production for consumption by their own families. The temptation for poor producers to sell everything is great, when they are faced with the pull of a free market economy; the efficiency of extraction of food from the rural areas in a totalitarian regime leaves them little choice.

There are those who say that the attitudes to population growth and hunger tend to be emotional and psychological, much influenced by personal dreams. On the other hand, the former Director-General of FAO, Dr. B.R. Sen, says: 'Hunger is more than a technical problem, it is also a social and moral problem, one that cannot be solved without drawing upon the ideas, skills and energies of whole societies.'

There is another school of thought that is deeply concerned that the rural peoples, exposed as they increasingly are to press, radio and other urban influences, may not have the patience to allow the economic sequence of events associated with planning and development to work themselves out. How long will they continue to bear considerable hardships for the sake of a theoretical agricultural revolution and a new era of ample and diversified nutrition for their families? There is already a sense of urgency to be seen. Is Hodson (1969) correct when he states that poverty, unemployment, and discontent are far more dangerous in a concentrated mass in the cities than when scattered over rural areas, villages and small towns? If so, the rural people had better be kept waiting; the present policy of urban-oriented production and distribution of food is correct.

But there is still another consideration of great political and economic significance. It is now recognized that there is a close relation between protein nutrition from conception to 5 years of age and the development of the brain (Chapter 11). The most significant question in nutrition research throughout the world is whether, as seems increasingly apparent, early protein deprivation is responsible for an impaired mental capacity subsequently to acquire and to use knowledge and experience. If so, we face a situation where the intellectual capacity of separate human individuals, with degree and variability controlled by genetic factors, may be promoted or hindered in full expression due to the nutritional environment in the critical periods of human life (Chapter 10).

We must await further reports of studies on the effect on chromosome abnormalities at mitosis in blood samples and bone marrow of an earlier period of advanced protein-calorie malnutrition in children (Armendares, Salamanca and Frenk, 1971), and whether malnourished children are abnormally susceptible to haematological malignancy. The possible relation between early malnutrition and the later behaviour of reproductive cells at and after meiosis must also be considered.

One may thus visualize something much more sinister than Tinker's 'broken-backed state', the term he proposed for an Asian situation where a democratic government persists without functioning effectively, and where the community falls back on the resources of tradition and religion (1969). Rather there is the possibility of vast populations of intellectually stunted and malleable human material. These would be ideal for manipulation by a ruling elite, in support of political systems and ideologies which they cannot possibly understand. Also, in the present context, it is not realistic to discuss new technologies and agricultural revolutions if rural cultivators do not have the level of intelligence required to appreciate and apply new techniques up to the necessary standard of economic efficiency.

Thus it can be seen that the ever-changing theories and fashions of economics and politics are out of place in a study on the long-term of the biology of food production and the ecology of rural nutrition. Quite a different approach would be needed to review the relation between human nutrition and the numerous Asian political and economic systems and ideologies, none of which yet appears to bear promise of being more successful than any other in coping with land/population problems.

A politico-economic study would show the relation between Asia and the rest of the world:

(a)   how the outside world looks at Asia, seen as misusing and misinterpreting the objectives of technical assistance and food aid, lacking sufficient effort and energy on the part of governments and people;

(b)   how Asia looks at the outside world, which it regards as losing interest in aiding developing nations; as having evolved a double standard for world nutrition by proposing the retirement of land from food production to human recreation in one part of the world, before it has been proved whether another part, namely Asia, can ever hope from its own resources to feed its children up to an acceptable nutritional level (Chapter 12).

The primary objective here has been to present the biological, ecological and anthropological factors that have operated to bring Asian nutrition to its present condition. Modern nutritional science has shown the targets which must be the aim of the future. Then those who talk in terms of biological maximal production will have to adjust their ideas and accept the constraints that operate, especially the economic and the human. It is essential to know far more about human ecology. If this book stimulates more intensive study of the nutritional ecology of the rural peoples of different ethnic and socio-economic groups in the manifold ecosystems of the monsoonal and equatorial environments, it will have achieved its purpose.

APPENDIX

Appendix

REGIONAL DIETARY PATTERNS

IT is the complex environmental pattern described in the main text that above all governs the practices and standards of rural nutrition in Asia. The characteristic diets of some 140 rural Asian communities have been assembled in this appendix. They have been classified on the basis of the most important food staple, contributing 60 to 90 per cent of the total food intake (see contents below).

In each case study, information is given, when it was available, regarding the foods of plant and animal origin which provide additional items in the diet; daily or other intakes; expenditure on food; and methods of preparation and cooking. Surveys made by nutritionists and doctors give details of nutrient intake, while those by anthropologists and workers only incidentally concerned with food are naturally less precise in this respect.

The geography of rural diets is affected by the type of land use and farming system, and the economic status and purchasing power of the rural people. The rural dietary patterns of Asia are governed by the ecology of the primary staple. Finally, and perhaps most important as far as balance in the diet is con-

FIG. A/1   Principal ethno-dietary zones of monsoon and equatorial Asia

cerned, are the ethnic and religious factors which divide the region into the western group of peoples, mainly of Caucasoid race, in the Indian subcontinent, the eastern Mongoloid group of peoples, and, in the south-east Asian and equatorial parts of the region, the Melanesian peoples (see Chapters 2 and 5).

The primary characteristics which have been considered in mapping these three main ethno-dietary regions (see Fig. App. 1) are:

(a)   *Western Monsoon Asia:* principal staples in order of importance are: rice, millets and wheat. Milk is acceptable and tolerated by most, especially in the north, when available. Flesh food (except beef) would be acceptable to a large proportion if economically available (especially mutton and chicken). Pulses play a regular part in the diet in the north, appear less frequently in the south, but are nowhere consumed in consistently adequate amounts. Consumption of vegetables and fruits is inadequate.

(b)   *Eastern Mainland and Insular Monsoon Asia:* principal staples in order of importance are: rice, wheat, sorghum, sweet potato, maize and barley. Milk becomes acceptable only after special training and adaptation from an early age, as in Japan. The preferred source of animal protein and that best adapted to east Asian agriculture is the pig; its use is severely limited for economic reasons. The soybean is an important source of plant protein, but its contribution has been greatly exaggerated. Vegetables are acceptable, with marked seasonal fluctuation in availability; intake per caput is small. The distinction between rural and urban diets so characteristic of the region does not apply to the farming community within access of the markets of urban Japan.

(c)   *South-East and Equatorial Asia:* the principal staple is rice, with some communities subsisting on cassava, maize, sweet potato and sago. Preferences for flesh foods have been influenced by the intrusion of Buddhist, Islamic and Chinese cultural traditions (Chapter 4). Most of Asia's 25 million families of shifting cultivators live in this region; these will eat most animals, fish and insects that they can hunt or trap. They will also forage for edible roots and plants in addition to the vegetables they grow. In contrast, wet rice farmers have little variety and inadequate balance in their diets. The only significant variety in the diets of the settled dry-land farmers may be in the form of secondary cereals and root crops. There is a small production of some of the Indian pulses and soybean, but again they play a quantitatively insignificant part in the diet. This is a difficult environment for the economic production of milk; consequently fresh milk is unavailable, unacceptable and not well tolerated, although there is a market for various forms of condensed and dried milk.

In the western section of Monsoon Asia, fish is consumed fresh in small amounts by coastal peoples, by communities along rivers and, in season, near lakes and large ponds. In the rest of Asia fish is acceptable fresh, dried, salted or fermented as a sauce. It is consumed along the coasts and rivers of China, Korea and Japan, but is most important in sector (c). Again, quantities consumed per caput are small.

Eggs are an expensive luxury to rural people, and almost universally sold. If the total estimated annual production of India or China is related to their total human populations, availability per caput is not more than twelve eggs per person per year — an artificial figure, since most of the eggs are consumed in urban areas. The figure for region (c) is even lower.

CASE STUDIES: REGIONAL DIETS

STAPLE FOOD	COUNTRY	STUDY NUMBERS
Rice, predominantly rice, rice and wheat, rice and millets, rice and maize, rice and barley, rice and cassava	India	1 to 15
	Nepal	16
	East Pakistan — Bangla Desh	17 and 18
	Ceylon — Sri Lanka	19 and 20
	Burma	21 to 24
	Malaysia	25 to 34
	Indonesia	35 to 43
	Thailand	44 to 52
	Cambodia	53 and 54
	South Vietnam	55 to 58
	Laos	59 to 61
	North Vietnam	62 and 63
	Philippines	64 to 76
	China	77 to 79
	Taiwan	80 and 81
	Okinawa (Japan)	83
	South Korea	84 to 86
	Japan	87 to 90
Sorghum and millets	India	91 to 101
	China	102 to 104
Maize, rice/maize	India	105 to 112
	Nepal	113
	Burma	114
	Indonesia	115 to 117
Wheat, wheat/bajra/rice	Pakistan	118
	India	119 to 124
	China	125
Barley	India	126
	South Korea	127
Sweet potato	Philippines	128
	Taiwan	129
	China	130
Sweet potato/millet/wheat	Okinawa (Japan)	131
Yams/bamboo shoots	Thailand	132
Cassava	Malaysia	133 and 134
	Indonesia	135
Sago	Malaysia	136
	Indonesia	137 and 138
Buckwheat	China	139
Pandanus/coconuts/roots/tubers	Andaman and Nicobar Islands (India)	140

LIST OF TABLES

| **1** | RICE | INDIA | KANTHER TERANG, ASSAM | SAIKIA, 1968 |

The Agro-Economic Research Centre for North-East India at Jorhat, Assam, has studied this village at five-year intervals. Economic data relate to the years 1960 and 1965, and the demographic data to March 1961 and March 1962. Shifting cultivation is primary occupation. Tribal villagers are unwilling to change; are apathetic towards educational and medical facilities available in urban centre in vicinity. Although yield from shifting cultivation low, diversity of crops remains attraction.

Consumption of rice per caput high, but food usually means boiled rice alone; other items not considered important ingredients. Adults take two meals a day, children take rice three or four times a day. A substantial part of the rice crop is used to prepare rice beer. Diet not adequate or balanced, but reasonable compared with rural areas nearby.

In 1965, most families used money obtained by selling other agricultural products to buy rice from market. They now grow and consume more maize than before. Pulses introduced; more vegetables than pulses consumed. Milk taken in tea at stalls. Some occasionally purchase fish or meat. No source of fruitful investment; earnings spent on food and 'fancy items'.

TABLE A/1

Food intake per head per day, Assam 1960 and 1965

	1960 *gm.*	*1965* *gm.*
Rice	582	750
Other cereals	15	53
Pulses	10	16
Sugar and gur	12	10
Mustard oil	—	6
Salt	22	20
Fish	15	21
Meat	12	10
Tea	2	3
Vegetables	101	117

| **2** | RICE | INDIA | JARA, NORTH-EAST FRONTIER AGENCY | CENSUS OF INDIA (1966c) |

Paddy husked for one or two meals at a time. Water entirely absorbed during cooking. Vegetables and meat cut into large pieces and boiled with chilli powder and salt. Each person consumes about 0.5 kg. food per day.

| **3** | RICE | INDIA | WEST BENGAL (AROUND CALCUTTA) | WEST BENGAL, 1968 |

TABLE A/2

Food intake per head per day
(in gm.)

	Howrah	Hooghly	Burdwan	Burdwan (Santhal)
Rice	260	400	403	503
Wheat	150	50	90	2
Bengal gram	10		1	0.2
Black gram			4	0.2
Green gram	10		5	0.6
Lentil	15	3	10	3
Leafy vegetables	80	156	51	57
Non-leafy vegetables	100	80	50	18
Roots and tubers		143	118	13
Fruits		5		9
Vegetable oil	55	21	10	7
Milk		65	75	15

Meat	2	3		1.7
Fish	15	17	40	30
Egg		0.2	1.3	
Crabs and snails			1	6
Sugar and jaggery	25	40	33	0.3
Condiments		9		
Toddy				4.5
Bread		1		

TABLE A/3

Nutrient intake per head per day
(in gm.)

Protein	50	45.7	62.1	43.2
Animal protein	3	5.4	9.7	6.6
Vegetable protein	47	40.3	52.4	36.6
Fat	60	27.3	18.9	11.8
Carbohydrate	373	428	521	419
Calories (number)	2237	2141	2505	1962

4	RICE	INDIA	SOUTHERN STATES	K.S. RAO, (1962)

Everywhere great deficiency of protective foods such as vegetables, meat and milk. Fishermen's children suffer from kwashiorkor because fish cash crop, all sold. Milk mostly sold, unless in areas remote from towns. In two villages, all used rice, wheat or millet.

Half had vegetables either daily or on alternate days, others less frequently. Two-thirds never used milk, remainder mostly only in tea. One-third used pulses daily or on alternate days. Cereal main source of protein. Contribution of pulses, meat and milk very small.

5	RICE	INDIA	MAYUR, KERALA	AIYAPPAN, 1965

In the coastal coconut belt, rice and other food must be bought; vegetables do not thrive in shade of coconut palms, and are little eaten. Colocasia, pulses, banana, tapioca and chillis grown. People entirely dependent on coconuts for cash and subsistence, and on

fish from backwaters. Coconut meat used for curries and sweets, coconut oil for cooking, its shell for fuel. Boiled tapioca disliked. Tea popular. Milk of cows, buffaloes and goats supplied to tea shops. Milk, eggs and soup eaten only on doctor's advice.

6	PREDOMINANTLY RICE	INDIA	MULAVUCAD, ISLAND BACKWATER, COCHIN	CENSUS OF INDIA, 1966e

Coffee and rice flour preparation for breakfast, rice or rice gruel for supper. Lunch rice with fish or meat and vegetables. Supper the same. Rice staple, with 17.89 per cent using tapioca as substitute. Coco-

nut, coconut oil, fish, meat and milk used by all, but in limited quantities. Few vegetables other than onions and potatoes.

7	PREDOMINANTLY RICE	INDIA	THEKKUMBHAGOM, NEAR ERNAKULAM, KERALA	CENSUS OF INDIA, 1966e

Three meals eaten daily.
Breakfast: Rice gruel, coffee or tea, with tapioca or rice-flour preparation.
Lunch: Rice, fish or meat.
Supper: Same.

50.39 per cent use only rice, others mix small amounts of tubers. 23.25 per cent vegetarians. Expenditure on milk, fish and vegetable oils higher than in other villages in region.

| 8 | PREDOMINANTLY RICE | INDIA | ERAVIPUM, QUILON, KERALA | CENSUS OF INDIA, 1964e |

Ragi, red gram, tapioca and plantain raised. Eggs exported.
Three meals customary, though 26.98 per cent have only two.

Breakfast　　　　: Rice gruel, tea or coffee, and dosai or pittu.

Lunch and Supper : Rice. 29.36 per cent add tapioca. Some fish or meat and milk bought.

Diets better than those of coir workers, and even of fishermen (in debt).

| 9 | PREDOMINANTLY RICE | INDIA | EDAMON, QUILON, KERALA | CENSUS OF INDIA, 1964e |

Rubber and tea plantation workers, receive three meals a day.
Boiled rice from supper kept overnight in cold water for breakfast. All non-vegetarian. 75.42 per cent use only rice, others mix tapioca.

Average income:　Rs. 44.15 to Rs. 135.75. Insufficient to meet rising costs.

TABLE A/4

Food prices in 1961

Food prices, 1961	n.p. per kg.	n.p. per litre
rice	64	
chilli	208	
coriander	137	
onions	22	
tapioca	7	
green gram	77	
black gram	68	
mutton	225	
fish	40	
cow milk		55
tea	474	
sugar	121	
coconut oil		251
dehusked coconut (per 100)	2,270	
kerosene	41	
firewood	231	
areca nut	335	
tobacco	357	

| 10 | PREDOMINANTLY RICE | INDIA | TANGASSERI, QUILON, KERALA | CENSUS OF INDIA, 1964e |

Rice staple, tapioca sometimes substituted. Anglo-Indians substitute wheat.
Fish, potatoes, onions, tapioca, coconut, milk and ghee main items.

Breakfast　　　　: coffee or tea and rice or wheat preparation.

Lunch and supper : Rice with meat or vegetables.

TABLE A/5

Percentage expenditure on food items

Food	Misc. industrial workers	Carpenters	Fishermen
Rice	38.65	41.42	41.54
Coconut	7.94	8.0	
Milk	7.13	5.37	
Meat and fish		8.49	
Fish	6.67		7.71 (own catch)
Wheat	3.46		
Tapioca	2.89	6.97	10.12

Monthly earnings of fishermen Rs. 25 to 50 (45.45 per cent); Rs. 51 to 75 (36.36 per cent) and Rs. 76 to 100 (remainder)

11	PREDOMINANTLY RICE	INDIA	THAZAVA, QUILON, KERALA	CENSUS OF INDIA, 1964e

Breakfast : Rice gruel or coffee, with tapioca or rice-flour preparation.

Lunch and supper : Rice and tapioca, coconut and fish or sometimes meat.

28 per cent have two meals, 52.8 per cent three meals.

Women who do not work, and children at home have only rice gruel for breakfast and lunch. Schoolchildren get school meals. On days when men unemployed, they also get only rice gruel.

TABLE A/6

Income per household

Income level	Percentage of households	Number of families	Class
Rupees per month			
less than 25	2.4		A
25 to 50	36.0	45	B
51 to 75	32.0	40	C
67 to 100	15.2	19	D
over 100	14.0	18	E

TABLE A/7

Expenditure for five income levels

Food item	A	B	C	D	E
	Rupees per month				
Rice	8.33	11.95	17.57	21.05	30.16
Other grains	0.25	0.55	0.86	1.16	1.93
Dhal	0.08	0.43	0.35	0.46	0.72
Tapioca	4.83	5.33	5.91	5.78	5.97
Coconut	2.66	3.82	5.08	6.04	8.64
Vegetables	0.42	0.56	0.74	0.88	1.75
Fish	2.08	2.84	3.75	4.42	6.0
Meat	0.33	0.18	0.75	1.13	1.97
Milk	0.42	0.81	1.46	2.23	3.75
Ghee	0.83	1.16	1.63	1.96	2.72
Chilli	0.75	1.06	1.49	2.01	2.68
Tamarind	0.22	0.26	0.34	0.4	0.56
Other	0.83	1.1	1.47	1.88	2.51

Purchase of onions, potatoes and other vegetables did not increase with higher income.

| 12 | RICE AND WHEAT | INDIA | UTTAR PRADESH | GOVIL, PRASAD AND PANT, 1958 |

During period 1949 to 1957, dietary surveys made by Provincial Hygiene Institute, Lucknow, on 596 schoolboys living in hostels and on 3,451 persons in 581 families living in the districts in the four divisions of the State: Himalayan hills and plateau; West Gangetic Plain; Central Plain; East Plain.

More rice than wheat eaten in East Plain, vice versa in Central Plain and West Plain, but diet usually of mixed cereals. Intake of grain legumes up to recommended levels. Four-fifths of total families deficient in protective foods, leafy vegetables, milk and milk products, meat, fish, eggs, fruits and nuts.

Calorie intake: schoolboys 2,863, families 3,079; animal proteins nil or grossly deficient; variety of cereal mixtures and cereal/grain-legume mixture may provide necessary protein; calcium intake low but highly variable, and grossly deficient in schoolboys; vitamin A deficient in families, more so in schoolboys, with 11 per cent incidence of xerosis conjunctiva, and 11 per cent dull, dry and rough skin; thiamine adequate, due to mixtures of cereals and use of home-pounded, parboiled rice; all diets deficient in riboflavine; vitamin C lost in cooking; iron and niacin adequate.

| 13 | RICE/MILLETS/CASSAVA | INDIA | TRIBES | ROY AND ROY, 1962 |

North-east (N.E.F.A.) and east India: Padam, Gallong, Minyong Abors of Abor Hills and Rang tribes of Tripura
Central India   : Bhumia, Baigis and Murias
South-west India: Uralis, Kanikkars, Malapantarams, Muthuvans, Ullatans (Kerala) Todas, Kotas, Irulas, Urali and Mulla Kurumbas (Nilgiri District, Tamil Nadu)

All depend on agriculture, except Todas and other tribes of Nilgiri hills. N.E.F.A. and Tripura tribes, and the Baigas practise shifting and settled agriculture. N.E.F.A. grow paddy and *Coix lacryma-jobi* by shifting cultivation; Tripura tribes grow paddy and tubers. Baigas grow millets by shifting cultivation. Murias of Bastar almost entirely settled cultivators. Todas pastoralists, with potatoes and cabbage grown by paid labourers.

Some tribals own land, some employed by State Forest Departments; these may raise some tapioca. Labour in plantations and forest departments basis of economy of tribes of Kerala and Nilgiris. Wherever possible, income supplemented by poultry raising, weaving and gathering forest products.

Staple of N.E.F.A., and Tripura tribes, the Murias of Bastar, the Mulla and Urali Kurumbas is rice; that of Bhumia Baigas of Madhya Pradesh and Muthuvans of Kerala different millets; of Irulas and Kotas, half rice, half millets, and of remaining Kerala tribes, tapioca.

Pulses eaten in quantity only by Murias and Kotas.

Kerala tribes have few vegetables; important in diets of other tribes. Food mostly cooked staple with boiled vegetables (brinjal, gourd, bean or radish, and in some areas, wild leaves and shoots). Bamboo shoots and mushrooms eaten. Dried vegetables. Large amounts of potato eaten in Nilgiris.

Meat appreciated by all but Todas, especially pork. Chicken rarely eaten. Abor hills depend on Esso, semi-domesticated animal with body like buffalo, but appearance of cow. Tripura tribes sacrifice buffalo, Murias cow or bull. Many depend on hunting for meat, while field rat, insects and grubs eaten. Flesh consumption very low. Fish liked, but few can get regularly. Hunted animals not always available. Domestic animals not killed. Only Todas' animals give enough milk.

Daily diet monotonous, mostly cooked cereal and boiled vegetables, sometimes chutney and pickles. Meat at festivals. Alcohol widely drunk, adding perhaps calories, proteins, minerals and B-group vitamins.

Gross deficiency of vitamins A, C and the B-complex, and calcium, except with Todas. South Indian tribes deficient in calories and total protein. Diets of many tribals low in animal protein, vitamin A, calcium and riboflavine. Todas lack vitamins A and C, and the Padam Abors lack animal protein and riboflavine, but both tribes have diets superior to non-tribal peoples in their States.

Seasonality of diet has not been studied among tribal peoples.

| 14 | RICE/CASSAVA | INDIA | ANKAMALI, ERNAKULAM, KERALA | CENSUS OF INDIA, 1966e |

Rice staple for 36.13 per cent; remainder mixed rice/cassava. All non-vegetarians.
Breakfast   :   Rice-flour gruel, pittu or dosai.
Lunch and supper: Staple with fish, ghee, chillis and other condiments, coconut, little dhal and onion. Few vegetables eaten.

TABLE A/8

Expenditure at different income levels
(Rupees per month)

Food item	25 to 50	Over 76	Over 100
Rice	14		
Dhal	0.28		
Cassava, potatoes vegetables	9.48		
Meat and fish	3		
Fish		4 to 5	
Meat			2.66
Milk		2	
Chillis/other condiments		2.25	3.42

15	RICE/CASSAVA	INDIA	KURICHY, KOTTAYAM, KERALA	CENSUS OF INDIA, 1966e

Breakfast: Coffee and boiled tapioca.
Lunch : Rice gruel and curry (fish, chilli, pulse, onion).
Supper : Rice and curry
Employed eat three meals daily. Labourer may have only two, or one in difficult times. Both rice gruel. Majority non-vegetarian. Fish eaten more than meat. One tribal group eats mice, rats, bandicoots and crocodile flesh.

16	RICE AND MAIZE	NEPAL	1 URBAN SITE AND 18 VILLAGES THROUGHOUT COUNTRY	BROWN, WORTH AND SHAH 1968a AND b

Dietary and clinical survey of 6,321 people in 957 households in eighteen villages and one urban site made during 1965/66 by team from Ministry of Health, Kingdom of Nepal, School of Public Health of University of Hawaii, and the Thomas A. Dorley Foundation. Geographic sample covered western, central and eastern mountains from 330 to 2,280 metres, and the eastern, mid-west and far-west Terai, 105 to 175 metres.

TABLE A/9

Nutrient intake per head per day for nineteen sampling sites

	Mean intake	Range
Calories	2440	1,930 — 3,550
Protein (gm.)	66	45.4 — 98.0
Fat (gm.)	35	20.4 — 47.9
Carbohydrate (gm.)	463	371 — 679
Calcium (mg.)	357	194 — 660
Iron (mg.)	12.6	9.1 — 19.6
Vitamin A (i.u.)	1960	3 — 10,643
Thiamine (mg.)	2.1	1.6 — 3.3
Riboflavine (mg.)	0.7	0.3 — 1.0
Niacin (mg.)	22	10.6 — 37.5
Ascorbic acid (mg.)	5	1 — 15

TABLE A/10

Food intake per head per day for nineteen sampling sites
compared with FAO recommendations

	Average intake gm./day	*FAO long-term target gm./day*	*Percentage of 19 villages above target*
Cereals	586	361	100
Beans and nuts	54	80	32
Vegetables and fruits	41	315	0
Meat, fish, eggs, poultry	22	104	0
Milk	122	140	37
Fats and oils	14	24	11

Mean nutrient intakes per caput varied widely among villages; calorie and protein intakes higher than reported for other areas of Far East. Virtually all protein contributed by grains. Calcium, riboflavine, vitamin A and ascorbic acid intakes low, but probably underestimated due to seasonal availability of vegetables and fruits. Thiamine and niacin intakes in general adequate, due to consumption of largely whole-grain cereals.

Dhal, meat and rice most favoured during pregnancy; milk and milk products not considered valuable at this time. Infant feeding related to caste. Vaisyas, predominant caste in Nepal, breast-feed for longer periods, add supplementary foods at a later age than most castes. Supplements rice with some high-protein foods; other castes choose rice or bread as supplements.

17	RICE	EAST PAKISTAN	GENERAL	MAQSOOD, 1961

TABLE A/11

Protein values of some diets and meals (per cent)

	Protein Calories per cent	*NPU (op) per cent*	*NDP Cals per cent*
East Pakistan diet	9.0	59	5.3
Rice/pulse/fish/vegetable curry	11.6	57	6.6
Rice/pulse/vegetable curry	10.4	63	6.6
Rice/pulse (khichri)	9.6	66	6.3

By end of second Five-Year Plan, energy value of diet higher, but protein content lower; Deficiency of minerals and vitamins owing to method of cooking rice.

18	RICE	EAST PAKISTAN	SEVENTEEN RURAL LOCATIONS	PAKISTAN GOVERNMENT, 1966.

85 per cent earned less than Rs. 200 per month, 5 per cent more than Rs. 300. Three meals daily, except in time of hardship when only two or even one taken. *Breakfast*: Rice or wheat preparation. Puffed rice, boiled rice or rice cakes, or leftover rice soaked in water overnight. Pulses might be added and cooked with spices to thick soup. Leafy green vegetables chopped to paste, highly spiced and fried in mustard, often with pulse-bread preparation. Wheat taken as chapathi, or less commonly, paratha.

Lunch: Large quantity of boiled rice with fish or vegetable curry. Sometimes meat (beef, mutton or poultry). In times of hardship, millet boiled with rice. Wheat chapathi may replace rice. Chillis and onions invariably eaten, either raw or in curry.
Evening meal: Same as lunch, often leftovers.
Rice generally parboiled. White potato frequently cooked with curry. Molasses main sweet item. Pulses and lentils prominent, usually eaten as dhal (masur, mung, lentils, black gram, Bengal gram). Vegetables

TABLE A/12

Food intake per head per day

	gm.
Cereals	536.9
Starchy roots	55.5
Sugars and sweets	7.4
Pulses and nuts	28.0
Vegetables	134.6
(Leafy green vegetables)	(15.8)
Fruits	10.2
Meat	5.7
Egg	1.6
Fish	32.8
Milk and cheese	17.3
Fats and oils	6.2
Miscellaneous spices	4.6

mostly colourless pumpkins and gourds in curries or fried. Green leafy vegetables generally mashed, fried in mustard oil and eaten with rice or chapathi. Unripe banana, papaya, jackfruit cooked and eaten as vege-tables. Unripe mango as condiment. Raw cucumber, onions, chillis and sometimes tomato used as salad on special occasions.

Milk curds popular in higher-income families. Fish only animal product regularly consumed by poorer households, freshwater preferred to dried or sea fish. Milk used in tea or for children and babies. Most live-stock products sold except when consumed at village feasts.

Nutritious leafy green vegetables only 12 per cent of total vegetable intake, thus inadequate. Daily meat intake inadequate in rural areas. Average chicken in-take 2.4 gm., beef 2.4 gm. and mutton 0.9 gm. per day. One duck or hen egg eaten each 22 days; con-sumption in lower-income families negligible, increas-ing sharply with income above Rs. 200 per month. Even poorest households consume approximately 28 gm. milk per head per day, though this drops during monsoon. (Cow milk 15 gm., goat milk 0.5 gm., curd 1.5 gm.). Milk consumption doubles with incomes over Rs. 300 per month. Milk production rises during fruit season, when cattle eat mango, papaya and jack-fruit peel. Protein intake below recommended level for over 60 per cent of households; most derived from cereals.

19	RICE	CEYLON	VARIOUS	CULLUMBINE, 1951

Survey of 1,307 families, 6,332 individuals, from families of urban, rural and estate populations in dif-ferent parts of the country, being Sinhalese, Ceylon Tamils, Indian Tamils and Ceylon Moors. Three eco-nomic levels distinguished, with income per adult per month in Rs.: less than 20, between 20 and 50, and above 50.

Quantity and quality of foods eaten depend on family income; in two lower-income groups, energy value of diet much less than in highest-income group. In lowest-income group, intakes of fat, calcium, phos-phorus, iron, vitamin A, the vitamin B complex and ascorbic acid absolutely and relatively low; findings related to a low intake of dairy products, eggs and meat, and relatively low intake of fish. Associated was high incidence of signs of undernutrition and mal-nutrition, skin lesions and anaemia. Diet of Moors was greatly inferior to other racial groups at all eco-nomic levels. Other racial groups showed individual differences in diet and close correspondence between average composition of the diet as calculated for each group and incidence of signs of nutritional deficien-cies. Urban families of lowest-income group ate more than similar rural families; at higher income levels, little difference between amounts eaten by urban and rural families. Estate population of Indian Tamils, ex-cept for four families, belonged to the middle-income group, diet superior in energy value and in most other respects to those of other groups.

(from abstract by L. Wills in *Nutrition Abstracts and Reviews*)

20	RICE	CEYLON	VARIOUS	BIBILE, CULLUMBINE, WATSON AND WICKREMANAYAKE, 1949

Survey of some thirty families of four different races from three areas in dry zone and two in wet zone. Three economic levels expressed as families with monthly income per adult consumption unit of Rs.: less than 20; 20 to 50, and more than 50. Majority belonged to middle-income category.

More than half of all families had not enough calo-ries; about 200 gm. per adult per day for all poorer families needed to correct this. Nearly all diets defi-cient in vitamin A; xerophthalmia and phrynoderma common, though the latter not closely correlated with intake of vitamin A. Majority of diets adequate in thiamine but not in riboflavine or nicotinic acid; phys-ical signs of deficiency rare.

Only two possible cases of scurvy seen; bases for calculating ascorbic acid content of diet were con-sidered probably to underestimate it. Intake of phos-phorus sufficient but calcium grossly inadequate. Signs of rickets rare, probably owing to ample sunlight. In-cidence of dental caries low. Intake of iron adequate for normal community, but hookworm infestation prevalent and haemoglobin values low.

(from abstract by E.M. Hume in *Nutrition Abstracts and Reviews*)

21	RICE	BURMA	EIGHT VILLAGES, SOUTH AND CENTRAL BURMA	ICNND 1963b

Nutrient	*Adequacy*
Calories	Between 2,000 and 2,300, one village having 15 per cent less.
Protein	Acceptable range, 19 per cent from animal sources.
Thiamine	Below acceptable range; 0.24 mg. per 1,000 calories, due to method of cooking rice, and limited use of pork and pulses.
Riboflavine	Below acceptable range; small intake of meat, milk and pulses.
Niacin	Low but acceptable.
Vitamin A	Low but acceptable by chemical analysis.
Vitamin C	Lowest limit of acceptable range by chemical analysis.
Calcium	Only two of five locations acceptable by chemical analysis.
Iron	High prevalence of anaemia.
Iodine	High prevalence of goitre.

TABLE A/13

Food intake per head per day
(in gm.)

Location	Rice	Vegetables	Sugar white	black	Pulse	Meat	Fresh fish	Ngapi
Indagaw	580	75	6.6	29.2	23	39	91	23
Kyee Taw	525	105	10.7	10.3	13	48	94	24
Shwe Daung	592	169	18	29	15	15	7	7
Lauk Sauk	472	102	4.5	5.7	13	28	13	8
Sé Bauk	473	154		22	4	22		11
Myaing-Gyi	580	184	15.5	17.1	31	39	7	20
Wet Wun	532	149	8.4	10.3	20	32	7	14
Ngayan Chaung	648	146	50	5	61	47	23	2

Location	Egg	Fruit	Misc.	Salt	Tinned milk	Dry fish	Fishpaste	Fresh milk
Indagaw	0.5	67	30	15	1	7	19	
Kyee Taw	9	52	32	18	2	8	4	
Shwe Daung	1	30	30	15		9		
Lauk Sauk	4	61	35	14	4	8	3	
Sé Bauk	4	59	35	14		2		
Myaing-Gyi	8	56	39	17	1	9		50
Wet Wun	9	39	42	20	2			32
Ngayan Chaung	7	58	49	31				11

Rice cooked either once daily (morning) or twice (morning and early afternoon). Curries and soups cooked once daily.

22	RICE	BURMA	NONDWIN, DRY ZONE VILLAGE NEAR MANDALAY	NASH, 1965

Annual expenditure on food (in kyat)	higher-income: 4,017.84	(1 kyat = 21 US cents)
	middle-income: 1,670.76	(1 viss = 1.62 kg.)
	lower-income: 708.6	(100 tics = 1 viss)

Staple: rice, with beans, oil and fish.

TABLE A/14

Monthly expenditure on major items of food in two income levels

Item	Price	per kyat	Middle-income		Lower-income	
			Amount	Total kyat	Amount	Total kyat
Cooking oil	4	viss	3.50 viss	14.00	1 viss	4.00
Firewood	3	cartload	1 cartload	3.00	0.5 cartload	1.5
Salt	0.5	viss	2 viss	1.00	2.5 viss	1.5
Sugar	2	viss	50 tics	1.00		
Rice	11	basket	300 baskets	33.00	200 baskets	22.00
Beans	11	basket	0.25 basket	3.00		2.00
Egg (chicken)	0.25	each				
Egg (duck)	0.25	each	8 eggs	2.00	4 eggs	1.00
Milk	0.75	viss	1.5 viss	1.25		
Fish	4	viss	2 viss	8	50 tics	2.00
Dried fish	10	viss	0.25 viss	2.50	0.25 viss	2.50
Chilli, dry	4	viss	0.5 viss	2.00	0.25 viss	1.00
Ngapi	2.50	viss	1 viss	3.50	0.50 viss	1.75
Beef	2	viss	1.50 viss	3.00		
Chicken	4	viss				
Pork	4	viss	1 viss	4.00	0.50 viss	2.00
Peanuts	8	basket				
Bananas	0.5	bunch				
Cabbage (Dec./May)	0.2	viss	1 head	0.1	0.5 head	0.05
Carrots (Dec./March)	0.5	viss	1 viss	0.2	0.5 viss	0.1
Onions	2	viss	0.5 viss	1.00	0.25 viss	0.5
Tomato	2	viss	3 viss	6.00	1 viss	2.00
Maize (Oct./Dec.)	1.25	100	500 ears	1.6	100 ears	0.3
Ngabyayei	2.5	viss	2 viss	5.00	1 viss	2.50
Average per month				139.23		59.05

23	RICE	BURMA	SOUTHERN CHIN HILLS	LEHMAN, 1963

Rice staple, few vegetables grown. Pumpkin, yam and taro during season of scarcity, after which wild tubers and calcareous fruits of some banyan eaten. Large white pumpkin most common. Few condiments used, mainly salt substitutes. Fishing in slack season.

24	RICE	BURMA	BURMESE SHANS, MOSTLY IN SHAN STATE, PLATEAU 1,000 m.	LEBAR, HICKEY AND MUSGRAVE, 1964

Primarily settled wet-rice agriculturists, with garden crops important and animal husbandry secondary. Gathering of wild products, but fish mostly purchased in markets. Irrigated terraces cut in mountain-sides, dry rice grown in upland areas. Crops include rice, tobacco, cotton, sugar cane and maize; garden plots produce peas, beans, okra, tomatoes, cucumbers. Oranges, bananas, melons and mangoes cultivated, and wild fruits, apples, pears and papaya gathered. Horses, water buffalo, pigs and chickens raised.

Staple diet is rice and vegetables, supplemented with fish, pork, beef and chicken. Pickled foods popular. Snails, frogs, larvae of certain beetles, wasps and bees eaten.

| 25 | RICE | MALAYSIA | OBSERVATIONS ON THREE ETHNIC GROUPS (MALAY, INDIAN, CHINESE) | WOLFF, 1962 |

Malay diet monotonous. Chinese spent more than other groups; diet slightly better but quantities still small. Only Indians ate parboiled rice. Almost every side dish cooked with chillis, pepper and salt. Chinese eat fresh or dried pork at most meals. Pork, fish or prawns generally cut into small pieces, then cooked with spices and vegetables in soup or sauce, Indian method similar. Eggs eaten infrequently by all groups, and in very small amounts; scrambled egg sprinkled over fish or cut hardboiled in curry. Pulses and grams eaten frequently by Indians and soybean by Chinese, less frequently by Malays. Vegetables used by Chinese at most meals, but usually those with least value; cucumber, cabbage. Malays eat little vegetable; their meals usually rice, fish and red pepper. Fruit (usually banana) snack rather than part of meal for all groups. Quantities of non-rice food small in all diets.

| 26 | RICE | WEST MALAYSIA | JENDRAM HILIR, SELANGOR | WILSON, P.J. 1967 |

Wealthier households eat more expensive food (meat, fish, poultry and vegetables) as lauk or side dishes; poor eat less. Average weekly household expenditure per week is M$3.20, often supplemented by home-produced fish, vegetables and occasionally eggs. $20 weekly income considered adequate to provide varied diet.

| 27 | RICE | W. MALAYSIA | PARIT DISTRICT, PERAK STATE | THOMSON, 1960 |

TABLE A/15

Nutrient intake per head per day as percentage of recommended allowances

	Intake found	*Recommended allowance*	*Intake as percentage of recommended allowance*
Calories	1,812	2,126	85.2
(Rice 1,064)			
Protein (gm.)	49	65	75.3
(animal protein 20 gm.,			
40 per cent; vegetable			
protein 29 gm., 60 per			
cent)			
Fat (gm.)	23		
Calcium (gm.)	0.57	1.1	51.8
Iron (mg.)	7	11	63.6
Vitamin A (i.u.)	1,988	4,275	46.4
Thiamine (mg.)	0.56	1.1	50.9
Riboflavine (mg.)	0.40	1.6	25.0
Nicotinic acid (mg.)	9.2	10.8	85.2
Ascorbic acid (mg.)	34	73	46.5

28 RICE WEST MALAYSIA PERAK KAMPONG, MALACCA KAMPONG McARTHUR, 1962

TABLE A/16

Two-week survey of consumption and expenditure in Perak kampong
(average of 30 households)

Number in family	Wage earners	Animal food per head per day (fresh raw) (gm.)	Milk purchased (sweetened condensed) (gm.)	Cost M.\$ Solids/animal	Milk
6	3	72.4		2.95	
4	1	87.8**		3.45	
3	1	91.0**		1.95	
6	2	61.3		2.40	
7	2	62.1		2.65	
4	2	82.2		2.05	
7	3	76.4	170.4	2.60	1.65 **
4	2	104.4	277.2	3.30	2.20
4	1	100.3	56.8	2.35	0.55
8	2	59.2	44.6	3.05	0.80
7	1	89.1		4.35	
7	2	100.3		3.20	
5	1	68.0		2.05	
7 *	2	75.6	56.8	2.60	0.6
5.55	1.9	84.7	100.5	2.89	1.25

*   1 child absent 5 days a week for one meal
**   family absent one whole day during survey

Food boiled rice with side dishes of animal or vegetable foods, or, if not available, a sambal made of chillis, salt and lemon juice always present. Flavourings — 'without them people could not eat enough rice to keep going'. Meat, fish or egg side dishes preferred to vegetables. Spices important.

	Early morning	*Afternoon*	*Evening*
Malacca	wheat flour, bananas	rice	rice
Perak	mostly rice, some wheat flour	rice	rice

Rice cooked twice daily; in Perak once early in morning and early mid-afternoon on return from fields. Evening meal cold leftovers. Side dishes prepared once daily, usually before lunch, some put aside. More coconuts available in Malacca (3 or 4 a week). More frying of food in Perak. In calculating nutritive value of foods, dried fish, prawns and belachan doubled. Animal protein intake from 30 to 50 gm. per head per day in Malacca, 25 per cent less in Perak. Households buying over 100 gm. animal protein per head were school teachers. Larger families did not buy more food for side dishes as they said it would not be eaten. Leafy greens: spinach, radish, Chinese chives, cabbage, mustard leaf, tops of papaya, sweet potato, tapioca, pumpkins. Snack buying widespread: rice, green gram porridge, biscuits, cakes, peanuts. Fruit not regular part of diet.

TABLE A/17

Two-week survey of consumption and expenditure in Malacca kampong
(average of 35 households)

Number in family	Wage earners	Animal food per head per day (fresh raw) (gm.)	Milk purchased (sweetened condensed) (gm.)	Cost M.\$ Solids/animal	Milk
7	2	47.8	85.2	3.70	1.50
4	1	89.1	85.2	5.25	1.55
9	1	86.4	85.2	6.25	1.65

7	1	62.2	227.2	4.35	4.45
4	1 *	43.9	66.3	0.80	1.05
5	2	31.2	113.6	0.65	2.05
6	2**	47.8		4.45	
9 ½	3	126.1	198.8	33.85	4.45
5	1***	123.0	367.0	11.78	6.60
6	4	67.3	113.6	4.55	2.15
4	2	79.4	142.0	1.88	2.75
8	2	46.0	170.4	3.85	3.05
7	3	65.7	56.8	3.64	1.00
3	1	144.9	227.2	10.9	4.55
6.2	1.7	68.5	175.9	7.20	3.61
				per week 3.60	1.80

*	at home 12 of 14 days
**	husband absent but contributed to support
***	at home 13 days

29	RICE	WEST MALAYSIA	MALACCA COASTAL PLAIN	BURGESS AND LAIDIN, 1950

Three groups: (a) smallholder agriculturists, Malays, with some Javanese and other Malaysians, one Chinese converted to Islam, living as Malays;
(b) fishermen, near agricultural community, all Malay;
(c) rubber estate workers from south India.

Diet essentially rice in all three communities, with small amounts of wheat, little fish, small amounts of vegetables, and a few highly flavoured foodstuffs. In earlier times of scarcity, other cereals and root crops used. Malays rarely eat legumes, though they are on sale. Eggs rarely eaten. Indians take milk, especially children. Indian cooking prolonged, Malay cooking swift.

Breakfast : coffee or tea; some eat leftovers, biscuits. Indians had no breakfast, and nothing eaten at this time in more than half the households.

Lunch and supper: main meals: rice, one or more side dishes.

TABLE A/18

Food intake per head per day in three communities
(in gm.)

	Smallholders	Fishermen	Plantation labour
Cereals	343	287	337
Legumes	2	0.5	27
Fresh fish	22	49	11
Dried fish	18	9	15
Prawn paste	7	7	
Meat	1	—	8
Milk	14	7	93
Leafy vegetables	16	9	19
Fruit and vegetables	11	12	47
Root vegetables	11	90	14
Sugar	18	31	45
Coconut oil	14	8	18
Fruit	5	1	7
Spices	8	7	10
Coconut flesh	9	4	8

| 30 | RICE | W. MALAYSIA | SUNGAI TEKAM, PAHANG | CHAPPELL AND JANOWITZ, 1965 |

Protein deficient in diet of most rural Malay families; 56 per cent have no meat, others rarely and in small amounts. Fish eaten by 90 per cent, usually dried, but in small quantities. Beans and spinach good source of protein, iron and vitamins A and B-complex, but consumption small. Infants under 12 months 56 per cent at breast, 44 per cent on sweetened condensed milk, with some overlap. Only 16 per cent receive powdered milk.

| 31 | RICE | W. MALAYSIA | RuMUDA, TRENGGANU, NORTH-EAST MALAYSIA | WILSON, C.S. 1970 a AND b |

Fishing village of 550 people, with sea as chief economic resource. Some rice grown. Little systematic agricultural effort apart from coconut growing. Food intakes observed in five families for about one week each. Diet of one young family, average in size, income and outlook given:

Meals : Flour pancakes with sugar
Rice noodles in coconut milk

Fish curry
Fish stew with spices
Rice
Snacks: Corn on the cob
Cakes
Banana
Green mango with soy sauce
Tea and coffee with sugar.

TABLE A/19

Nutrient intake per head per day of a Trengganu family

	Age Years	Calories	Protein gm.	Calcium mg.	Iron mg.
Othman	32	1188	33.3	326	4.8
Me' Ngah	30	1089	23.5	65	3.3
Fatimah	12	899	22.6	76	3.6
Ramlah	9	930	20.3	74	3.6
Zabeda	7	1065	24.2	91	4.5
Rohema	3	1098	24.3	97	4.8

Between-meal snacks not included. Othman (husband) daily in coffee shop, others took snacks of cakes and probably received an additional 750 to 1000 calories from drinks with condensed sweetened milk.

| 32 | RICE/CASSAVA | WEST MALAYSIA | JAKUN, DWELLING ON UPPER REACHES OF RIVERS IN SELANGOR, MALACCA, NEGRI SEMBILAN, JOHORE AND SOUTHERN PAHANG | LEBAR, HICKEY AND MUSGRAVE, 1964 |

Agricultural patterns range from swidden farming accompanied by periodic shifting of settlements through combinations of settled plantation farming with upland swiddens to wet-rice farming in permanent settlements. Rice, maize, cassava, sweet potatoes, chillis, beans, cucumbers, bananas and tobacco cultivated. Diet supplemented by hunting, fishing and gathering. Wild hogs, deer, mouse deer, monkeys, snakes, frogs, wild pigeon, partridge and pheasant hunted.

| 33 | RICE | EAST MALAYSIA | DUSUN, SABAH | WILLIAMS, 1965 |

Rice from swidden and padi supplemented with sweet potato, yam and tapioca. Adult takes three half-coconut shells per day of uncooked rice, child two. Adult requires 27 litres, child 18 litres rice per month. Household of three adults and two children requires 1,350 litres rice per year, plus 900 litres for animals, seed, ritual and social purposes.

Most families cultivate gardens and plant trees, sweet potato, greater yam, tapioca, bottle gourd, mung bean, garlic, elephant's ear, tomato, melon, squash, chilli, onion, ginger, betel, cowpea, corn mustard, peanut, pineapple, watermelon, eggplant, sugarcane, cabbage. Sago also used for food, also coconut, breadfruit, banana, mango, papaya, malay apple, durian, lime and other citrus fruits, and coffee beans.

Hunting and gathering from primary jungle. Most animals considered edible, especially pig, deer, anteater, bear, gibbon, orang-utan and other monkeys, and rats. Fishing by bamboo traps in streams, irrigation channels and padis; also by nets, lines and poles. Fruits and vegetables gathered from jungle. Vegetables, and occasionally dried and pickled meat may be marketed. Chicken, duck and some geese kept. Chicken, pig and kerabau important in ritual, subsequently eaten.

| 34 | RICE | EAST MALAYSIA | RUNGUS DUSUN, SABAH | APPELL, 1968, 1969 |

Dried, salted and fresh fish eaten several times a week. Eggs, vegetables and fruits eaten regularly. Rice taken increasingly to Chinese shops for polishing.

| 35 | RICE | INDONESIA | KUTUGAMBER, NORTH SUMATRA | SINGARIMBUN, 1967 AND 1968 |

Three meals daily, mainly rice and gulén (vegetables cooked in coconut milk), chillis and salt, or vegetables and meat/dried meat/dried fish, or meat/fish without vegetables. Occasionally gulén and fried salted fish. Crickets, locusts and other insects eaten. Hunting and fishing expeditions. Tangerines, coconut and other fruits eaten in season. Eggs and chickens kept for ceremonies and home consumption. Pigs and water buffalo for sale and important ceremonies.

| 36 | RICE | INDONESIA | SUNGEI PUAR, CENTRAL SUMATRA | FREEDMAN, 1954 |

Matrilineal Minangkabau village at 1,000 m. elevation, 9 km. from Bukit Tinggi. Sawahs support village for two months of year; other industries fill gap. Minangkabau favour meat and dislike green vegetables, considered 'fit only for goats'. However consume spinach, cabbage, long green beans, eggplant, cucumber, type of celery, Chinese cabbage, young cassava leaves. Cassava flour crisp eaten with meat, fried or boiled. Haricot beans, onions, potatoes, groundnuts, sweet potato, green gram, tomatoes used, but rarely soybean. Animal food from buffalo, Zebu cattle, goat, sheep, chicken, fish and fish paste. Beef and fish (dried or fresh from sawahs and ponds) most common. Eggs used, duck eggs preferred. Despite liking for meat, little eaten. Top-income group buys meat once a week, the lowest once a month. Buffalo beef rupiah 15 per kg., Zebu beef rupiah 17 per kg. Liver, a favourite food, rupiah 30 per kg. Household rarely buys more than 0.5 kg. meat at a time; poor spend 4 to 5 rupiahs a time.

Banana only common fruit; others eaten in season. Cream cheese from buffalo milk used for ceremonies. Early morning meal tea or coffee and snack of leftovers. Rice cooked twice daily, at 9 to 10 a.m. and 4 p.m., and eaten barely warm. Poor eat rice, chillis and grilled small fish; if they can afford, fish fried in coconut oil and onions or garlic. Cooked vegetables may be eaten on alternate days. Fresh fish available twice weekly at market, and in sawahs. Snacks of less significance than in Java.

| 37 | RICE | INDONESIA | KAMPONG UTAN, NEAR JAKARTA, JAVA | FREEDMAN, 1954 |

Meat, usually water buffalo bought by group, eaten only on feast days. Eggs rarely, and milk never consumed, except by those who keep cows. Fresh fish seldom bought because expensive; some obtained from ponds, padis and rivers. Dried fish cheap and easily available. Rice not generally highly milled because of cost. Cassava used for snacks and cakes; during times of crisis, it becomes rice substitute. Sweet potato and gadung used, latter as staple in dead season. Young papaya and jackfruit, tree fruits, few berries and beans used as vegetables, also onion, garlic and chillis. Less often spinach, beans and bean shoots. Soybean preparations too costly. Banana and other fruits used in season.
Standard meal: rice, dried fish, sour vegetables and tamarind.
Rice cooked only in morning, heated for evening. Quantity of fish very small, 30 to 50 cents per day spent for whole family. Rice considered essential for life and health; other foods as flavouring or seasoning.

| 38 | RICE | INDONESIA | PATJET, WEST JAVA | POSTMUS AND VAN VEEN, 1949 |

Diet satisfactory, with more animal products than most places in Java. One group 36.7 gm. and another 26 gm. per head per day, mostly salted dried fish and other fish products. One man consumed average of 850 gm. raw rice per day. Vegetables abundant but mostly sold; intake low. *Pithecolobium lobatum* or djengkol bean pulse preferred. Festivals added to food intake. Rice provided 90 per cent of calories, 74 per cent of protein, and 19 per cent of fat.

TABLE A/20
Food and nutrient intakes per head per day

Animal protein	*gm.*	*Plant products*	*gm.*	*Nutrients per day*	
meat	5.90	rice	550.00	calories	2,100
dried meat	0.20	roots and tubers	15.00	animal protein	9 gm.
fresh fish	10.20	pulses	30.00	vegetable protein	42.5 gm.
dried, salted,		coconut oil	3.60	fat	8.8 gm.
other fish	19.86	leafy vegetables,		vitamin A	1470 i.u.
milk and eggs	0.47	young pulses	20.00	thiamine	1 mg.
		other vegetables	24.00		
		fruits	24.00		

| 39 | RICE | INDONESIA | PATARUMAN AND PISANGAMBO, NORTHWEST JAVA | POSTMUS AND VAN VEEN, 1949 |

TABLE A/21
Food intake per head per day in area with vitamin A deficiency diseases
(in gm.)

	PATARUMAN		*PISANGAMBO*
	Group with xerophthalmia	*Group without xerophthalmia*	
Rice	406	583	585
Green vegetables, young pulses	8.4	13.3	24.1
Fruits with provitamin A	1.6	1.3	4.8
Animal protein	4.3	11.2	4.2
Vegetable protein	33.8	49.5	46.8
Fat	7.7	16.3	9.2
Calories	1,528	2,317	2,096
vitamin A i.u.	557	1,104	1,515
thiamine	0.75	1.2	1.1
Average family size	5.3	5.7	6.5

40   RICE   INDONESIA   RARAK,   GOETHALS, 1967 AND 1969
                                                        SUMBAWA VILLAGE

Three meals daily, although housewives during lean season took two to save food for others. Breakfast often tea or water and plain rice, with very little 'soup' or vegetable water. From August to beginning of wet season when men work hard to clear swiddens, they eat small bowl of rice before work; at 11 a.m. a heavier meal of rice and vegetables and/or meat; third meal early in evening on return to settlement, again boiled rice with salt, boiled vegetables (frequently overboiled), chilli; when possible, bits of meat. Deer hunted in dry season; deer meat, dried and salted, most relished meat. No report that wild boar eaten or sold when killed. Goats and water buffalo killed for ceremonies during dry season. Goethals thought betel chewing among women and smoking among men 'psychological surrogates for adequate diet and nutrition.'

41   RICE   INDONESIA   BONTORAMBA,   CHABOT, 1967
                                                        SOUTHWEST SULAWESI   AND 1968

Meals usually rice, vegetables and soup made from meal of meat few days previously. Occasionally better meal would provide a little egg or meat. Evening meal largest of day. Most had two meals daily, poorest only one. Wealthiest start day with tea or coffee. Fruit taken as snack. Goats kept for milk, and slaughter for ceremonies. Chickens and eggs for sale and subsistence. Buffaloes slaughtered at important ceremonies; some sold to slaughterhouse at Macassar.

42   RICE   INDONESIA   TELANG, NORTH OF BANDJARMASIN,   HUDSON AND
                                       KALIMANTAN   HUDSON, 1967

Household size 5.27 members. Rice and fish, animals and birds from jungle, though little shot available for rifle. Crops raised in swidden: cassava, eggplant, banana, pineapple, sugarcane, red pepper, variety of gourds and squashes, and a few leafy vegetables. Durian, rambutan sold to Muslim traders. Chickens and domestic pigs killed only for ceremonies and feasts. Meat rarely eaten because only one rifle available for hunting.

43   RICE   INDONESIA   FISHING   KRISHNANDHI, 1969
                                                        VILLAGES

Rice consumption 90 kg. per caput per year, or 360 kg. for family of four. Income from fishing equivalent to only 410 kg. rice. Consumption of fish averages 11.4 kg. per caput per year, and less in Java, where incomes are lower and prices higher.

44   RICE   THAILAND   SERIES OF FAO   ANDERSON, 1960
                                                        REPORTS

Minburi, near Bangkok (1949): Calories sometimes inadequate; low animal protein and fats, general lack of essential nutrients.
80 families in rural areas (1951): Thiamine/calorie ratio low; frequent signs of malnutrition.
North, northeast, Central Plain and south (1951–3):

Both urban and rural areas had high carbohydrate consumption, low protein intake, low fat intake, low essential vitamins.
Cholburi, 4 villages (1952): One of most prosperous provinces. 84 per cent of calories from rice. Pulse consumption very low.

| 45 | RICE | THAILAND | RURAL GENERAL | DE YOUNG, 1955 |

In north, onions, garlic, cabbage and groundnuts grown after rice harvest for home consumption and sale. Vegetables grown in compound year round, requiring daily watering. Pigs not slaughtered, for economic and religious reasons. Poultry eaten more in north and south than central Thailand. 4 to 5 chickens eaten per year; most chickens, ducks and eggs sold. Thai fish consumption highest in South-East Asia. Each family fishes. Dried fish bought. Some of catch fermented. Families contribute enough food to monastery to support an extra family member.

| 46 | RICE | THAILAND | MALAY VILLAGE, SOUTH THAILAND | FRASER, 1966 AND 1968b |

Morning meal glutinous rice, garnished with fish or shrimp sauce. Main meal includes about 15 to 20 cm. length of fish per person. Once a week, joint of chicken per person. More rarely mutton or beef. Estimated 4—6 oz. condensed milk per person per day in tea or coffee. Half fish catch reserved for home consumption. Rice grown during monsoon when fishing impossible.

| 47 | RICE | THAILAND | CENTRAL | BERTHOLET AND BENCHADISWAT, 1958 |

Meat eaten not more than three times a week; many never eat.

Food	Frequency of consumption
Pork	18 gm. per caput in 5 weeks.
Buffalo	57 gm. per caput in under one week.
Beef	70 gm. per caput in under one week.
Poultry	Once week if money available (88 gm. chicken per head per week)
Duck	Once in seven weeks.
Hen egg	Three times in four weeks. 20 gm. per head per time.
Duck egg	Once in four weeks. 20 gm. per head per time.
Fish	Once daily, or more. *Small fish* from tanks, streams and padis during wet season. Two or three times weekly during cold season, very little at beginning of hot season. Average of 15 gm. per head eight times a week, or 120 gm. per week during wet season and 30 gm. per week during cold season. *Large fish* 47.5 gm. eight times a week.
Frog	Throughout wet season (July to November) 480 gm. per head per week.
Insects	25 gm. per head when available.
Silkworm	20 to 30 worms per head three or four times per week, mixed with fish.
Snails	During rainy season.
Shrimps	Once or twice when fields flooded.
Crabs	30 gm. per head about seven times during rainy season.
Rice	200 gm. per person per meal (glutinous)

Vegetable and fruit consumption probably overestimated by villagers.

| 48 | RICE | THAILAND | BANG CHAN, CENTRAL THAILAND | HAUCK, RAJATASILPIN, CAMPBELL AND THORANGKUL, 1958 |

Food mostly home-produced; important factor number of productive hands available. Rice a first essential in every meal, only minority using home-pounded grain. Fresh or preserved fish next in importance, and chillies and spices more commonly grown and used than vegetables and fruit. Swamp cabbage most common vegetable, growing wild in canals. Cash expenditures small; during busy work seasons, farmers bought fish, as well as usual purchased foods: onion, garlic, limes, coconut, palm sugar and small amounts of vegetables. Tilapia and mushroom culture regarded primarily as source of cash. Adults took two meals daily, except during busy work seasons when third meal might be taken. 90 per cent of school children ate snacks, mostly sweets and fruits. Rain water preferred for drinking, but canal or fish pond water used for three or four months each year.

Rice contributed four-fifths of calories and over half protein of groups studied. Animal foods, chiefly fish, provided two-fifths of protein. Intake of fats and sugars small. Higher caloric intake during heavy work season chiefly from rice. Highest protein intake during post-harvest season, when fish ponds drained.

APPENDIX

TABLE A/22

Comparison of calories and nutrients available to group A (some showing signs of malnutrition)
and group B (generally healthy), with estimated allowance

	Estimated amounts available [1]		Allowance	
	Group A	Group B	Group A	Group B
Food energy, calories	1731	2009	1935	1955
Protein (gm.)	50	59	59	59
Fat (gm.)	14	22	—	—
Carbohydrates (gm.)	342	384	—	—
Calcium (mg.)	129	194	650	650
Phosphorus (mg.)	847	895		
Iron (mg.)	6.9	8.4	8.7	8.8
Vitamin A (i.u.)	2047	1340	2522	2548
Thiamine (mg.)	0.68	0.76	0.93	0.96
Riboflavine (mg.)	0.37	0.28	1.073	1.06
Niacin (mg.)	11.3	11.5	9.3	9.6
Ascorbic acid (mg.)	27	23	24	24

[1] Estimates based on values for edible portion without allowance for cooking losses.

TABLE A/23

Contributions in terms of calories and nutrients of selected foods commonly[1] eaten by groups A and B

Foods	Frequency of use	Wt.	Calories	Protein	Fat	Carbohydrates	Ca	P	Fe	Vit. A	Thiamine	Riboflavine	Niacin	Vit. C
		gm.		gm.	gm.	gm.	mg.	mg.	mg.	i.u.	mg.	mg.	mg.	mg.
Group A														
Rice		399	1,440	28	3	316	28	634	3.5	(0)[2]	0.54	0.14	7.5	(0)
Eggs	9	4	8	1	1	0	3	8	0.1	48	0.01	0.01	0	0[2]
Fish, fresh	31	57	58	10	2	0	19	124	0.6	0	0.03	0.04	2.4	0
Fish, dried	8	6	12	3	0	0	4	2	0.2	0	0	0.02	0.2	0
Fish, fermented	2	2	2	0	0		19			0	0	0.01	0	
Fish soy	5	2	0	0						0	0	0	0.1	
Shrimp paste	33	3	3	1	0					0	0	0	0.2	
Swamp cabbage	4	20	3	0	0	1	9	6	0.3	750	0.01	0.01	0.1	4
(2) Phag (2) kacheed	4	3	1	0	0		6		0.1	204	0	0.01	0	2
sweet basil		4	4	0	0	1	3	2	0.1	504		0.09		0
Calabash	3	11	2	0	0	0	1	2	0.1	8	0	0.01	0.1	1
Chilli, fresh	17	4	1	0	0	0	0		0	126	0	0	0	8
Eggplants	10	13	3	0	0	1	2	5	0.1	4	0.01	0.01	0.1	1
Radish, white	5	7	2	0	0	0	0	6	0	1	0	0	0	1
Sweet potato	1	18	22	0	0	5	5	9	0.1	74	0.02	0.01	0.1	4
Banana	2	3	3	0	0	1	0	1	0	14	0	0	0	0
Coconut milk[3]	22	144	30	0	2	2								
Coconut oil	2	15	0	2	0	0	0	0	0	0	0	0	0	0
Lard	—	4	0	0	0	0	0	0	0	0	0	0	0	0
Sugar, palm	6	22	0	0	0	5	5	2	0.6	0			0	
Total			1,637	43	10	332	104	799	5.8	1,733	0.62	0.36	10.8	21
Total from all foods			1731	50	14	342	129	847	6.9	2,047	0.68	0.37	11.3	27

Group B

Rice		438	1,579	30	3	345	29	654	3.7	(0)	0.56	0.15	7.4	(0)
Glutinous rice		8	30	1	0	7	1	12	0.1	(0)	0.01	—	—	(0)
Eggs	7	5	9	1	1	0	3	10	0.1	58	0.01	0.01	0	0
Fish, fresh	32	72	75	13	2	0	25	158	0.7	0	0.04	0.05	3.0	0
Fish, dried	10	12	22	5	0	0	7		0.3	0	0.01	0.03	0.5	0
Fish, fermented	2	4	5	1	0		46			0	0	0.01	0	
Fish soy		3	2	0	0					0	0	0	0.1	
Shrimp paste	28	2	3	1	0					0	0	0	0.1	
Swamp cabbage	5	9	2	0	—	1	6	4	0.2	542	0.01	0.01	0.1	3
(2) Phag (2) kacheed	2	3	1	0	0	0	6		0.1	198	0	0.01	0	2
Calabash	1	10	2	0	0	0	1	2	0.1	7	0	0.01	0.1	1
Chilli, fresh	8	3	0	0	0	0	0		0	48	0	0	0	6
Eggplants	3	5	1	0	0	0	1	2	0	2	0	0	0	0
Radish, white	2	12	3	0	0	0	4	3	0.1	3	0	0	0	2
Coconut milk[3]	16	76	52	1	4	3								
Coconut oil		3	27	0	3	0	0	0	0	0	0	0	0	0
Lard		3	30	0	3	0	0	0	0	0	0	0	0	0
Sugar, palm		11	43	0	0	11	9	4	1.3	0			0.1	
Total			1,886	53	16	367	138	849	6.7	858	0.64	0.28	11.4	14
Total from all foods			2,009	59	22	384	194	895	8.4	1,340	0.76	0.28	11.5	23

[1] All items were eaten by 25% or more of the participating families. Under 'frequency of use', the number of times the item was used as a main ingredient of a 'with-rice' dish is indicated for 24 survey days for Group A and 20 survey days for Group B.

[2] ( ) means imputed value; 0 means none or insignificant amount; — means no values available, but probably contains measurable amount; blank space means that no information was found.

[3] Different values were used for the calculation of nutrient content of coconut milk for Groups A and B.

49	RICE	THAILAND	NEAR CHIANGMAI, NORTH THAILAND	GERHOLD, 1965

TABLE A/24

Food intake per head per day
(in gm.)

	Families purchasing all food	Families producing and also purchasing food
Rice (glutinous)	567	553
Vegetables	125	125
Meat	24	20
Fish	14	15
Egg	negligible	5.3
Fat	0.3	0.4
Groundnuts	31.3	20.4

50	RICE	THAILAND	NORTH	THANANGKUL, WHITAKER AND FORT, 1966

Highly-polished rice used (glutinous); even soaked overnight and water discarded. Meagre portions of fried pork, beef, chicken, fish and vegetables, primarily to give flavour to rice. Eggs considered luxury. Fruit also considered luxury (except banana) though abundantly grown. Dairy products neither available nor appreciated.

**51   RICE   THAILAND   CHIANGMAI, CHIANGRAI, UBOL, UDORN   RAMALINGA-
                                      NORTH AND NORTHEAST[b]   SWAMI, 1956**

Glutinous rice consumed in north, ordinary rice in central and south Thailand. 60 per cent of thiamine in glutinous rice, and 75 to 90 per cent in ordinary rice lost in preparation. Foods used to supplement rice do not provide sufficient amounts of nutrients in which rice is deficient. Intake of green and leafy vegetables variable; meat and fish intake low; pulses and eggs not consumed regularly nor in significant amounts. Milk not part of diet.

**52   RICE   THAILAND   LUA' AND SKAW   KUNSTADTER,
                                           KAREN PEOPLE,   1968
                                           MAE HONG SON
                                           PROVINCE, NORTH-
                                           WEST THAILAND**

Marked difference in amount of protein intake between two groups, due to religious differences. Lua' make many more animal sacrifices: large animals (pig or buffalo) at least three times a year, household sacrifices of pig and chicken at least twice a year, and 'preventive medicine' sacrifices once a month in households with children as well as curing ceremonies when required. Tendency to combine to buy animal for butchering whenever long period elapses since last meat consumption. Karens use more chickens than other animals; their curing ceremonies are less frequent and there is no stress on protecting young. Vegetable protein comes largely from rice, little from beans.

53   RICE   CAMBODIA   KALAB, 1969

Basis of diet rice, with fish, dry or as fermented paste. An above-average meal of merchant includes boiled rice, soup with fish or meat, another preparation of fish or meat, possibly a salad, and fruit. Rural people gain merit by eating the leavings of monks at pagoda feasts. Sufficient food of great variety is prepared, and a few hundred of the faithful may feast richly on the leavings. Dietary standards depend less on wealth and class than on general lack of interest in food preparation; if children are not around in time for their breakfast of rice porridge, they have to go without.

There appears to be adequate protein from fish (few people below 45 or 50 years of age actually abstain from killing), plus crabs, frogs, mussels and other rarer delicacies like a kind of hairy spider. The virtuous do not break eggs, but perhaps the younger people are not so strict. In any case, the shopkeeper may always crack a shell 'a little on purpose' and all is well. Chinese salted eggs accepted by the virtuous and in pagoda feasts. Meat, pork and beef available in markets; ducks and chicken always sold live. Cambodians do not milk cattle, but becoming accustomed to condensed milk and dry milk powder, at least for coffee. The Japanese have started a dairy farm in Kompong Cham province. Most Cambodians eat some fruit, and there is great variety; also salads, and cooked vegetables made with fish or meat.

**54   RICE   CAMBODIA   PEASANTS, GENERAL   DELVERT,
                                                                    1961**

Rice	600 to 700 gm. per head per day
Fish	20 kg. per head per year (unevenly dis-
Prahoc (fermented fish sauce)	70 kg. per family per year where little fresh fish available
Beef	1.5 kg. per head per year
Pork	4 to 6 kg. per head per year
Chicken	1 to 4 chickens per head per year.

| 55 | RICE | SOUTH VIETNAM | HENDRY, 1959 |

TABLE A/25

Major expenditures on food per day

	Upper-income		Middle-income		Lower-income	
	$VN	*per cent*	*$VN*	*per cent*	*$VN*	*per cent*
Rice	12.6	20	16.1	34.8	18.9	40.3
Meat and eggs	16.1	25.6	7.7	16.7	10.5	22.4
Fish	8.4	13.3	6.3	13.6	6.3	13.4
Fish sauce (nuoc nam)	2.8	4.4	2.8	6.1	2.8	6.0
Other sauces	1.4	2.2	1.4	3.0	1.4	3.0
Vegetables	3.5	5.6	2.8	6.1	2.1	4.5
Fruits	3.5	5.6	1.4	3.0	1.4	3.0
Other items	14.7	23.3	7.7	16.7	3.5	7.5
	63.3		46.2		46.2	

| 56 | RICE | S. VIETNAM | RURAL, TWELVE AREAS | ICNND 1960 |

TABLE A/26

Protein consumption by different groups (percentage)

		Land animal	Fish, seafood	Vegetables and grains
Vietnamese				
Highland:	Khu Trung Luong	10.4	35.8	53.8
	Phyong Qui	13.9	41.2	44.9
	Tung Nghia	10.3	9.3	80.4
	La Bui	4.5	56.5	39.0
Coastal:	Hai Chau	6.1	32.2	61.7
	My Khe	1.9	21.0	77.1
Delta	Long Thanh	9.5	20.8	69.7
	Thuong Thanh	12.5	28.5	59.0
Highlanders				
Kontum:	Kom Trang Monay	0.7	14.6	84.7
	Lang Kom Ho Ring		10.9	89.1
Dalat:	Lat	3.2	28.9	67.9

Calorie intakes generally attained, but do not greatly exceed calculated requirements for Vietnamese. Protein, fat, carbohydrate and salt adequate. Low intakes of vitamin A. Iron intake satisfactory, calcium generally so. Low vitamin C intake. Niacin intake satisfactory, but thiamine and riboflavine intakes low with most groups.

| 57 | RICE | S. VIETNAM | KHANH HAU MEKONG DELTA | HICKEY, 1964 |

Food for family after harvest kept in bins or piles on floor. Half population raises fruit and vegetables; 22 per cent neither. Most common among upper-income groups. Local tuber boiled and served in soup. White-stemmed Chinese cabbage popular vegetable; also preserved in brine and consumed in soup. Prickly balsam pear used in soup or stuffed with ground meat and steamed. Red chilli used in most meals. Carrots pickled in brine, usually added to fish as condiment. Several onions and green leafy vegetables consumed daily. Boiled maize as snack. Yams low-prestige food, used rarely as rice substitute. 80 per cent raise poultry, keeping two-thirds for home consumption. Eggs not sold. Beef eaten at family celebrations, together with lettuce, tomato, green beans and potato. Fresh and dried fish readily available.

| 58 | RICE | S. VIETNAM | VIETNAM CHAMS OF SOUTH-CENTRAL COASTAL PLAIN AND BORDER WITH CAMBODIA | LEBAR, HICKEY AND MUSGRAVE, 1964 |

Cham agriculture historically dominated by market gardening rather than paddy agriculture; area occupied by this group not amenable to extensive paddy cultivation. Both paddy and upland rice cultivated, also sugar cane, maize, coconut, banana and other fruit trees, green beans, peas, eggplant, cucumbers, millet, sesame, peppers and areca and betel leaves (both used for alcoholic drink). Cassava and groundnuts also grown.
Buffalo, ducks, chickens and goats domestic animals. Due to their Brahman origins, cattle not raised, and pigs rare, even among non-Muslims.

| 59 | RICE | LAOS | RURAL GENERAL | HALPERN, 1964 |

Vientiane area: 250 kg. rice per head per annum required for all purposes. Hunger not uncommon before harvest, and malnutrition prevalent, often in extreme forms. When rice is inadequate, Meos and to a lesser extent Lamet and Khmu use maize. Lamet and Khmu gather forest plants, especially bamboo shoots and tubers. Roots, greens, flowers, frogs and insects from the forest are in Lao diet, especially before harvest. Three meals of glutinous rice daily, with chillis and padek; sometimes curries or other vegetable dish. Fish occasional, meat rare. Morning and evening meals freshly cooked, lunch leftovers. Meat consumption usually ritual and ceremonial; hunting only when field work slack. Lao and Meo sometimes smoke pork and salt and dry beef; easier in cooler, mountain air. Lao, Meo and Khmu resemble Chinese in not using fresh milk or milk products. Canned evaporated milk sometimes added to tea, coffee or cocoa as luxury. Not used by pregnant mothers or children.

| 60 | RICE | LAOS | RURAL GENERAL (BASED ON INTERVIEWS) | ORR, 1967 |

Breakfast: glutinous rice, dried meat, egg and chiau (sauce of pepper and salted fish) and raw vegetables.
Noon: Bamboo shoot soup, fried meat, Lao caviar, tartar steak with vegetables such as mustard, cucumber, eggplant, lettuce.
Evening: Pounded fish, chicken in coconut milk, chicken soup, fish sauce and vegetables.
(Composition of meals obviously represents most appreciated items, and is not attained in practice).
One interviewee mentions malnutrition 'because people cannot buy fruit, vegetables and meat'. Most in rural areas obtain these from their surroundings. When food is scarce they get just rice and fish sauce.
Adult consumes 634 gm. uncooked milled rice a day. Meat not eaten regularly: about ten people may buy and share a buffalo, and each may further subdivide and sell. Fish caught in padis and streams; saltwater fish unknown. Fish abundant during rains and some dried or made into padek. Each family requires two jars containing 50 to 60 kg. padek a year. Vegetables planted only in wet season; too dry during rest of year. Forest leaves used.

| 61 | RICE | LAOS | SAUGKHALOK | GERHOLD, 1965 |

Average family 4.8 members. Home-pounded glutinous rice staple. Edible plants gathered from forest; fishing. Rice cooked once daily, eaten cold, kneaded to form scoop and dipped into sauces and stews.
Breakfast : sticky rice, egg, meat or fish
Lunch and supper: same, with highly spiced fish and/ or meat stew with vegetables. some salad
Meat and fish used in combination. Padek (fermented salted fish kept several months before use) usually used as seasoning, spoonful as basis of sauce or stew. Some families had two meals, some three. Fruits, often unripe, snacks between meals. Even those who took no breakfast often gave rice to monks.
High rice consumption may be due to fact that it absorbs less water. Cooked glutinous rice is 1.5 times the dry weight, and ordinary rice 2.5 to 3 times; up to 90 per cent of thiamine lost in preparation. Protein requirements met in most families, according to WHO recommendations. Vitamin C most deficient nutrient. Only one out of seventeen families had adequate vitamin A. Consumption of fruits and vegetables very low.

TABLE A/27

Food intake per head per day

	Families purchasing all food gm.	Families producing and also purchasing food gm.
Rice (glutinous)	700	850
Vegetables	64	109
Meat	67	59
Fish	45	39
Egg	15	9
Padek (fish sauce)	14	20

62	RICE	N. VIETNAM	RED TAI OF MUONG DENG AREA, THANH HOA PROVINCE, NORTH VIETNAM	LEBAR, HICKEY AND MUSGRAVE, 1964

Glutinous rice staple, with salt and vegetables. Meat consumed only at festivals or sacrifices, or after successful hunt. Only well-to-do regularly have meat and spices with rice. Eleven kinds of fish caught from rivers and padies. Porcupines, squirrels, turtles, monkeys, rats, snails and toads eaten; sweet chestnuts, palm shoots, bamboo pods and shoots, wild banana roots and latania palm fruit gathered.

Rice grown wherever possible in irrigated rice fields, and maize, cotton, cassava, sweet potatoes, taro and bananas also cultivated. Domestic animals include buffalo, horses, some goats, chickens and bees.

63	RICE	N. VIETNAM; KWANGSI, CHINA	THO OF NORTH AND NORTHEAST RED RIVER DELTA	LEBAR, HICKEY AND MUSGRAVE, (1964)

Glutinous and non-glutinous rice cultivated in paddy fields and by swidden methods on valley slopes. Hunting and fishing more for sport than food supply. Maize and buckwheat also cultivated. Watercress planted along edges of paddy fields. Sugar cane, cassava, mulberry trees and betel cultivated in small plots, and sweet potatoes, tomatoes, string beans, eggplant, lettuce, ginger and peppers grown in kitchen gardens. Cattle and buffalo kept as draft animals and for occasional sacrifice.

64	RICE	PHILIPPINES	FIFTY-FOUR BARRIOS, MEAN POPULATION 658.5	BUSTRILLOS, 1961

Meals generally deficient in vitamins A and C, proteins, fats and oils. Supper best meal of day, breakfast poorest; one-third of people took only carbohydrates and beverages. One-third of population had no animal protein in any meal. Meals: polished rice, succulent vegetables and mongo beans. Fruits sold rather than eaten. Meat eaten only occasionally — fresh pork at weekends. Dried fish and canned goods usual substitute for fresh fish. Farmers tend to have poorer diets than teachers and carpenters.

| 65 | RICE | PHILIPPINES | SOUTHERN TAGALOG, REGION, LUZON | PHILIPPINES, FNRC 1965 |

TABLE A/28

Food intake per head per day
(in gm.)

Total intake	700	
Rice (90 per cent polished) and maize	350	
Root crops	44	
Vegetables (21 per cent leguminous pods, 9 per cent leafy or yellow)	97	
Fruit (mostly banana and tomato)	54	
Fish, meat, poultry	67	
Coconut milk	27	
Sugar, sweets	26	
Fat, oil	10	
Egg	6	
Salt, spices, vinegar, drinks	31	

Breakfast Boiled or fried rice and leftovers; dried salted fish fried or toasted, or fresh fish simmered in vegetables and salt. Coffee with brown sugar.

Lunch and supper: Boiled rice, fish and vegetables cooked and served as one dish.

Cereals provide 57 per cent of total protein. Protein, minerals (except iron) and vitamins (except niacin) deficient.

| 66 | RICE | PHILIPPINES | CAGAYAN VALLEY, BATANES REGION, LUZON (RURAL AND URBAN) | PHILIPPINES, FNRC 1963b |

TABLE A/29
Food intake per head per day

	gm.
Rice (4 per cent unpolished)	267
White and yellow maize (ground)	71
White sweet potato and white and purple yam (6 per cent of total)	41
Sugars and syrups	20
Beans, nuts, seeds (too small to be significant)	13
Leafy and yellow vegetables (squash fruit, leaves and flowers, swamp cabbage, malunggay leaves, taro and sweet potato leaves, bittermelon and jute leaves; much smaller amounts of Chinese cabbage, yardlong bean leaves, malabar nightshade, onion leaves, chilli leaves, mustard, ferns, sponge gourd leaves)	24
Vitamin C-rich foods: Tomato	12
Mango	12
Others (papaya, pomelo, lime, orange, mandarin, kalamansi, Spanish plum, guava, etc.)	37
Other fruits (two-thirds banana)	65
Other vegetables (eggplant, bottle gourd, bamboo shoot, cabbage, leguminous pods, green papaya, sponge gourd, bittermelon, onion. Lesser used: banana heart, pepper, okra, unripe jackfruit, seaweed, yam bean, young coconut, garlic, ginger, tamarind leaves and flowers, taro petioles, mushroom etc.).	96
Poultry, meat, fish: pork	15
chicken	6
carabao	3
beef	1
organ meats	4
tinned meat	1

fresh fish	11
processed or canned fish	22
dried fish	3
Hen egg	4.5
Duck, turkey and ant egg	0.5
Milk	13

Household average 6.2 members. Daily per caput cost of food: 43 centavos. Only cereals, fruits and vegetables adequate. Meat and fish 68 per cent of requirement. Adequate amounts purchased only where daily per caput expenditure reaches 70 centavos. Two thirds spent less than 50 centavos, the remainder from 0.50 to 1.49 pesos per head per day. Only with profes-sional, managerial, administrative and office workers were requirements for meat, fish, poultry and eggs met. Manual workers, labourers, farmers, fishermen and hunters received lowest ratings. 90 per cent engaged in some form of home production, but those not producing had better diets.

TABLE A/30

Consumption of different nutrients as percentage of requirements

	Percentage of requirement
Iron, niacin, ascorbic acid	100
Calcium	39
Riboflavine	41
Calories	81
Protein	87
Vitamin A	64
Thiamine	65

Biochemical tests revealed no signs of protein malnutrition. Serum albumin acceptable, globulin good, albumin/globulin ratio acceptable.

| 67 | RICE | PHILIPPINES | 'TARONG', NORTH-WEST LUZON | NYDEGGER AND NYDEGGER, 1966 |

Study of Ilocos barrio. Three full meals per day when children attend school. Other families take two full meals and one or two snacks. Breakfast may be cold rice, but rice freshly cooked for noon and evening meals, served with vegetable sauce, flavoured and salted by pickled fish, fresh ginger or hot peppers. Most add meat or fish to the vegetable sauce three to five evenings a week. When small birds, fish or frogs collected, or a chicken is killed, roasted on a spit for special meal. An extra dish of fried or boiled vegetables served when plentiful. May be sliced tomatoes or squash blossoms with pickled fish. Salads rarely served raw; if a food cannot be peeled, it is boiled for few minutes. Fresh fruit may be served at dinner. Rice is rolled into a small ball and dipped into sauce. Chief difference between higher and lower-income groups is that latter rarely buy meat and rely more on wild foods; difference largely in quantity consumed. Saltwater fish costly; fresh fish comes chiefly from padis (mudfish which bury themselves in dry season). Snails and frogs eaten during wet season. Beetles, locusts, crickets and ants roasted during short season available, providing occasional titbit. Pork, beef or carabao bought in amounts from 450 to 900 gm., and part cured to keep. Sliced thin, washed in vinegar and sun-dried; diced and fried on use. Frogs may be dried. Seaweed, mongo beans and maize similarly treated. Tiny fish pickled in vinegar and salt, sealed in large containers and aged.

| 68 | RICE | PHILIPPINES | TINGLAYAN, BONTOC REGION, NORTH LUZON | QUIOGUE, 1966b |

TABLE A/31

Food intake per head per day
(in gm.)

Rice	800
Leafy vegetables	303
Other vegetables	365
Animal protein (mostly fish, no eggs)	28
Sugar	12

| 69 | RICE | PHILIPPINES | MAKAYAN, BONTOC REGION, NORTH LUZON | QUIOGUE, 1966b |

TABLE A/32

Food intake per head per day

	gm.	*Per cent of total*
Cereals (rice 43 per cent unpolished)	363.99	48.15
Sweet potato	163.86	21.68
Dried beans	19.57	2.59
Leafy and yellow vegetables	18.45	2.44
Tomato and papaya	5.22	.69
Other fruits and vegetables	107.94	14.28
Meat, poultry and fish	29.54	3.90
pork	6.21	
beef	1.31	
chicken	.14	
carabao and goat	.04	
canned and processed meat	4.18	
fresh fish	2.49	
dried fish	3.41	
crustaceans and molluscs	5.39	
snails	2.15	
dried canned squid	2.70	
Hen egg	2.05	
Evaporated whole milk	5.53	

Cereals provide 89 to 90 per cent of calories, 61 to 71 per cent of protein, 71 to 72 per cent of thiamine, 77 to 83 per cent of niacin. Animal protein provides 8 to 15 per cent of total protein. Sweet potato main source of vitamin A and vitamin C.

Requirements met in cereals, sweet potato. Diet deficient in quantity and quality. Adequate only in iron, thiamine, niacin and vitamin C. Lack of fat makes probable a deficiency of vitamin A. This village, being near small town, has access to highly processed, less nutritious foods which are costly.

70	RICE	PHILIPPINES	ILOCOS REGION, NORTH LUZON	PHILIPPINES, FNRC 1963a

TABLE A/33

Food intake per head per day
(in gm.)

Cereals (rice, 80 per cent polished; with rice products 96 per cent, remainder maize and bread and bakery products)	409
Sweet potato (mostly white)	44
Yellow and mung beans	10
Other beans: pigeon pea, cowpea, snap bean, peanut, lima bean, soybean, sprouted mung	10
Leafy and yellow vegetables: squash, carrots, sweet potato tops, taro leaves and petioles, swamp cabbage, mustard, black nightshade, leeks, celery, jute leaves, squash leaves and flowers, ferns, spinach, lettuce, water lily leaves, watercress	15.02
Tomato	9
Mango	22
Other vitamin C-rich fruits	10
Other fruits and vegetables:	
banana	17
pineapple, avacado, jackfruit, watermelon, sapodilla, black plum, eggplant, bamboo shoots, bottle gourd, cabbage, horse-radish, snap bean, yardlong bean, cowpea, sweet pea	61
Meat (mostly pork)	24.67
Fresh fish	16
Processed and canned fish	19
Salted fermented fish	14
Hen egg	6

Average household 5.9 members. Diet predominantly rice and vegetables.

Protein 71 per cent plant (58 per cent cereal, 7 per cent bean) and 29 per cent animal.

Bean intake adequate; meat, poultry and fish less than 75 per cent of requirement; other foods range between one-third and one-half of requirement, except milk (one-eighth of requirement) and fats (one-fifth).

	Ilocos	*Igorot*
Breakfast:	Broiled fish, fresh or dried, boiled mixed vegetables or boiled dried beans. Boiled rice, coffee with milk and sugar.	Broiled fish, sweet potato tops, rice or sweet potato, coffee or tea with sugar.
Lunch:	Vegetables or beans, rice, fruit	Breakfast leftovers
Supper:	Vegetables, rice and fish or stewed May beetles	Boiled mixed vegetables and rice or sweet potatoes.

| 71 | RICE | PHILIPPINES | ILOCOS VILLAGE, NORTH LUZON | PHILIPPINES, FNRC 1963a |

TABLE A/34

Food intake per head per day

	gm.	per cent of total
Rice (73 per cent unpolished)	486	
Sweet potato	494	78
Boiled sweet potato tops	dish	
Dried beans	42	3.33
Rice wine	54	
Pork	5.92	
Chicken	1.88	
Carabao and goat	2.15	
Fresh fish	3.74	2.37
Dried fish	1.0	
Snails	12.24	
White snap beans	35.49	
Black beans	2.75	
Green mung beans	2.45	
Yellow bean	1.18	

Requirements met for cereals, sweet potatoes, beans, leafy and yellow vegetables. Diet adequate except in calcium and riboflavine.

| 72 | RICE | PHILIPPINES | LUZON AND VISAYAS | U.S.A. D n.d. |

TABLE A/35

Food intake per head per day, compared with recommended allowances

	Food group	Per caput food intake gm.			Recommended allowance	Per cent sufficiency
		Luzon 4 regions	Visayas 2 regions	Average		
I.	Cereals	342	325	334	318	105·0
II.	Starchy roots and tubers	36	75	55	70	78·6
III.	Sugars and syrups	24	13	19	33	57·6
IV.	Dried beans, nuts and seeds	10	6	8	20	40·0
V.	Leafy & yellow vegetables	16	18	17	68	25·0
VI.	Vitamin C-rich foods	36	17	26	87	29·9
VII.	Other fruits and vegetables	120	65	93	94	98·9
VIII.	Meat, fish & poultry	79	72	75	108	69·4
IX.	Eggs	7	3	5	14	35·7
X.	Milk & milk products	38	14	26	168	15·5
XI.	Fats & oils including fats from coconut	10	4	7	29	24·1
	TOTAL	718	612	665	1,009	65·9

TABLE A/36

Nutrient intake per head per day, compared with recommended allowances

Nutrient	Per caput nutrient intake			Recommended allowance	Per caput intake in per cent RDA
	Luzon	Visayas	Average		
	4 regions	2 regions			
I. Calories	1,774	1,568	1,672	2,193	76.2
Fats (gm.)	27	15	21	—	—
Carbohydrates (gm.)	331	312	321	—	—
II. Protein (gm.)	47.7	45.4	46.6	54.4	85.7
III. Calcium (gm.)	.34	.36	.35	1.00	35.0
IV. Iron (mg.)	10	9	10	8	125.0
V. Vitamin A (i.u.)	2,097	1,700	1,900	3,772	50.4
VI. Thiamine (mg.)	.84	.76	.80	1.19	67.2
VII. Riboflavine (mg.)	.60	.43	.52	1.36	38.2
VIII. Niacin (mg.)	15	13	14	12	116.7
IX. Ascorbic acid (mg.)	68	72	70	70	100.0

(No allowance make for losses in cooking.)

73	RICE	PHILIPPINES	WESTERN VISAYAS	PHILIPPINES, FNRC, 1968

Nutrition survey of 3,485 individuals in 512 households, 1 February to 30 May, 1964, complete with dietary, clinical and biochemical phases.

Polished rice predominant cereal, supplemented by maize in proportion of 3:1; sweet potato and cassava principal starchy roots, taro and potato constituting one-tenth. A teaspoon of mung beans per day. One-quarter of vegetables were of leafy type; of foods rich in vitamin C, tomatoes contribute half, mango, papaya and others half. 70 gm. meats and fish consumed by more than three-fourths of group; eggs half a teaspoon; four teaspoons of milk and milk products, of which two-thirds were evaporated filled milk and condensed milk.

Food intakes per caput adequate only with cereals and 'other fruits and vegetables'. Intakes of all other food groups were 12 to 66 per cent of allowance; total food intake only 63 per cent of all foods recommended for adequate nutrition. Calories and all nutrients except iron and niacin insufficient. Quantity and quality of food intakes related to economic status, educational level, size of household, home food production and location (urban or rural), etc.

The biochemical phase covered 1,753 individuals in 318 households; carotene deficient; serum vitamin A, urinary thiamine and riboflavine low; haemoglobin variable; serum vitamin C and serum total protein acceptable; pregnant mothers have low serum albumin value; pregnant and nursing mothers very high serum globulin.

The most prevalent clinical signs of deficiency were those suggestive of vitamin A, riboflavine, niacin, ascorbic acid, iodine, thiamine and vitamin D deficiencies. Incidence of intestinal parasitism was 91.5 per cent (*Ascaris, Trichuris* and hookworm).

| 74 | RICE/MAIZE | PHILIPPINES | EASTERN VISAYAS | PHILIPPINES, FNRC, 1969 |

Nutrition survey of 1,951 individuals in 306 households, from 24 April to 4 June, 1965. This is maize-growing region; 15 per cent of total households had rice/maize mixture, the rest either rice or maize. Starchy roots important; 60 per cent sweet potato, remainder mostly cassava and taro. Half teaspoon a day of dried beans. Less than half vegetables (40 gm.) were leafy and yellow; fruits (25 gm.) two-thirds banana, one-third fruits rich in vitamin C. 70 gm. meat, fish and poultry, half total being fish, meat one-fifth, and rest dried and processed fish, crustaceans and molluscs. Half a teaspoon of egg; one teaspoon of milk (three-fifths filled, two-fifths whole). Fats and oils less than one teaspoon; tuba (alcoholic beverage from fermented coconut sap) forms three-quarters of 'miscellaneous foods' group (total 72 gm.)

Breakfast: boiled rice, fried dried fish; coffee with sugar
Lunch : boiled maize, boiled fish with ginger, green onions, tonglad.
Supper : boiled maize, left-over boiled fish, boiled vegetables.
Snacks : Fruits in season, if any

Food intakes per caput adequate only in starchy roots and tubers; all other groups supply 3 to 42 per cent of recommended allowances, while total intake only 59 per cent of all foods recommended.

Inadequacy in calories and all nutrients, except apparently iron and ascorbic acid, the absorption of which is in doubt. Calories 32 per cent and protein 30 per cent below recommended allowances; fats very low, did not contribute to calorie value and also aggravate marked deficiency of vitamin A.

Biochemical phase studied on 56 per cent of total subjects; low mean haemoglobin values for males and females in 1 to 6 years age group, and among pregnant women; total serum protein and albumin/globulin ratio acceptable and normal respectively, except for pregnant women; mean serum vitamin C, serum vitamin A, urinary thiamine and urinary riboflavine all low; serum carotene deficient.

Clinical signs of nutritional deficiencies of vitamin A, riboflavine, ascorbic acid, niacin, thiamine, iodine and vitamin D.

Of 1,665 subjects, 88.8 per cent positive for intestinal parasitism; highest in age-groups 7 to 12, 1 to 6 and 40 to 59 years; prevalence in infants below 12 months 23.3 per cent. *Ascaris, Trichuris* and hookworm.

| 75 | RICE AND MAIZE | PHILIPPINES | 187 HOUSEHOLDS NORTH-EASTERN MINDANAO | PHILIPPINES FNRC (in press) |

TABLE A/37

Food intake per head per day

	gm.		gm.
Total intake	672.02	*Total recommended*	996
Rice and rice products (90 per cent polished)	249.87		
Maize and maize products	84.57		
Other cereals	16.98		
Starchy roots and tubers (mostly sweet potato)	36.71		
Sugars and syrups	20.68		
Dried beans, nuts and seeds	5.21		
Leafy and yellow vegetables	20.57		
Vitamin C-rich foods	9.08		
Other fruits and vegetables (41 gm. banana)	74.13		
Meat, fish and poultry	82.76		
(fresh fish, 31.17; fresh meat, 16.09; canned and processed fish, 13.05; dried fish, 7.24)			
Eggs	3.47		
Milk and milk products (13.82 gm. whole milk)	14.99		
Fats and oils	7.51		
Miscellaneous (19 gm. fermented palm sap)	45.49		

76	RICE AND MAIZE	PHILIPPINES	225 HOUSEHOLDS SOUTH-WESTERN MINDANAO	PHILIPPINES FNRC (in press)

TABLE A/38

Food intake per head per day

	gm.		*gm.*
Total intake	662.49	*Total recommended*	*1,013*
Rice and rice products (98 per cent polished)	231.41		
Corn and corn products	102.02		
Other cereals	12.60		
Starchy roots and tubers	27.23		
Sugars and syrups	14.22		
Dried beans, nuts and seeds	4.93		
Leafy and yellow vegetables	21.97		
Vitamin C-rich foods	17.04		
Other fruits and vegetables	67.19		
Meat, poultry and fish	77.17		
(fresh fish, 40.14 gm; canned and processed fish, 12.53; poultry, 5.63; fresh meats, 5.29; crustaceans and molluscs, 6.88)			
Eggs (mostly hen)	2.81		
Milk and milk products (whole milk, 20.09 gm.)	20.15		
Fats and oils	5.09		
Miscellaneous (fermented palm sap, 36 gm.)	58.66		

77	RICE	CHINA	KWANGTUNG PROVINCE, SOUTH CHINA	YANG, 1959

Adult male consumes about 600 gm. food per day, with heavier consumption during hard work, less during slack season. Rice staple, with whatever vegetables and occasionally meat that can be afforded. 250 kg. rice required per year. Poor eat plain boiled rice with boiled fresh vegetables (cabbage or eggplant) from own land, of inferior quality which cannot be sold. Meat eaten at festivals only. Higher income-group family eat meat and vegetables with rice as staple, with pork, eggs, fresh or salted fish, large dish of vegetables and soup in addition to rice. On the 1st and 15th of each month, chicken, or duck and roast pork eaten.

78	RICE	CHINA, BURMA, THAILAND, LAOS NORTH VIETNAM	LÜ OF THE SIP SONG PANNA, CENTERING ON THE MEKONG, EXTREME SOUTHERN YUNNAN	LEBAR, HICKEY AND MUSGRAVE, 1964

Primarily wet-rice plains farmers. Glutinous rice staple, with beans, vegetables and meat from domestic animals, and fish from rivers and canals. Insects, maggots, grubs, and wild leaves and fruits gathered for food. Some dry rice grown on valley sides and slopes. Beans, peppers, maize, vegetables, sugar cane, cotton and tobacco grown. Cattle, buffalo, horses, chickens, pigs, ducks, dogs and cats kept as domestic animals, with pork most popular meat, followed by beef, chicken and duck.

79	RICE/BUCKWHEAT	CHINA, THAILAND BURMA	LISU, MOSTLY WESTERN YUNNAN	LEBAR, HICKEY AND MUSGRAVE, 1964

Among northern Lisu, diet primarily buckwheat cakes and porridge, supplemented with vegetable soup to which occasionally chicken or egg may be added. Southern Lisu eat mainly steamed rice, served in a curry with vegetables. Meat in the form of pork, chicken, wild fowl and game relatively rare, except among those who keep pigs and make frequent animal sacrifices. Wild honey important adjunct to diet. Alcoholic beverages made from maize or millet consumed in large amounts.

Irrigated rice grown on artificial terraces in tropical valley bottoms in Yunnan border area. Higher up, swiddens are planted to upland rice, maize, barley and millet, and still higher, buckwheat is chief crop. Additional crops include beans, yams, sweet potatoes, melons, gourds, chard, peppers, tobacco, cotton and hemp. Most raise opium poppies.

80	RICE	TAIWAN	RURAL GENERAL	TAIWAN, JCRR 1968a

Six bowls rice per head per day.
Breakfast: rice, pickles, vegetables, peanuts: higher-income groups might add salted fish, soybean curd or egg.
Lunch   : Same as first meal, plus fried vegetables and soup, and perhaps pork bones, organ meats.

Supper   : Rice, invariably fish or meat, added to vegetables and soup.
Egg, when used, is made into 'custard', cooked with onion or other vegetables. Fresh fish may be eaten three times a week.

81	RICE/SWEET POTATO	TAIWAN	HSIN HSING, NORTH TAIWAN	GALLIN, 1966

Rice, dried or steamed fish, fresh vegetables and pickles normal diet. Many substitute sweet potato, steamed when fresh or shredded dried and steamed, mixed with rice, at other times. Many feasts throughout year, when additional food is pork, or fresh fish and soup. Chicken, duck, goose or even a pig may be slaughtered for important occasions.

82	RICE/SWEET POTATO	TAIWAN	100,000 ABORIGINAL PEOPLES	JOLLIFFE AND TUNG, 1959

Rice, sweet potatoes, chestnuts, taro and millets staple.

83	RICE/SWEET POTATO	OKINAWA	'TAIRA', NORTH-EAST OKINAWA	MARETZKI AND MARETZKI, 1966 MARETZKI, T, 1968

Breakfast: boiled sweet potato, soybean soup
Lunch   : noodle soup, fried cabbage, dried cabbage, perhaps rice, always sweet potato
Supper   : Rice, bean paste or noodle soup.
Meat rarely eaten. If goat or pig killed for festival, it is fried or put into soup. More rice eaten in mid-summer after harvest, and at end of year after second harvest. Small amounts of fish mixed with condiments, eaten with rice. Whale meat eaten two or three times a year. Young sweet potato leaves, onions, giant radish, beans and cabbages used as vegetables. Some wheat used. Only fifteen families out of 141 self-sufficient in rice; remainder had to buy.

| 84 | RICE/BARLEY | SOUTH KOREA | THROUGHOUT RURAL AREAS | CHAI, 1967 |

33 different groups surveyed, both industrial and rural. 55 per cent of food intake rice and barley. Animal foods 3.5 per cent; foresters received only one-quarter to one-fifth that of towns. Small amounts of wheat products eaten. Small amounts of grain legumes, soy-sauce, soypaste and vegetable oil consumed.

TABLE A/39

Food intake per head per day
(in gm.)

Group	Fish	Other animal food	Cereals and tubers	Vegetables
Agriculturists	24	1.7	1,259.2 (mostly rice)	406
Fishermen	91.5	0.4	1,000.9 (other grains and potatoes)	259
Foresters	11.5	0.4	1,045.2 (other grains and potatoes)	330

| 85 | RICE/BARLEY | S. KOREA | SUWON | CHAI, 1967 |

Slum study, some people coming from farms. Combination of rice and barley 54 per cent of total food for 110 households. Combination of rice, barley and red beans 12 per cent of all dishes; wheat flour kneaded and sliced into soup 9 per cent of total; wheat flour noodle 7 per cent; white potato 7 per cent.

Side dishes: 36.4 per cent Korean Kimchis (pickled cabbage or radish); 20.9 per cent thin stew of pumpkin, cabbage, white potato and meats; 8.9 per cent boiled vegetables and fish; 11 per cent roasted side dish; 9 per cent Jorim, (hard-boiled side dish with salty liquid); 8 per cent soup; 8 per cent cooked vegetables; less than 8 per cent raw vegetables.

Soup usually made of soybean sprout, cabbage, potato, tangle and dried cabbage or radish leaves. Common animal foods dried or salted small sardines and salted shrimps in both soups and Kimchi. Net consumption per caput very small.

Grains provide 90 per cent of calories and 76 per cent of total protein. Animal food provides 0.98 per cent of total intake, 3.6 per cent of protein. Vegetables 40 per cent of total intake (including beans and potatoes).

| 86 | RICE/BARLEY | S. KOREA | 282 HOUSEHOLDS SUWON | YOUNG, 1968 |

90.7 per cent mixed rice with other grains. 97 per cent of those with income below 6,000 won* per month. Farm households had higher proportion of grains other than rice. Barley, Italian millet, millets, red beans and other beans and potatoes cooked with rice, according to season. Principal addition was barley followed by Italian millet and potatoes. In autumn, when price of rice and beans falls, more eaten. Farmers eat barley alone in summer, and 33 per cent barley in autumn and winter. Beans are 33 per cent of farm diet in autumn and 66.7 per cent in winter, because they produce their own.

*100 S. Korean won = US$0.250

87	RICE	JAPAN	FARMERS IN GENERAL	JAPAN, MINISTRY OF AGRICULTURE AND FORESTS, 1968

TABLE A/40

Food intake by farmers, per head per year (in kg.)

	1960	1961	1962	1963	1964	1965
Polished rice	156.4	150.4	155.5	158.8	150.9	150.4
Milled wheat or barley	16.6	14.3	11.7	9.4	7.0	6.0
Wheat flour and noodles	14.4	12.7	11.4	11.5	11.0	10.7
Potatoes	34.2	34.6	28.7	24.2	23.8	20.4
Soybean and azuki	2.9	3.1	2.8	2.8	2.7	2.2
Vegetables fresh and pickled, green and yellow	16.5	17.1	16.6	17.7	17.3	17.9
Other vegetables and pickles	92.0	90.1	93.8	98.2	91.6	90.5
Fish and shellfish	17.6	19.1	21.0	22.1	22.2	23.9
Meat	1.4	1.8	2.3	3.4	3.6	3.7
Hen eggs	3.9	5.1	5.9	6.5	7.9	7.9
Cow milk	11.4	10.7	11.0	11.6	12.0	12.0
Soybean paste	9.5	9.2	9.2	9.3	8.8	8.4
Soybean sauce	13.4	13.5	13.5	11.3	9.6	9.5
Edible oil	1.4	1.6	1.6	1.6	1.9	2.0

TABLE A/41

Nutrient intake by farmers, per head per day

	1960	1961	1962	1963	1964	1965
Calories	2,325	2,301	2,331	2,404	2,354	2,434
Protein (gm.)	62.42	62.87	64.36	66.76	65.22	67.69
Fat (gm.)	18.78	19.97	20.72	22.45	23.39	25.78
Calcium (mg.)	387	397	406	427	432	442
Vitamin A (i.u.)	1,053	1,114	1,104	1,181	1,209	1,157
Thiamine (mg.)	0.98	0.95	0.99	1.0	0.97	0.99
Riboflavine (mg.)	0.81	0.83	0.86	0.89	0.85	0.8
Vitamin C (mg.)	90	92	91	94	96	88
Ratio of animal protein (per cent)	19.5	20.7	21.9	23.1	24.2	25.3

88	RICE	JAPAN	OKAYAMA PREFECTURE, VILLAGE ON INLAND SEA	NORBECK, 1967

Consumption of meat, eggs and dairy produce increased threefold in past decade.

Breakfast: steamed rice, slice of pickled radish, soup of bean paste, little onion, sometimes small pieces of fish. Increasingly, boiled or fried egg.

Lunch : simple except during school holidays. Noodles or leftover rice, hot bean soup and cooked vegetables.

Supper : mixture of 'western and Japanese' vegetables, boiled and seasoned, with soup, rice, pickles, tea. Boiled or broiled fish in small quantity four or five times a week.

Rice no longer mixed with barley, as in past. Grandparents rarely ate fish in past. Fruit still considered luxury. Snacks usually sweet potato. Tempura, pork and beef few times per year. (See p. 89.)

| 89 | RICE/BARLEY | JAPAN | NIIIKE, OKAYAMA PREFECTURE | BEARDSLEY, HALL AND WARD, 1959 BEARDSLEY, 1968 |

Rice and barley staple foods, proportion of barley down to one-sixth of total just after new year harvest. At peak periods of work, rice alone may be consumed. Late in year before harvest, barley may be the only food grain, with taro and sweet potato. Largest food expenditure fish (one-fifth of total); usually minute cuts of sardine and mackerel bought from pedlar. Only at special feast does each person get more than a couple of bites. Villagers beginning to purchase items formerly made at home, such as noodles (often of buckwheat, for soup), and sauces. Roots chopped into soup or cooked separately as vegetables to supplement cereals. Fish, meat and eggs rarely used, as flavouring rather than food. Miso standard ingredient of breakfast soup, tofu common extender of soups and stews. Soysauce common. New taste for milk developing among children, who get it at school. Always choice of fruits and vegetables. Three meals taken daily, except during harvest, when five are eaten.

| 90 | RICE/BARLEY | JAPAN | YAMANASHI PREFECTURE, TWO VILLAGES 'S' AND 'Y' | NAGAMINE ET AL, 1963 |

32 families out of 48 in secluded villages took less than recommended level of calories, and 31 families less protein. Little pork eaten. Chief foods wheat, rice, barley, maize, radish and turnip leaves.

TABLE A/42
Food intake per head per day
(in gm.)

	Rice	Barley	Wheat	Other cereals	Potato	Miso*
S. Village	190	108	98	49	179	32
Y. Village	258	72	120	20	110	38

	Fresh fish	Dried fish	Processed fish	Egg	Goat milk
S. Village	12	14	13	19	42
Y. Village	17	6	20	21	40

	Fresh vegetables	Other vegetables	Fruit
S. Village	106	81	18
Y. Village	45	87	71

* Little other soybean or pulse products taken.

| 91 | SORGHUM AND MILLETS | INDIA | RAJASTHAN | BOSE AND MALHOTRA, 1964 |

Study of Banjaras, nomads who sell salt. Bajra, or in its absence barley, and dhal staples. Vegetables rarely eaten. Milk and ghee obtained from their own animals.

| 92 | SORGHUM AND MILLETS | INDIA | DAULATPUR HIRA, PILIBHIT DISTRICT, UTTAR PRADESH | CENSUS OF INDIA, 1965g |

70.8 per cent non-vegetarians. Bajra eaten from November to March, and mixture of barley and gram from April to October. Few eat wheat, rice occasionally. Roti, dhal are daily food, vegetables when possible. Quantities of green and powdered chillis used. Domestic fowl eaten occasionally, goat meat, eggs and fish when available. Milk and ghee inadequate. Melon, water melon and mango in season.

Breakfast: Matha and chapathis
Lunch   : Roti, dhal and vegetables
Supper   : Roti, dhal and vegetables.

| 93 | SORGHUM AND MILLETS | INDIA | CHAPNU VILLAGE, JAUNSAR-BAWAR AREA, UTTAR PRADESH | CENSUS OF INDIA, 1965h |

Village of 16 households in Himalayan foothills. All non-vegetarian. Mandua, jhangora and rice staples. Mandua and jhangora grown locally. It is considered mandua has virtue of staying long in stomach, as it is slow to digest and therefore satisfies hunger for longer. Wheat, barley and maize occasionally used for chapathis. Sattu of maize eaten with curd and salt. Vegetables and pulses grown locally and eaten.

| 94 | SORGHUM AND MILLETS | INDIA | VILLAGE IN JAUNSAR-BAWAR AREA UTTAR PRADESH | SAKSENA, 1962 |

Village grows enough food for needs; also commercial crops, including potatoes, turmeric and ginger. Upland terraces produce kharif crop of mandua, inferior millets, maize and pulses; during rabi season, wheat, barley and mustard. Wet farming in low-lying valley produces rice, wheat, potatoes, tobacco, barley, tomatoes and onions. Shifting cultivation producing wheat and barley in rabi season and mandua, chaulai and pulses during kharif. Mandua and jhangora preferred staples. Cattle, goats and sheep kept. Cattle provide manure, milk and meat. Goats and sheep provide wool for weaving local cloth.

| 95 | SORGHUM AND MILLETS | INDIA | THAPLI VILLAGE, GARHWAL DISTRICT, UTTAR PRADESH | CENSUS OF INDIA, 1964b |

Lunch : boiled rice or jhangora and lentils or curry.
Supper: chapathi (mandua or mandua/barley) and dhal, or local vegetables if in season.
An edible root, tairu, also eaten. Milk only for higher-income families; meat and fish luxury items.

| 96 | SORGHUM AND MILLETS | INDIA | CENTRAL UTTAR PRADESH CENTRAL MADHYA PRADESH | ICMR, 1951 |

Millets boiled to consistency of cooked rice, or porridge, or boiled in excess water and taken as gruel; boiled with pulses into khichri; or as chapathi. Skimmed milk not drunk by producers in milk tract of Jubbulpore. Kodo millets, kurthi and maize consumed with millets. Poorest take dry mahua flowers (*Bassia latifolia*), boiled, as substitute for cereals. Mahua flour may be made into dough with Bengal gram powder, cooked as chapathis. (Also practice among aboriginals and very poor of Bihar). Principal pulses: Bengal gram, lentil, green gram, khesari (used as dhal or ground into flour for chapathis). Bengal gram flour mixed with wheat flour also used for chapathis. Vegetables consumed in small quantities, as most are sold. Consumption of fruits negligible.

| 97 | SORGHUM AND MILLETS | INDIA | AURANGABAD (MAHARASHTRA) NIZAMABAD (ANDHRA PRADESH) RAICHUR (MYSORE) | ICMR 1951 |

TABLE A/43

Food intake per head per day in three states
(in gm.)

	Aurangabad		Nizamabad	Raichur (Alampur)	
Rice		8.5	570	14	88
Wheat		3.0	40		12
Millets	660	715	136	720	515 (jowar)
Pulses	17	30	57	37	80
Leafy vegetables	6	3	3	3	6
Non-leafy vegetables	3	6	65	3	12
Fruits					12
Ghee			6		6
Vegetable oils	1.2	6	14	3	6
Milk, buttermilk		21	110	60	250
Meat, fish, eggs	6	12	8.5	14	3
Sugar, jaggery			8.5		3

| 98 | SORGHUM AND MILLETS | INDIA | CENTRAL PENINSULAR INDIA | ICMR 1951 |

Wide belt across peninsular India from Bijapur District, Maharashtra, Kolhapur, Mysore, and parts of Tamil Nadu, where cholam (jowar) is staple. Cholam ground into flour and boiled or steamed into small balls. In Tamil Nadu, fish consumed along coastal belt by lower social classes. Pulse and vegetable intakes very low, condiments, especially chillis and tamarind, important. Consumption of milk negligible, though buttermilk popular with higher-income groups.

Andhra Pradesh — jowar staple except in northeast, north and south. Animal food intake negligible, milk rarely consumed. Amaranth, fenugreek, roselle, radish, carrot and vegetable marrow grown.

| 99 | SORGHUM AND MILLETS | INDIA | DISTRICTS IN TAMIL NADU | CENSUS OF INDIA, 1964d |

Millet staple for 18 per cent; millet/rice/wheat staple for 30 per cent; and rice, 51 per cent. Milk taken mostly in tea or coffee; average consumption 51 gm. (those who take twice daily receive 135 gm., once daily, 73 gm., and if taken only at foodstall, 20 gm.) Some receive none. Koilpatti, Sankarankoil, Perambalur and Bhavani consume cumbu, locally grown millet.

Chingleput: Millets staple for labourers, rice for remainder. Ragi most popular millet, followed by varagu, cumbu and cholam. Total consumption 575 gm. per head per day. Agricultural labourers take gruel with pickles and chillis in the morning and at noon, and rice and sambar in the evening.

North Arcot: Ragi widely used, also cholam, varagu, cumbu and samai. Gruel or porridge morning and noon, and rice eaten in evening.

Salem: Cholam, ragi and cumbu cooked in solid form, with pickles and sambar added for breakfast and noon. Rice with sambar or rasam eaten at night. Those who take millets and rice daily have total intake of 650 gm., while those eating only millets have 530 gm. daily.

Nilgiris: Mixed grain total intake 450 gm. per head per day, millets only 225 gm. per head per day. On plantations rice part of diet, elsewhere ragi and samai. Labourers take solid ragi, pickles and chutney for breakfast, boiled rice and sauce for lunch, and evening meal same as breakfast.
Madurai: Breakfast: cholam leftovers; lunch; cholam; supper: rice. Even in rice-growing areas, labourers take rice only at night.
Kanyakamari: Rice staple. 54 per cent take three meals; lower-income groups two (27 per cent) or only one (19 per cent). Rice supplemented by tapioca.

TABLE A/44

Consumption of pulse per head per day
by different income groups

Income, Rs. per month	Daily pulse consumption (gm.)
0 to 25	27
26 to 50	31
51 to 75	37
76 to 100	46
101 to 150	42

Tamil Nadu requires 7.7 lakh tons of pulses per year, and only 4.9 lakh tons are available.

Intake of protective foods varies according to district. Fish consumption averages 12 gm. per day; more eaten on coast. Vegetable consumption low, particularly among lower-income groups. In Nilgiris, consumption 24 gm. per head per day, becoming satisfactory only in towns (Coimbatore 140 gm.; Madras 130 gm.). Chillis and onions important in diet.

TABLE A/45

Consumption of milk per head per day
by different income groups

Income group (Rs. per month)	Milk consumption (gm.)
0 to 25	20
26 to 50	30
51 to 75	50
76 to 100	90
101 to 150*	112

* Only this group could afford meat, receiving 28 gm. per head per month; no eggs eaten.

TABLE A/46

Households in different income groups

Income group (Rs. per month)	Per cent
0 to 25	22.3
26 to 50	43.0
51 to 75	12.7
76 to 100	11.6
101 to 150	4.9
151 to 200	2.7
201 to 400	1.8
401 and above	1

Cost of balanced diet estimated at Rs. 123. Only those with Rs. 400 income per month are able to afford balanced diet. 89.6 per cent had income of less than Rs. 100 per month.

100	SORGHUM AND MILLETS	INDIA	CLOSEPET, MYSORE	ICMR
			TEHRI GARHWAL VILLAGES	1951
			UTTAR PRADESH	

TABLE A/47
Food intake per head per day
(in gm.)

	Mysore, Closepet		Tehri-Garhwal Barkot	Narendranagar
Rice	70	48	440	190
Wheat			20	480
Millets	700	680		
Other			110	
Pulses	60	43	54	70
Leafy vegetables	37	14	14	45
Other vegetables	25	24	132	65
Ghee/vegetable oil	3	6	6	14
Milk products	53	28	26	178

Sources of protein	per cent
Cereals	72.3
Pulses	16.2
Vegetables and fruits	3.2
Milk	2.3
Animal products	4.2
Condiments	1.9

No fruit, meat, fish, eggs, sugar or jaggery eaten.

101   SORGHUM AND MILLETS   INDIA   'GOPALPUR',   BEALS,
                                                            MYSORE   1962

Sorghum basis of every meal. All try to have a few mango and tamarind trees, and small garden for onions, leafy vegetables and eggplant. Green mango only fresh plant food during dry season. All try to keep female buffalo for milk.

Breakfast: cold leftovers.

Lunch   : chilli, beans, leafy vegetables, tamarind and salt simmered slowly together and placed on sorghum chapathi. Sometimes also rice, mango pickles or yoghurt mixed with water. Ghee if buffalo is in milk.

Supper   : Cold meal.

---

102   MILLETS   CHINA   LIU LING, NORTHERN   MYRDAL, 1966
                                                    SHENSI

Millet staple. Wheat considered luxury — 'there's no strength in it'. Potatoes, various millets, buckwheat and maize eaten; maize and oats chiefly for fodder. 'Milk harmful to others than infants'. Country people buy very little of their food. Each family receives a quota of grain from the labour group to which it belongs. They produce all else that is required on their private plots, mostly vegetables, beans, tobacco. They could buy vegetables, pork, sweetmeats on the market.

Meat eaten at New Year; perhaps at three or four other occasions during year. Meat might be bought in market for guests. Goat preferred to mutton. Vegetables are dried in spring: mustard root, beans, maize and potatoes. Sticky millet wine made in December. Bean curd made at New Year.

Menu for one family, 20 August 1962

Breakfast: Millet porridge, maize bread and a vegetable dish of fried tomatoes, beans and potatoes, spiced with chilli. Watered gruel (no water or tea)

Dinner   : Steamed millet, same vegetables as morning, broth of vegetable water.

Supper   : Millet porridge

Tuesday, 21 August 1962

Breakfast: Millet porridge with pumpkin. Potato chips fried in oil

Dinner   : Bean flour and wheat meal noodles; fried tomatoes, beans and potatoes. Chive, pepper and salt sauce

Supper   : Millet porridge

Wednesday, 22 August 1962

Breakfast: As Tuesday

Dinner   : Steamed millet, fried beans

Supper   : Millet porridge

Thursday, 23 August 1962

Breakfast: Millet porridge, turnips, maize bread and fried vegetables

Dinner   : Thick maize porridge made with potatoes and fresh cabbage

Supper   : Millet porridge (watermelon and small yellow melon eaten this day)

Friday, 24 August 1962

Breakfast: As Thursday

Dinner   : Wheat noodles with sauce and tomatoes and cabbage

Supper   : Millet porridge, maize cobs and steamed pumpkin

Saturday, 25 August 1962

Breakfast: As Tuesday

Dinner   : Steamed cakes of finely chopped potato kneaded with wheat flour. Fresh green beans, onion and garlic (taken at all meals)

Supper   : Millet porridge. Maize cobs. Steamed pumpkin

Sunday, 26 August 1962

Breakfast: Millet porridge and maize bread

Dinner   : Steamed wheaten bread with beans and tomatoes

Supper   : Millet porridge, maize cobs and steamed pumpkin

---

103   SORGHUM/MILLETS/RICE/WHEAT   CHINA   LICHUNG   WANG, 1947

Those investigated (May, 1945) were officials, institution workers, farmers, labourers, merchants, students and others. Most families had two meals per day. Calories sufficient only with farmers. Quantity sufficient for farmers and labourers, but quality poor. Fat inadequate in all diets. Phosphorus and iron sufficient; calcium adequate only for farmers and labourers; vitamin A deficient in farmers' diets.

104   SORGHUM AND MILLETS   CHINA   FANGCHENG PREFECTURE,   *JAPAN TIMES*
                                                      HEILUNGKIANG   1970a

The Sungari River region was formerly regarded as one of the most fertile in Manchuria. The characteristically objective *Japan Times* publishes an account of an interview with a group of farm settlers who have returned to Japan after some thirty years in Manchuria, in recent years in people's communes. The account is regarded as being nearer the truth than the reports of Japanese visitors to China, who have been shown model communes located near urban centres and designed as showpieces for visiting foreigners.

The returning group came with only the clothes on their backs:

and a couple of bundles of pitiful goods to show for their years of hardship and suffering . . . the people's commune system was put into effect in 1958, when (the family) farm of 8 hectares was confiscated . . . . The family was then assigned to the First Production Unit of the Tsomu Battalion of the Paohsing People's Commune in Fangcheng Prefecture. The production unit consisted of sixty families of 300 people. The units made up one battalion. Work started at dawn and ended at dusk. . . . .

Each working peasant received an average of one yuan (about 150 yen in Japanese currency or less than 50 U.S. cents) per day, or an annual income of 200 to 300 yuan. In addition each worker received a ration of about 150 kg. grain per year, sufficient to feed a family for four months. The balance had to be purchased.

Kaoliang (sorghum), maize, millets, rice and wheat, soybeans and vegetables were cultivated. After the failure of the Great Leap Forward, the peasants were in 1961 permitted to cultivate private plots at about 20 ares per family. These were cultivated during lunch breaks, were better managed and produced more than the common plots. Each family managed to keep one or two pigs and thirty or forty chickens, but for sale, since revenue was more important than food.

There was not much to eat and the returnees said they were hungry a great deal of the time. Rice was a treat reserved for New Year's Day and the few other festive occasions. Meat in the form of Chinese ravioli could be afforded only three or four times per year. Clothing was under strict rationing, enough for one cotton-padded winter suit every four years. All other essentials were also rationed. No household had bath facilities.

There was equality in the sense that everyone indiscriminately shared the same hardship and suffering.

---

105   MAIZE   INDIA   KAILASHPURI,   CENSUS OF INDIA, 1967a
                                        RAJASTHAN

Bhils (tribal people), Rajputs and Muslims non-vegetarian. Maize, barley and jowar staples. Local green vegetables eaten; pulses and onions common, peas and potatoes rare. Birds and animals hunted.

---

106   MAIZE   INDIA   PEEPAL KHOONT,   CENSUS OF INDIA,
                                        RAJASTHAN   1965a

Population chiefly Bhils. Maize staple; during times of scarcity, kodra eaten, also koori and batti. None of these rot during years of storage. Wheat, rice and meat eaten at festivals or community feasts. Pulses only occasionally. Bread (roti) eaten with buttermilk or maize flour boiled in buttermilk, or with chutney made by grinding salt and chillis together. Paniya is a special Bhil preparation, made of well-kneaded maize flour, flattened into a slice, placed between two leaves of dhak, close-stitched with straw and baked on a cowdung cake fire. Mangoes, mahua and other fruits eaten in season. Fish, fowl, partridge, sheep and goat eaten when available.

Breakfast: boiled leftovers
Lunch   : maize loaves
Supper   : same, or maize porridge. If meat available, eaten at this meal.

107	MAIZE	INDIA	DONGARPUR, RAJASTHAN	ICMR 1964

TABLE A/48

Food intake per head per day or per week

	gm. per caput per day	Number of families	Percentage of population
Rice	up to 57	171	29.4
	170	286	49.2
	255	20	3.4
Wheat	up to 57	1	0.2
	170	69	11.9
	up to 255	115	19.8
	312	134	23.1
	369	90	15.5
	425	17	2.9
Maize	up to 57	5	0.9
	170	48	8.3
	255	87	15.0
	312	144	24.8
	369	99	17.0
	425	43	7.4
	510	104	17.9
	624	14	2.4
	737	25	4.3
Millet	up to 57	26	4.5
	170	181	31.2
	255	48	8.3
	369	28	4.8
	425	12	2.1
Pulses	nil	32	5.5
	up to 57	540	93.1
Milk	nil	372	64.0
	up to 43	91	15.7
	85	77	13.2
	gm. per caput per week		
Meat and fish	nil	344	59.2
	up to 14	34	5.8
	43	136	23.4
	85	65	11.2
	142	2	0.3
Leafy vegetables	14	6	1.0
	57	415	71.4
	113	98	16.9
	326	57	9.8
Other vegetables	up to 57	342	58.9
	113	160	27.5
	326	54	9.3

108	MAIZE	INDIA	KHAJOORA, RAJASTHAN	CENSUS OF INDIA, 1964a

The staple of this Bhil village is maize, though kodra (*Paspalum scrobiculatum*), koori and batti also used. Rice eaten only on festive occasions. Wheat rarely used except to entertain guests. Chapathis and panya eaten. Gram and urud pulses taken; green vegetables and gram leaves. Spices or salt used. Radbi (boiled flour in buttermilk)common food. Mutton, hare, deer or other animals and birds caught in forest. Tea taken strong, with cow or goat milk, sugar, or more commonly jaggery. However, low economic status makes tea drinking rare.

---

109   MAIZE   INDIA   KALATH,   CENSUS OF INDIA,
                              SIMLA DISTRICT   (1965d)

Maize staple, with wheat, rice and koda (kharif millet). From May to August, wheat is staple, occasionally alternating with maize or rice. Maize chiefly eaten from September to April, with occasional substitutions. Koda taken by Untouchables and the poor in December and January. Cereals taken as chapathis, rice sometimes as small baked balls, with pulse or boiled butter-milk pottage. Pulses or vegetables cooked twice a day; buttermilk, onion, chillis fried in ghee and ginger. Milk consumed in small quantities. Meat prepared four to five times a month in Rajput households; Untouchables eat only once or twice a month. Pheasants, quail, partridge and wild goat may be hunted; mutton purchased from nearby communities. Three meals a day in summer, only two in winter. Sweet dishes prepared once a month. Kheroo, a type of stew, made from butter-milk and gram flour, cooked as vegetable. Rehru, another soup, prepared by boiling stale butter-milk and adding salt and chillis, as substitute for vegetables, taken with boiled rice.

Typical menus

May to August

7 a.m.	Tea and leftovers with butter
10 a.m.	Wheat chapathis and mash pulse (July — August)
	Wheat bhatooras (fermented chapathis) (May — June), or occasionally curry and rice, or wheat or rice flour chapathis
1 p.m.	Maize satoos with butter-milk, sauce, salt and pickles
5 p.m.	Tea
8 p.m.	Same as lunch
9 p.m.	Milk (those who have milch cattle in milk)

September to April

8 a.m.	Tea and leftovers with butter
11 a.m.	Maize chapathis, sarson sag and pulse, alternating occasionally with wheat or rice
4 p.m.	Heavy workers get leftovers from lunch Tea
8 p.m.	Same as lunch

---

110   MAIZE   INDIA   GOSHEN, HIMACHAL   CENSUS OF INDIA,
                              PRADESH   1967b

In this Gaddi village, staples are wheat, barley and sarswan (mustard-like oil seed) in winter; in summer; maize, millet and upland rice, also cholla (*Fagopyrum esculentum*). On poorer soils, *Phaseolus aureus* and bhares grown instead, but not favoured as food.

Among beans are ma (possibly *Dolichos biflorus*), mung, and brown beans. Potatoes, cucumbers, tomatoes, pumpkins, peppers, green chillis and apples eaten. Honey and toadstools gathered in jungle.

---

111   MAIZE   INDIA   NORTH BIHAR   ICMR 1964

Maize staple for two or three months per year, as chapathis or baked. Vegetable consumption low. Bengal gram popular in many forms; also red gram, lentils, *Lathyrus*, horse gram and green gram. Flesh consumption very low. Aboriginals also eat rats, crocodile and immature red ants. Sweet potato eaten by poor. Milk consumption negligible even in milk-producing tracts, as all sold. Butter-milk drunk by ghee makers.

---

112   MAIZE   INDIA   DARJEELING/KALIMPONG   WEST BENGAL,
                              DISTRICTS   1969

Maize staple, with dhal made of soybean. Maize may be made into gruel with milk and banana if available. Maize boiled with vegetables or pork when afforded. Many make butter, giving butter-milk to children and pigs. Piece of hard cheese sucked during heavy work.

In evening, fermented drink made of buckwheat, maize and millet taken with warm water. In morning, tea or coffee and a biscuit taken; at midday in the fields, chapathi and tea with salt eaten.

---

113   MAIZE   NEPAL   'BANYAN HILL'   HITCHCOCK,
                              1966

Maize and millet main dryland crops. Wheat, barley and upland rice of secondary importance. Rice grown on irrigated land. Livestock used for cash, sacrifice and festivals. Scheduled Castes eat buffalo; leather-workers eat beef if animal has died natural death.

| 114 | MAIZE | BURMA | NORTHERN CHIN HILLS | LEHMAN, 1963 |

Maize staple, though agricultural system depends on farming several crops: rice grown only in warm fields with particular soil. Rice considered superior food, is scarce and rarely eaten. Millets figure in ritual for grain increase, and were apparently staple before maize. If crops fail, mixture of millets and yams taken, though disliked. If maize fails, everything fails. Millets can be stored for considerable periods, as also un-hulled sulphur beans. Only poor eat these regularly, since taste disliked; hulling and elaborate leaching necessary to remove toxic factors. Fruits grown but eaten only sporadically, usually green with salt, es-pecially by children.

Hunting and fishing important; fish prominent in diet. Legumes, peas and runner beans eaten. Also melons, mustard greens, pumpkins, yams and taros, potatoes, bottle gourds, cucumbers. Sesamum seed used for cooking oil. Leeks, onions, garlic, chillis and indigo grown in kitchen gardens; spices (turmeric and roselle) on margins of swiddens.

| 115 | MAIZE, RICE/MAIZE | INDONESIA | EAST JAVA VILLAGES | BAILEY, 1961 AND 1962 |

Tengger: at 1,700 to 1,900 metres. Maize staple; im-mersed in water for a week, sun-dried and pounded into fine flour, steamed in banana leaf and eaten with soup, vegetables (carrot and cabbage) and potatoes.
Talang Agung: on Malang plains. Rice and maize cooked and eaten together with beans.
Sukodai: 700 metres, overlooking Malang. Maize staple.
Djimbaran: 700 metres. Maize staple, cassava grown for sale.
Patemon: Madura. Rice and maize eaten in equal pro-portion. Meat and fish frequently eaten, but small quantities. Vegetables relatively scarce.

Tjerme: 30 km. from Surabaya. Rice and maize mixed in equal proportion, salted. Fish and tempeh frequently used. During shortage, dried cassava used.

TABLE A/49

Nutrient intake per head per day

		Calories	Protein (gm.)	Iron (mg.)	Carotene (i.u)	Thiamine (mg.)	Vit. C (mg.)
A	Djatiredjojoso-Sitiredjo	1,211	32.5	8.9-9	934	789	12.8
	Tengger	1,186	32.0	7.9-8	1,662	996	38.8
	Talang Agung	1,158	33.3	10.9-11.1	566	808	11.6
	Sukodai	1,597*	35.2	13.2	2,770	1,224	23.0
B	Djimbaran	1,205	35.1	9.4-9.8	2,590	1,767	34.4
	Patemon	1,099	30.3	5.8-7.1	1,561	905	29.2
	Pademawu Barat	1,259	35.2	7.2-7.6	2,981	904	37.1
C	Tjerme	927	25.5	6.1-6.2	1,569	826	12.6
	Timbulhardjo	615?	13.8?	4.2-4.6	251	494	4.1
	Kedungsari	660?	11.4?	4.8-6.2	1,485	393	20.6
	Triwidadi	318?	6.5?	2.2-2.5	313	251	4.6
D	Madura (hinterland)	917	19.3	8.6-9.3	3,990	344	242.7
	Sempol	1,094	20.0	5.1-9.1	1,681	570	28.6
	Wonogiri	1,579	19.8	5.3-12.6	237	645	4.0
	Gunung Kidul	1,350	15.6	4.6-11.7	539	522	7.2

* Result considered too high.
? Total considered unreasonably low.

TABLE A/50

Calorie and protein intakes of groups of villages

Village group	Calories	Protein (gm. per day)
A	1,100 to 1,500	30 to 35
B	1,000 to 1,300	30 to 35
C	900	20 to 25
D	1,000 to 1,500	15 to 20

---

116   MAIZE   INDONESIA   CENTRAL AND EAST JAVA   POSTMUS AND VAN VEEN, 1949

More maize and rice, sometimes maize and cassava, eaten here than elsewhere in Java. Rice alone may be eaten after harvest, then rice and maize, then maize alone till next harvest. If crops grew normally, 400 gm. food grains available per head per day; if one crop fails, half this amount available. Region too densely populated for land available. Houses have only small compounds for growing protective foods. Study undertaken because oedema had appeared, following crop failures over two years.

TABLE A/51

Food and nutrient intakes per head per day of families with and without oedema

Foods	Families with oedema (gm.)	Families without oedema (gm.)
Meat, fish	11	10
Rice	227	221
Maize	40	94
Dried cassava (40 per cent root)	34	33
Pulses and tempe	6	9
Green leafy vegetables and young pulses	22	17
Other vegetables	14	27
Fruit	1	
Nutrients		
Calories	989	1,164
Animal protein (gm.)	3.9	3.6
Vegetable protein (gm.)	22.8	27.8
Fat (gm.)	5.1	8.3
Provitamin A (i.u.)	1,258	1,036
Thiamine (mg.)	0.5	0.6

---

117   MAIZE   INDONESIA   SOBA, WEST TIMOR   CUNNINGHAM, 1967

Hilly, loose-soiled terrain, very heavy rains December to March. Shifting cultivation practised by increasing population and increase in cattle numbers (700,000) contribute to what the geographer Ormeling has called a 'deteriorating environment'.
Different types of maize of varying maturation planted; first ready in March 'for the children' to break period of hunger. Rice and corn of longest maturation ready in April.
Wet season, marked by dwindling food supplies, called *lapar biasa* – 'the usual hunger'.
Households grow piper betel, areca nut, banana and coconut. Some plant tomato, garlic, cassava or spring onion for market.

| 118 | WHEAT | WEST PAKISTAN | GENERAL | MAQSOOD, 1961 |

TABLE A/52

Protein values of diets and meals

	Protein Calories (per cent)	NPU (op) (per cent)	NDpCals (per cent)
West Pakistan diet	13.3	51	6.8
Wheat/pulse/meat curry	14.5	52	7.5
Wheat/pulse/vegetable curry	14.2	52	7.4

By end of second Five-Year Plan, energy value of diet higher, but protein content lower.

| 119 | WHEAT | INDIA | RANG MAHAL, GANGANAGAR DISTRICT, RAJASTHAN | CENSUS OF INDIA, 1965b |

Brahmins, Jats and Kumhars vegetarians, remainder non-vegetarian. Daily food: sogra (thick bread of bajra baked hard); rab (flour diluted in buttermilk, cooked at night for next morning); khich (husked bajra mixed with pulse in proportion of four to one, boiled thick in water); chapathi; dalia (coarse grain flour boiled thick).

Onions and pulse only vegetables; occasionally tree pods used. Salt and chillis used as flavouring. 65 families ate three times, 18 twice a day. Jats keep cattle and take milk and ghee. When cattle in milk, children given milk twice daily. Occasionally a goat or ram killed for festivals.

| 120 | WHEAT | INDIA | LUDHIANA PUNJAB | BANERJEE AND SAHA, 1968 |

Study of vegetarians and non-vegetarians, athletes and non-athletes, same ethnic origin, similar economic and social background.

TABLE A/53

Heights, weights and food intakes of vegetarians and non-vegetarians

	Males		Females	
	Vegetarian	Non-vegetarian	Vegetarian	Non-vegetarian
Height (cm.)	167.6	170	156	156
Weight (kg.)	72.9	51.75	71	50.8
Food intake (gm. per day)				
Carbohydrate	264	270	155	155
Protein	81	115	51	86
Fat	59	77	36	42
Calories (number)	1,916	2,236	1,154	1,343

| 121 | WHEAT | INDIA | VILLAGE 90 MILES NORTH OF DELHI IN UTTAR PRADESH | MINTURN AND HITCHCOCK, 1966. MAHAR, 1969 |

Breakfast: chapathis; some take milk only
Lunch : chapathis, rice and pulses: during slack season men return from fields, otherwise children take food in pots to field.
Supper : same
Milk important in diet, mostly as curds and ghee. Wo-

men are vegetarians; men wanting meat obtain and cook it in their separate quarters. Men and boys eat goat, duck, chicken and fish at least four times a month. Tender leaves of papaya regular part of diet. Little fresh fruit except for guava and mango in season. Other fruit too costly. Popcorn and sugar snacks.

122   WHEAT   INDIA   SAROJINI NAGAR, UTTAR PRADESH   MALAVIYA, SEN GUPTA, SRIVASTAVA AND PRASAD, undated.

Survey of boys and girls in six basic primary schools in the area of the Rural Health Centre, Department of Social and Preventive Medicine, King George's Medical College, Lucknow, with supervision of Nutrition Section, Provincial Hygiene Institute, Lucknow; situated at 16th kilometer on Lucknow/Kanpur road; 516 students aged 4 to 15 years. A dietary survey conducted in 46 families of these children showed that the intake of protective foods was far below Indian Council of Medical Research Institute standards; deficiencies marked for animal protein, calcium, vitamin A, ascorbic acid, riboflavine and niacin; iron and thiamine satisfactory.

Some 79 per cent had one or more nutritional defects; 54 per cent showed one or other of the clinical signs of vitamin A deficiency in eyes and skin.

Other manifestations were, in percentage of the children:

rickets   14.34   spongy, bleeding gums 11.29
caries   50.77   goitre   2.71
and to a less extent papillary hypertrophy and angular stomatitis.

123   WHEAT   INDIA   BILASPUR, SAHARANPUR DISTRICT, UTTAR PRADESH   CENSUS OF INDIA, 1965f

Wheat, gram and barley staples from April to October. Dhal and vegetables eaten. Urd preferred to arhar as pulse. Potato, cauliflower, brinjal, lauki, karela, pumpkin and several other vegetables eaten. 72 families vegetarian, 78 non-vegetarian. Milk and ghee unavailable unless cattle are owned. Fruits eaten when available; water melon and musk melon in summer, mango in rainy season. Gur common, but little sugar. 79 per cent take two meals, 21 per cent three. Staple diet: loaf of wheat bread (roti) and bajra taken with urd. Chilli much used. Rice only occasionally.

124   WHEAT/BAJRA/RICE   INDIA   GUJARAT, RURAL AND POOR URBAN AREAS (NEAR BARODA)   RAJALAKSHMI AND NANAVATY (UNDATED)

Survey from 1958 to 1964 among different socio-economic groups. Most poor families in both rural and urban areas composed of 4 to 5 members, and at least 50 per cent of income spent on food. Most had two main meals daily, with a cup of tea early in the morning and late afternoon. Children had some leftover food in early morning. Most meals either roti with dhal or vegetable, or a rice and dhal preparation, with butter-milk soup or vegetable. Jowar, maize, varagu and ragi also used in addition to staples in rural areas. While a number of cereals are used, generally only one is used at a time, and not always with a legume. Fruits generally consumed only by children. Cooking methods lead to losses in nutrient value: rice and dhals washed, and vegetables steeped in water before cooking, and cooked for prolonged periods in an open pan.

Percentages of those who restricted food intake for reasons other than economic were lower than those given by the *Diet Atlas of India* (58 per cent), being 23 per cent in one survey, and only 9 per cent in another.

The average diet was inadequate in poorer groups, and there was no awareness of the special needs of infancy, growth, pregnancy and lactation, while food-sharing practices aggravated the inadequacies for these groups. Calorie intakes low, and protein intakes for poor families low and unbalanced. When pulses used, they were in combination with cereals at a proportion of 10:1, whereas 4:1 is probably desirable. Chief deficiencies are carotene, riboflavine, calcium and iron for adults, and also for children and nursing mothers, who also lack protein. All groups appear to suffer from a calorie deficiency.

TABLE A/54

Food intake per head per day

	Mean consumption per caput (gm.)	Range (gm.)	No. of families consuming less than mean value
Cereals	326.0	140-570	35
Pulses	28.0	2.8 -159	68
Milk	53.9	0-510	74
Sugar and jaggery	21.2	2.8-40	85
Oils	14.0	2.8-85	94

| 125 | WHEAT | CHINA | NORTH-WEST YUNNAN | LEBAR, HICKEY AND MUSGRAVE, 1964 |

Nakhi, Tibeto-Burman speaking tribal people, within loop of Yangtze. Unleavened wheat bread, roasted barley meal, yak butter and tea staple foods.

| 126 | BARLEY | INDIA | BHADKAR UDARHAR, ALLAHABAD DISTRICT, UTTAR PRADESH | CENSUS OF INDIA, 1964c |

Bejhar (mixture of barley and gram) staple from April to October, bajra from November to March. Dhal and vegetables supplement staple. Wheat used for festive occasions. Spice used by all. Mustard oil for cooking. 65.4 per cent vegetarians. Meat and fish taken by others when available. Milk and ghee greatly valued. Milk purchased for sick, but seldom for growing children. Fruits eaten when available; melons and water melon in summer, and cheap variety of mango in rainy season.

Breakfast consists of leftovers; some take gram with salt. Only higher-income families take fresh chapathis in morning. Each household has midday and evening meal.

| 127 | BARLEY | SOUTH KOREA | GENERAL | YANG, T.H. 1966 YOUNG, 1968 CHAI, 1967 KWON ET AL, 1967 |

FAO Report TA 2236 (Yang, 1966) refers to survey of 1958 by College of Medicine, Yonsei University, covering 20 farm families, 118 persons, in typical rural area. Shortage of calories in winter and especially spring. Bean consumption low. Vitamin A intake low. Angular stomatitis in children throughout year.

Young (1968). In Suwon, average consumption of grains 19 litres per month, lower-income groups taking greater proportion of barley mixed with rice. Higher-income group had more rice and added soybeans. Consumption of livestock products increase with income.

Chai (1967). Animal food 3.5 per cent of total intake; forestry and mining areas received one-quarter to one-fifth animal protein intake of town dwellers, agricultural areas one half. Protein deficiency indicated by consumption surveys and biochemical examinations, particularly among pregnant and lactating women.

Kwon et al. (1967). Survey in urban slum. Staple rice/barley for 54 per cent; 12 per cent took rice/barley/small red bean; 9 per cent wheat flour kneaded and sliced in soup; 7 per cent wheat flour noodle, and 7 per cent white potato. Only 4.6 per cent took rice alone as staple.

Side dishes	*Per cent*
Kimchi (pickled cabbage or radish)	36
Tchige (boiled food), pumpkin, cabbage, white potato	21
Bokkum (roasted side dish with no fluid), cabbage, pumpkin, leek	11
Jorim (hard boiled side dish with salt, i.e. beef/soybean sauce)	9
Soup (soybean sprout, cabbage, potatoes, radish leaves, etc.)	8
Cooked vegetables: bean sprouts	8

Most important animal food dried small sardine, salted sardine, salted shrimp cooked with soup and kimchi. Only 11 per cent of households used fish, shells and meats, and only occasionally in very small quantities. 35 gm. soysauce, 17 gm. soybean paste and 7 gm. pepper paste consumed per head per day. Grains provided 90 per cent of calories and 76 per cent of total protein. Vegetables, beans and potatoes provided 20 per cent of total protein (11.41 gm.). Animal foods (7.95 gm. per head per day) provided 3.6 per cent of total protein.

| 128 | SWEET POTATO | PHILIPPINES | MAYAOYAO, MOUNTAIN PROVINCE, CENTRAL LUZON | GUTHRIE, G.M. 1964 |

Based on interviews with Crate Larkin, American physician who lived in Ifugao tribal village for several years.

Terraced mountains and shifting cultivation on unterraced slopes. Strong concept of conservation and value of forest in water conservation. Anyone cutting forest in catchment area at top of mountain regarded as a criminal. Terraces used for rice with other crops as admixtures. Fourteen to sixteen varieties of rice grown: hard white, red and glutinous, the last type being used for rice wine, which takes 50 per cent of crop.

Very little food imported and virtually none exported. Diet varied, but deficient in protein and iodine. Foods introduced from lowlands often upset dietary habits and do more harm than good. After weaning, young children show marked signs of protein deficiency; their diet does not improve until they are big enough to compete for the adult ration.

Staple is sweet potato, consumption 360 kg. per caput per year. Rice first for wine, then as food. Maize eaten, but much fed to chickens. Peas grown on trees. String beans; no melons; plant resembling watercress, and rich in iron, collected in mountain streams. Sugar cane grown on edges of swidden.

Coffee grows around settlements, and is used, also tea. Areca nut actively cultivated and chewing common.

Pigs and chickens eaten only at sacrifice, divided among rich and poor equally. Few fish in terraces, including eels. Frogs and two types of snail eaten. Flying ants fried at certain seasons. Locusts in occasional swarms. Grubs and beetles. Deer meat kept, eaten partly decomposed. Wild pigs, bats, flying fox, small migratory birds hunted.

Health threatened not only by new diseases, but also by new foods and population pressure. Civilization will bring more polished rice, less good sources of protein as bugs and bats become disdained, with consequent deterioration of diet.

---

129   SWEET POTATO   TAIWAN   SOUTH TAIWAN   BLACKWELL, 1961

TABLE A/55

Summary of nutritional surveys in area where blackfoot disease prevalent

Quality of diet	Poor
Variety	Limited
Caloric intake	Adequate
Protein intake	Barely adequate
Amino-acid intake	Barely adequate, marginal methionine
Fat intake	Low
Main source of calories	Sweet potato, secondly rice
Main source of protein	Fish
Ability of diet to support rat growth	Inadequate

Families from agricultural, salt-producing and urban areas, and fishing villages. Poorest families could afford fresh vegetables only for a few meals a month. From December to June sweet potato eaten fresh, main source of vitamins. Higher-income families eat no sweet potato, but majority eat appreciable quantities.

Ice fish cheapest and most commonly eaten. Fishing village families ate small amounts of crabs, shrimps and oysters. Pork too expensive for poor; bought ten times a year for special occasions. Higher-income families ate a few times a month. Soybean eaten in small amounts because of cost; curd, fermented curd, salty bean paste, and small amounts of oil, to add taste and palatability to staple. Agricultural people consumed some of their products. Fishing and salt-producing areas grew less; vegetables expensive to buy. Chinese cabbage, cucumber, garlic, scallions and Welsh onions eaten. Sweet potato leaf and wild grasses may be used. Fruit luxury item. Dried sweet potato eaten between July and November, but also throughout the year, because easier to digest than when fresh.

TABLE A/56

Comparative distribution of caloric intake (in per cent)

Nutrient	Average of Blackfoot area	Taiwan average 1951	Taiwan average 1958
Carbohydrate	84	76	75
Fat	7	12	12
Protein	9 (4 to 15)	12	12
Calories (total mean)	2,740	2,650	2,700

TABLE A/57

Food intake per head per day (in per cent)

	Average of Blackfoot area	*Taiwan average 1951*	*Taiwan average 1958*
Rice	46	66	57
Sweet potato	44	11	11
Wheat			7
Beans	2	8	8
Vegetable oil	2	2	3
Vegetables and fruits	—	4	4
Animal foods	4	7	9
Miscellaneous	—	2	1

TABLE A/58

Protein consumption per head per day (in per cent)

	Average of Blackfoot area	*Taiwan average 1951*	*Taiwan average 1958*
Rice	44	57	44
Sweet potato	19	—	4
Wheat flour			6
Beans	4	13	13
Vegetables and fruit		6	6
Animal protein	32	20	26
Pork	3	8	9
Fish	29	10	14
Other		2	3
Miscellaneous	1	4*	1
Total intake per adult man	60 gm.	67 gm.	68 gm.

* Includes sweet potato and wheat flour.

130	SWEET POTATO	OKINAWA	'TAIRA', NORTHWEST OKINAWA	MARETZKI AND MARETZKI, 1966

Sweet potatoes planted throughout most of year. Less popular than rice, but wholly utilized. Large tubers given to adults, small to pigs, leaves used as vegetables, with older leaves for pigs. Forms staple with rice. Wheat, beans and vegetables additional subsistence crops.

131	SWEET POTATO, MILLET, WHEAT	CHINA	TAITOU, SOUTH-WESTERN SHORES OF KIAOCHOW BAY, OPPOSITE TSINGTAO	YANG, 1945

Population at this time divided into four groups: lowest level had sweet potato as staple; next had combination of sweet potato and millet, third group millet and wheat, and top group only wheat. All classes eat garden vegetables when available. The two poorest groups rarely have any animal food, the last two only occasionally.

The poor eat sweet potato at every meal throughout the year — from harvest until spring, fresh, and then dried slices. This is supplemented with gruel of barley flour and peanut powder, and a hash of chopped turnips and soybean juice, and pickles.

During busy season food more plentiful. Steamed millet or millet bread takes place of sweet potato slices, and green vegetables cooked in fat added. Soybean oil and peanut oil used in cooking, while richer households use pork fat. A poor woman tastes sugar only when she delivers a child.

As economic condition improves, millet, barley, soybeans, wheat and other kinds of cereal added to sweet potatoes. In winter and early spring, sweet potato mainly used. Quality of food improves in busy season, when a *morning meal* might consist of steamed millet and soybean powder bread, boiled sweet potatoes, barley gruel, turnip and soybean hash, salted fish and pickles. *Noon meal* steamed millet bread, steamed wheat bread, dish of green vegetables, gruel of millet and rice, salted fish and pickles. *Evening meal* resembles morning meal. During wheat harvesting more wheat bread is served, and a stew of pork and green vegetables often served, while wheat flour noodles and salted fish and pickles eaten regularly.

Protein consumption high at New Year. From tenth month to last part of twelfth (lunar calendar), people suffer calorie deficiency and complain of monotony of diet. Wealthy families have better food throughout year.

| 132 | YAMS/BAMBOO SHOOTS | YUMBRI, NOMADIC GATHERERS OF NORTHERN THAILAND | LEBAR, HICKEY AND MUSGRAVE, 1964 |

Bamboo shoots staple for part of year, otherwise wild yams and other edible roots. Wild fruits, berries, leaves, wild sago palm, snails, caterpillars, crabs, lizards, frogs, turtles, mice, rats, squirrels, honey and birds' eggs part of diet. Small animals such as porcupines and rodents, and occasionally barking deer or wild pig are caught. Meat roasted over an open fire or boiled in a length of green bamboo, usually eaten half raw. Roots, herbs and shoots are baked on hot coals or boiled in bamboo container. Occasionally they may obtain rice by trade or theft, and they then season it with salt and wild chillis and peppers. Jungle produce — wild honey, wax, rattan, firewood, mats and baskets — traded for tobacco, rice, salt, meat, secondhand clothing and knives with Meo, Yao, T'in and Khmu peoples.

| 133 | CASSAVA | W. MALAYSIA | TEMIAR OF KELANTAN | SLIMMING, 1958 |

Tapioca staple, with rice occasionally. Marrows, bananas, sugarcane, maize also grown. Hunting and fishing supplement diet; no eggs eaten.

| 134 | CASSAVA | E. MALAYSIA | MURUTS OF SABAH | LEY, 1967 |

Hill paddy and tapioca staples, with sweet potato, maize, local spinach, edible fungi, bananas, jungle fruit. Hunters supply wild fowl, deer, pig and fish. Fish and meat often salted and stored in bamboo containers with rice and herbs for 6 to 9 months.

| 135 | CASSAVA | INDONESIA | VARIOUS AREAS | BAILEY, 1961 AND 1962 |

Tjelapar, south central Java
Lunch and supper gruel of cassava with side dishes. Goats raised as meat for feasts.
Pademawu Barat, few km. from capital of Madura
Cassava supplement or substitute for maize and rice for half year during dry season.
Kedungsari, near Jogjakarta, Java
Non-irrigated rice fields give low yield. None landless. Half coconut crop sold to supplement income. Cassava and other root crops grown, since nothing else possible on poor clay soil matted with coconut roots and other trees. Taro, canna, arrowroot and yams grown, even under bamboo. One meal rice, one meal cassava.
Madura hinterland
Cassava staple, eaten fresh, grated and steamed. Uprooted as required daily. Maize grown, but in poorer villages, enough for only few days' consumption. Considerable numbers of cattle, though no pasture. Many fish in shallow waters. Smaller ones sun-dried and taken inland for export to Java, salted then dried. Important both in economy and diet; half price of those in Java, thus pressure to sell less heavy. In absence of fish, meat might be used, or no animal food. Meat always on sale in markets. Common legumes, lima and field beans, pre-cooked, mixed and steamed again with grated cassava.
Sempol, Malang Regency, east Java
Situated at 500 m. elevation. Income from coffee, sugarcane and livestock. Cassava flour basic staple, especially for poor, also some rice and maize.

| 136 | SAGO | EAST MALAYSIA | MELANAU COMMUNITY, SARAWAK | MORRIS, 1953 |

First meal : Coffee and sago biscuits and dried fish, or, if money available, water biscuits made of wheat flour from Singapore

Midday meal : Meat if any, more usually dried fish eaten with boiled rice and few vegetables and sauce, eaten more as relish than as a separate dish.

Evening meal : Coffee, sago biscuits and dried fish. If any boiled rice left over from lunch, this may take the place of sago biscuits.

TABLE A/59

Food intake at seventy-six meals, covering twenty-seven days

Item	No. of times eaten
Sago biscuits	43
Rice	28
Fresh fish	23*
Dried fish	51
Salt fish	11
Tinned fish	1
Peanuts	27
Fowl	2
Cucumber	7
Kankong	6
Split peas	2
Sundry leaf vegetables	2

* More fresh fish than usual, since material collected during fishing season, during January and February.

In times of hardship, less rice is available and more sago biscuits eaten.

| 137 | SAGO | INDONESIA | CERAM | POSTMUS AND VAN VEEN, 1949 |

Sago flour, prepared from *Metroxylon* spp., staple. Sago woods distant from villages, cultivation near village. Fish along coast. People not industrious, but sago does not make them energetic. Permanent or temporary immigrants work hardest. Other crops: cassava, sweet potatoes, taro, yams, rice and maize (last infrequent). Sugarcane, bananas and leafy vegetables grown, mostly after main swidden crop. Coconuts available on coast. Hunting important in mountainous areas.

Main foodstuff sago as porridge or cakes, with smaller but not inconsiderable quantities of tubers; latter so frequently washed that only taro and sweet potato retain minerals and vitamins. Immigrants eat cassava and maize as staple.

TABLE A/60

Food and nutrient intakes per head per day
(in gm.)

	Coastal villages	Mountain villages
Animal food	90 to 113	12 to 43
Coconuts	45 to 85.6	
Vegetables	160 to 200	160 to 200
Calories	1,600 to 1,700	2,000
Protein	9 (up to 26)	9 (up to 24)

Mountain area took three meals daily, coastal villages two. Since tuber or sago staple, protein intake low, despite relatively high intake of animal food. Thiamine is deficient in sago diets. Fresh sea and shellfish readily lose thiamine content, while dried fish has none. Vitamin A adequate, the mean intake of pro-vitamin A being 1400 to 1600 i.u. daily in coastal villages, and 4800 to 13,000 in mountain regions where yellow sweet potato eaten. Despite deficiencies, evidence of malnutrition rare. However under stress, deficiency diseases occur (malaria and fevers accompanied by oedema and beri beri). Those who do heavy work for prolonged periods in the jungle show deficiency diseases on return.

| 138 | SAGO | INDONESIA | 'ALLANG', AMBON, MOLUCCAS | COOLEY, 1967 |

Land far back in steep, heavily wooded areas, some not cultivated. Well-suited to nutmegs and cloves, former being most important cash crop. Fish chief source of protein, with fowl and wild game on special occasions. Staple diet sago flour, tubers, cassava, coconut, few leaves of vegetables and trees, nuts and fruits. Rice occasionally used. Sago baked into biscuits or boiled to form viscous jelly, eaten hot.

| 139 | BUCKWHEAT | CHINA | MOUNTAINS OF SOUTHWEST SZECHUAN | LEBAR, HICKEY AND MUSGRAVE, 1964 |

Nosu, tribal people inhabiting Ta'liang Shan and Hsiao-liang Shan. Buckwheat cakes, unleavened maize cakes and sour vegetable soup staples. Bean curd, green vegetables and boiled potatoes occasional luxury. Beef, pork, mutton and poultry eaten only by tribal aristocracy, and then only on special occasions. No milk used.

| 140 | PANDANUS/COCONUT/ ROOTS AND TUBERS | INDIA | ANDAMAN AND NICOBAR ISLANDS | (1) ROY AND ROY, 1969 (2) SANGAL, 1971 |

(1)   Joint scientific expedition in which seven departments belonging to five Ministries of Government of India participated, February to May 1966. Great Nicobar (865 sq. km.), largest island of Andaman and Nicobar group in Bay of Bengal; hilly and covered with forests. Two tribes inhabit the island, Nicobarese and Shompens; only 139 individuals Nicobarese, of which 48 surveyed for food sources, dietary habits and nutrient intakes.

Staples pandanus (red and white varieties), coconut and marine fish, animals; other plant foods bananas, yams, taro, papaya and some wild fruits. Octopus consumed daily in large amounts, also shark, ray, prawns and shellfish, pomfrets, turtles. Wild and domestic pig not important source of meat. Insect larvae, fowls, crocodiles, wild birds and honey also consumed. Beverages: fermented coconut toddy, fresh milk of green and ripe coconuts.

The pandanus, coconut, foods of animal origin and fermented toddy provide about 35, 28, 23 and 10 per cent respectively of the daily calorie intake of 3050 per consumption unit. The nutrient content of the diet is satisfactory, rich in animal protein (103 gm. per person daily), high in fat. In fact, of all the population groups so far surveyed in the Indian Union, the Nicobarese have the best diet.

(2)   Forest tribal population of Andaman and Nicobar Islands consume animal products (chiefly pig, also oysters, freshwater fish and prawns, turtle eggs, bird eggs, jungle cat, bats, water lizards and grubs, honey and bee larvae), roots and tubers, stem cores, fruits, seeds, leaves and buds.

Bibliography

ABDON, I.C. (1969). 'Coconut as a source of protein.' *Philippine J. Nutrition* 22, 103–113.

ADAMS, A.R.D. *and* MAEGRAITH, B.G. (1964). *Clinical tropical diseases* (4th ed.), Blackwell Scientific Publications. Oxford. 582 pp.

AGARWAL, K.N., MANWANI, A.H., KHANDUJA, P.C., AGARWAL, D.K. *and* GUPTA, S. (1970). 'Physical growth of Indian school children.' *Indian Pediat.* 7, 146–55.

AGARWAL, J.R., SHETH, S.C. *and* TIBREWALA,' N.S. (1969). 'Rickets – a study of 300 cases.' *Indian Pediat.* 6, 792–8.

AGUILLON, D.B. *and* VALDECANAS, O.C. (1969). 'Bridging the gap between nutrition research and its application.' *Philippine J. Nutrition* 22, 43–7.

AIRD, J.S. (1968). *Estimates and projections of the population of mainland China, 1953–86.* U.S. Bureau of Census Series P–91: 17, Washington. 73 pp.

AIYAPPAN, A. (1965). *Social revolution in a Kerala village: a study in culture change.* Asia Publishing House, Bombay. 183 pp.

ALABASTRO, V.Q., BAUTISTA, A.P., TULIO, A.R., LINGAO, A.L. *and* RODRIGUEZ, N.C. (1970). 'Family food plans for Western and Eastern Visayas, South-west and North-east Mindanao.' *Philippine J. Nutrition* 23, 17–32

ALEID, R. (1960). *Report to the Government of the Federation of Malaya on home economics.* F.A.O. E.T.A.P. Report no. 1274. mimeo. Rome. 14 pp.

ALLCHIN, B. *and* ALLCHIN, F.R. (1968). *The birth of Indian civilization.* Pelican. Penguin Books, Harmondsworth. 365 pp.

ALLCHIN, F.R. (1969). 'Early domestic animals in India and Pakistan'; 'Early cultivated plants in India and Pakistan.' In *The domestication and exploitation of plants and animals* (ed. P.J. Ucko and G.W. Dimbleby), pp. 317 – 22 and 323 – 9. Duckworth, London.

ALLEN, D.M. *and* DEAN, R.F.A. (1965). 'The anaemia of kwashiorkor in Uganda.' *Trans.Roy.Soc.Trop. Med.Hyg.* 59, 326–41.

ANDERSON, E.N., Jr. (1970). 'Lineage atrophy in Chinese society.' *Amer.Anthropol.* 72, 363–5.

ANDERSON, M.M. (1960). *Report to the Government of Thailand: nutrition education program.* F.A.O. E.T.A.P. Report no. 1276. mimeo. Rome. 23 pp.

ANAND, D. *and* RAO, A.R. (1962). 'Feeding practices of infants and toddlers in Najafgarh area.' *Ind.J.Child Health,* April. 172–81.

APPELL, G.N. (1968) Personal communication.

—————————— (1969) Personal communication.

ARMENDARES, S., SALAMANCA, F. *and* FRENK, S. (1971). 'Chromosome abnormalities in severe protein calorie malnutrition.' *Nature, Lond.* 232, 271–3.

ASHWORTH, A. (1969). 'Growth rates in children recovering from protein-calorie malnutrition.' *Brit.J. Nutrition* 23, 835–45.

———— *and* WATERLOW, J.C. (1969). 'Improved rates of recovery in malnourished infants as a result of increasing their calorie intakes.' *West Indian Med.J.* 18, 251—52.

AUTRET, M. *and* PAUL-PONT, I. (1971). 'Planning for better living.' *Nutrition Newsletter 9 (3), 40—45.*

———— *and* PERISSE J. (1970). 'Indicative World Plan for Agricultural Development: nutritional digest.' *Nutrition Newsletter* 8 (2), 8—16.

————, PERISSE, J., SIZARET, F. *and* CRESTA, M. (1968). 'Protein value of different types of diet in the world: their appropriate supplementation.' *Nutrition Newsletter* 6 (4), 1—29.

AYKROYD, W.R. *and* DOUGHTY, J. (1964). *Legumes in human nutrition.* F.A.O. Nutritional Studies no. 19, Rome. 138 pp.

———— *and* ———— (1970). *Wheat in human nutrition.* F.A.O. Nutritional Studies no. 23, Rome. 163 pp.

———— *and* PATWARDHAN, V.N. (1960). *The nutritive value of Indian foods and the planning of satisfactory diets.* (5th ed.). Indian Council of Medical Research Health Bulletin no. 23. New Delhi.

————, GOPALAN, C. *and* BALASUBRAMANIAN, S.C. (1966). *The nutritive value of Indian foods and the planning of satisfactory diets.* (6th ed.). Indian Council of Medical Research Health Special Report Series no. 42. New Delhi. 257 pp.

BAGCHI, K., HALDER, K., CHOUDHURY, S.R., SANYAL, B. *and* SEN, P.C. (1960). 'A study of nutritional and non-nutritional factors in the incidence of kwashiorkor in a rural area of West Bengal.' *Indian J. Med. Assoc.* 34, 441—49.

BAILEY, K.V. (1961a). 'Rural nutrition studies in Indonesia. III Epidemiology of hunger oedema in the cassava areas.' *Trop. Geogr. Med.* 13, 289—302.

———— (1961b) 'IV Oedema in lactating women in the cassava areas.' *Trop. Geogr. Med.* 13, 303—315.

———— (1962a) 'V Field surveys: procedure and background.' *Trop. Geogr. Med.* 14, 1-10.

———— (1962b) 'VI Field surveys of lactating women.' *Trop. Geogr. Med.* 14, 11—19.

———— (1962c) 'VII Field surveys of Javanese infants.' *Trop. Geogr. Med.* 14, 111—20.

———— (1962d) 'VIII Field surveys of Javanese school-age boys.' *Trop. Geogr. Med.* 14, 121—28.

———— (1962e) 'IX The Gunung Kidul problem in perspective.' *Trop. Geogr. Med.* 14, 238—58.

BALASINGAM, E., LIM, B.L. *and* RAMCHANDRAN, C.P. (1969). 'A parasitological study of Pulau Pinang and Pulau Perhentian Kechil, off Trengganu, West Malaysia. II. Intestinal helminthiasis.' *Med.J. Malaya* 23, 300 — 304.

BANERJEE, B. *and* SAHA, N. (1968). 'Influence of diet and physical activity on serum cholesterols.' *Med.J. Malaya* 22, 332—34.

BANIK, N.D.D., NAYAR, S., KRISHNA, R., RAJ, L. *and* GADEBAR, N.G. (1970). 'Skeletal maturation of Indian children.' *Indian J. Pediat.* 37, 249—54.

———— , KRISHNA, R., MANE. S.I.S., RAJ, L. *and* TASKAR, A.D. (1970). 'A longitudinal study of physical growth of children from birth up to 5 years of age in Delhi.' *Ind. J. Med Res* 58, 135—42.

BARDHAN, P.K. (1970). 'Chinese and Indian agriculture: a broad comparison of recent policy and performance.' *J. Asian Studies* 29, 515—37.

BARNETT, K.M.A. (1967). 'A bang— or a whimper?' *Far Eastern Econ. Rev.* 29 June, 710—13.

BASHAM, A.L. (1954). *The wonder that was India: a survey of the culture of the Indian sub-continent before the coming of the Muslims.* Sidgwick and Jackson, London. 568 pp.

BASSIR, O. (1962). *Biochemical aspects of human malnutrition in the tropics.* Monographiae Biologicae V, fasc. 3—4. Junk, The Hague. 122 pp.

BAYLESS, T.M. *and* ROSENSWEIG, N.S. (1966). 'A racial difference in incidence of lactase deficiency.' *J. Amer. Med. Assoc.* 197, 968—72.

———— (1967). 'Incidence and implications of lactase deficiency and milk intolerance in white and negro populations.' *Johns Hopkins Medical J.* 121, 54—64.

BEALS, A.R. (1962). *Gopalpur, a south Indian village.* Holt, Rinehart and Winston, New York, Toronto, London. 99 pp.

BEARDSLEY, R.K. (1968) Personal communication.

————, HALL, J.W. *and* WARD, R. (1959). *Village Japan.* University of Chicago Press. 498 pp.

BEGUM, A. *and* PEREIRA, S.M. (1969). 'Calcium balance studies on children accustomed to low calcium intakes.' *Brit.Med.J.* 23, 905–11.

————, RADHAKRISHNAN, A.N. *and* PEREIRA, S.M. (1970). 'Effect of amino acid composition of cereal-based diets on growth of preschool children.' *Amer.J.Clin. Nutrition* 23, 1175–83.

BELAVADY, B. (1963). *Studies on human lactation.* Indian Council of Medical Research Special Report Series no. 45. 17 pp.

———— (1969). 'Nutrition in pregnancy and lactation.' *Indian J. Med. Res.* 57, 63–74.

BENDER, A.E. (1971). *Report to the Government of Nepal on food and nutrition policy.* Nutrition Consultants Reports Series no. 22. F.A.O., Rome. 26 pp.

BENGOA, J.M. (1969). *Recent trends on prevalence of protein-calorie malnutrition.* Paper to VIIIth Inter. Congress on Nutrition, Prague. Protein Advisory Group document 1.2.1/1. mimeo. 14 pp.

———— (1970). *Curative aspects of malnutrition and rehabilitation of the malnourished child.* Paper to Eastern Mediterranean Region Food and Nutrition Seminar. F.A.O., Rome. 17 pp. 9 tables.

————, JELLIFFE, D.B. *and* PEREZ, C. (1959). 'Some indicators for a broad assessment of the magnitude of protein-calorie malnutrition in young children in population groups.' *Amer. J. Clin. Nutrition* 7, 714–720.

BERNSTEIN, T.P. (1968). 'Problems of village leadership after land reform.' *China Quarterly* 36, 1–22.

BERTHOLET, C.J.L. *and* BENCHADISWAT, (1958). 'Housing and food patterns in eleven villages in northeast Thailand.' Thailand U.N.E.S.C.O. Fundamental Education Centre, mimeo. 118 pp.

BETEILLE, A. (1969). *Caste, class and power: changing patterns of stratification in a Tanjore village.* California University Press, Berkerley and Los Angeles. 238 pp.

BHARGAVA, V., GHOSH, S. *and* BHARGAVA, S.K. (1970). 'Survival, growth and development in babies weighing 2000 gms. or less.' *Indian Pediat.* 7, 139–45.

BHATNAGAR, D.P., GOVIL, K.K. *and* PRASAD, B.G. (n.d.) 'Haematological studies in healthy adults.' (Reprint, no journal or page numbers given).

BIBILE, S.W., CULLUMBINE, H., WATSON, R.S. *and* WICKREMANAYAKE, T. (1949). 'A nutritional survey of various Ceylon communities.' *Ceylon J. Med. Sci.* 6, 15–69.

BLACKWELL, B.N., BLACKWELL, R.Q., YU, T.T.S., WENG, Y.S. *and* CHOW, B.F. (n.d.). 'Further studies on growth and feed utilization in progeny of underfed rats.' mimeo. 11 pp. plus tables.

BLACKWELL, R.Q. (1961). 'Speculations on the etiology of blackfoot disease.' *J. Formosan Med. Assoc.* 60, 460–72.

BLAIR, H.W. (1971). 'The green revolution and 'economic man': some lessons for community development in South Asia?' *Pacific Affairs* 44, 353–67.

BLANKHART, D.M. (1962). 'Measured food intakes of Indonesian children.' *J. Trop. Pediat.* 8, 18–21.

———— (1967). 'Individual intake of food in young children in relation to malnutrition and night blindness.' *Trop. Geogr. Med.* 19, 144–53.

BOERMA, A.H. (1971). 'Address to First Asian Congress of Nutrition.' *Nutrition Newsletter* 9 (1), 1–7.

BOLIN, T.D. and DAVIS, A.E. (1969). 'Asian lactose intolerance and its relation to intake of lactose.' *Nature, Lond.* 222, 382–3.

BOSE, A.B. *and* MALHOTRA, S.P. (1964). 'Some characteristics of occupational castes in central and lower Luni in western Rajasthan.' *Eastern Anthropol.* 17, 137–56.

———— *and* SAXENA, P.C. (1965). 'The diffusion of innovations in a village in western Rajasthan.' *Eastern Anthropol.* 18, 138–51.

———— and ———— (1966). 'Opinion leaders in a village in western Rajasthan.' *Man* 46, 121–30.

BOSE, C. (1966). 'Lactation and feeding practices of mothers in urban area.' *Alumni Assoc. Bull. All-India Institute of Hygiene and Public Health, Calcutta.* 16, 11–13.

BOTHA-ANTOUN, E., BABAYAN, S., *and* HARFOUCHE, J.K. (1968). 'Intellectual development relating to nutritional status.' *J. Trop. Pediat.* 14, 112–15.

BOWERS, J.B. (1966). 'Educational processes and problems in combatting malnutrition in the pre-school child.' In Proc. International Conference on Prevention of Malnutrition in the Pre-School Child, Washington, December 1964. *Pre-School Child Malnutrition* (ed. U.S. Academy of Sciences). pp 272–278. U.S. National Academy of Sciences, Washington.

BOYNE, A.W., AITKEN, F.C. *and* LEITCH, I. (1957). 'Secular changes in height and weight of British children, including an analysis of improvement of English children in primary schools, 1911–1953.' *Nutrit. Abst. Rev.* 27, 1–18.

BRADFIELD, R.B., JELLIFFE, E.F.P. and JELLIFFE, D.B. (1972). 'Assessment of marginal malnutrition.' *Nature, Lond.* 235:112.

BRANT, C.S. (1954). 'Tagadale: a Burmese village in 1950.' Southeast Asia Program Data Paper no. 13. Cornell University, Ithaca. mimeo. 41 pp.

BROCK, J.F. *and* AUTRET, M. (1952). *Kwashiorkor in Africa.* W.H.O. Monograph Series no. 8. Geneva. 78 pp.

BROOKS, C.E.P. (1949). *Climate through the ages.* (2nd ed.) Ernest Benn, London. 395 pp.

BROTHWELL, D., *and* BROTHWELL, P. (1969). *Food in antiquity.* Thames and Hudson, London. 248 pp.

BROWN, M.L., WORTH, R.M. and SHAH, N.K. (1968a). 'Food habits and food intake in Nepal.' *Trop. Geogr. Med.* 20, 217–24.

———— and ———— (1968b). 'Health survey of Nepal.' *Amer. J. Clin. Nutrit.* 21, 875–81.

BULATO-JAYME, J., DE LA PAZ, D. *and* GERVASIO, C.C. (1971). 'Recommended height and weight standards for Filipinos.' *Philippine J. Nutrition* 24, 161–77.

———— *and* MADLANGSACAY, R.M. (1965). 'Infant feeding and weaning practices in the Philippines. II: Northern Luzon, southern Tagalog and western Visayas.' *Philippine J. Pediat.* 14, 330–9.

————, PADLAN, A.A., ALCANTARA, E.O. *and* BAILEY, K.V. (1966). *Baseline surveys of the Philippines Applied Nutrition Program. I. Clinical.* mimeo. W.H.O., Manila. 34 pp.

————, RAMILLA, E., ALEID, R. *and* BAILEY, K.V. (1966). *Baseline surveys of the Philippines Applied Nutrition Program. II. Dietary.* mimeo. W.H.O., Manila. 27 pp.

————, VILLEGAS, N.M. and MIRANDA, N.E. (1970). 'The nutritional reevaluation of the Bayambang Applied Nutrition Project II. Dietary survey.' *Philippine J. Nutrition* 23, 59–66.

BURGESS, A. and DEAN, R.F.A. (1962). *Malnutrition and food habits.* Macmillan, London and New York. 210 pp.

BURGESS, R.C. and LAIDIN, A.M. (1950). *A report on the state of health, the diet and economic conditions of groups of people in the lower income levels in Malaya.* Institute for Medical Research, Malaya, Report no. 13. Kuala Lumpur. 80 pp.

BURHAMZAH. (1970). 'An economic survey of Maluku.' *Bull Indonesian Econ. Studies* 6(2), 31–45.

BURKHARDT, V.R. (1953). *Chinese creeds and customs* I. South China Morning Post Ltd., Hong Kong. 180pp.

BURLING, R. (1965). *Hill farms and padi fields.* Prentice Hall, New Jersey. 180 pp.

BUSTRILLOS, N.R. (1961). *Food management practices and homemaking in the rural areas of Quezon City.* Community Development Research Council, University of the Philippines. 185 pp.

CAMCAM, G.A. (1968). 'Ascorbic acid metabolism of some Filipinos.' *Philippine J. Nutrition* 21, 137–47 and 148–62.

———— (1969). 'The heights and weights of school children in relation to socio-economic status.' *Philippine J. Nutrition* 22, 11–24.

CENSUS OF INDIA (1964a). *Rajasthan: Khajoora. A village survey.* Manager of Publications, Delhi. 59 pp.

———— (1964b). *Uttar Pradesh: Village Thapli, District Garhwal.* Manager of Publications, Delhi. 76 pp.

———— (1964c). *Uttar Pradesh: Village Bhadkar Udarhar, Allahabad District.* Manager of Publications, Delhi. 36 pp.

———— (1964d). *Madras, Food habits in Madras State.* Manager of Publications, Delhi. 96 pp.

———— (1964e). *Kerala: Village survey monographs: Quilon District.* Manager of Publications, Delhi. 282 pp.

———— (1965a). *Rajasthan: Village Peepal Khoont.* Manager of Publications, Delhi. 68 pp.

———— (1965b). *Rajasthan: Village Rangmahal.* Manager of Publications, Delhi. 44 pp.

———— (1965c). *Punjab: Village Mahsa Tibba, Ambala District.* Manager of Publications, Delhi. 93 pp.

———— (1965d). *Punjab: Village Kalath, Simla District.* Manager of Publications, Delhi. 83 pp.

———— (1965e). *Uttar Pradesh: Village Bankati, District Dheri.* Manager of Publications, Delhi. 45 pp.

———— (1965f). *Uttar Pradesh: Village Bilaspur, District Saharanpur.* Manager of Publications, Delhi. 88 pp.

———— (1965g). *Uttar Pradesh: Village Daulatput Hira, District Pilibhit.* Manager of Publications, Delhi. 38 pp.

———— (1965h). *Uttar Pradesh: Village Chapnu, District Dehra Dun.* Manager of Publications, Delhi. 36 pp.

———— (1965i). *Madras: Todas.* Manager of Publications, Delhi. 147 pp.

———— (1965j). *Madras: Village Hallimoyar.* Manager of Publications, Delhi. 100 pp.

———— (1966a). *Tripura: Village Kamalghat.* Manager of Publications, Delhi. 58 pp.

———— (1966b). *Manipur: Village Thangjing Chiru.* Manager of Publications, Delhi. 20 pp.

———— (1966c). *North-East Frontier Agency: Village Jara.* Manager of Publications, Delhi. 57 pp.

———— (1966d). *Waromung (an Ao Naga Village).* Manager of Publications, Delhi. 211 pp.

———— (1966e). *Kerala: Village Survey Monographs: Ernakulam and Kottayam Districts.* Manager of Publications, Delhi. 296 pp.

———— (1967a). *Rajasthan: Village Kailashpuri.* Manager of Publications, Delhi. 32 pp.

———— (1967b). *Himachal Pradesh: A study of Gaddi – Scheduled Tribe.* Manager of Publications, Delhi. 104 pp.

———— (1967c). *Madras: Village Arkavadi.* Manager of Publications, Delhi. 168 pp.

CENTRAL TREATY ORGANIZATION. (1968). *Proc. conference on combating malnutrition in pre-school children, Islamabad, Pakistan.* C.E.N.T.O., Ankara. 164 pp.

CENTRO INTERNACIONAL DE MEJORAMIENTO DE MAIZ Y TRIGO (CIMMYT). (1970–71). *Report on maize and wheat improvement.* CIMMYT, Londres, Mexico. 114 pp.

CHABOT, H.T. (1967). 'Bontoramba: A village of Goa, South Sulawesi.' In *Villages in Indonesia* (ed. Koentjaringrat). pp. 189–209. Cornell University Press, Ithaca.

———— (1968). Personal communication.

CHAI, Re Suk. (1967). 'Studies on the nutrition of the Koreans.' *J. Nat. Acad. Sci.* 7, 129–79.

CHAMPAKAM, S., SRIKANTIA, S.G. *and* GOPALAN, C. (1968). 'Kwashiorkor and mental development.' *Amer. J. Clin. Nutrit.* 21, 844–52.

CHAN, L.K.C., LEE, K.L. *and* TAN, S.E. (1967). 'A recommended diet for West Malaysian pregnant women.' *Med. J. Malaya* 22, 95–98.

CHANDLER, R.F. (1969). 'Improving the rice plant and its culture.' *Nature, Lond.* 221, 1007–10.

CHANDRAPANOND, A., RAJATASILPIN, A., TUNSUPASIRI, S. and PUNGPAPONGSE, V. (1969). 'Nutritional status among schoolchildren in Bang Khen study area. (1968).' *J. Med. Assoc. Thailand* 52, 915–32.

CHANDRASEKHAR, S. (1967). 'Marx, Malthus and Mao.' *Current Scene, Hong Kong,* 5(3), 1–24.

CHANG, Jen-hu. (1971). 'The Chinese monsoon.' *Geogr. Rev.* 61: 370–95.

CHANG, Kwang-chih. (1966). 'Excavations in Formosa.' *Asian Perspectives* 9, 140–9.

———— (1968a). *The archaeology of ancient China.* (2nd ed.). Yale University Press, New Haven. 483 pp.

———— (1968b). 'Archaeology of ancient China.' *Science* 162, 519–26.

————— (1968c). *Settlement archaeology.* National Press, Palo Alto. 229 pp.

————— (1970). 'The beginnings of agriculture in the Far East.' *Antiquity* 44, 175—85.

CHAPPELL, J.E. Jr. (1970). 'Climatic change reconsidered: another look at 'The Pulse of Asia.'' *Geographical Review* 60, 347—73.

CHAPPEL, J.N. *and* JANOWITZ, E.R. (1965). 'Health review of rural Malay population, F.L.D.A., Sungai Tekam, Pahang.' *Med. J. Malaya* 19, 191—200.

CHASE, H.P., LINDSLEY, W.F.B. Jr. *and* O'BRIEN, D. (1969). 'Undernutrition and cerebellar development.' *Nature, Lond.* 221, 554—5.

CHEN, C.S. (1970). *The agricultural regions of China.* American Institute of Crop Ecology, Silver Spring, Maryland. 47 pp.

CH'EN, J.S. *and* LI, O.L. (n.d.). *Composition of Chinese foods.* Department of Biochemistry, National Defense Medical Center, Taipei, 38 pp.

CHEN, Nai-ruenn. (1966). *Chinese economic statistics — a handbook for mainland China.* Edinburgh University Press. 539 pp.

CHEN, P.C.Y. (1969). 'Spirits and medicine-men in rural Malaya.' *Far East Med. J.* 5, 84—87.

————— (1970). 'Effects of the trained midwife on traditional domiciliary midwifery in a Malay rural community.' *Southeast Asian J. Trop. Med. Pub. Health* 1, 212—14.

CHEN, S.S.C. (1948). 'Study of seasonal changes in calcium utilization of adult men in Chungking.' *Chinese J. Nutrition* 2, 8—13.

CHEN, S.T. *and* DUGDALE, A.E. (1970). 'Weight and height curves for Malaysian schoolchildren.' *Med. J. Malaya* 25, 99—101.

CHENG, L. (1968). '*Contribution à l'étude du développement somatique des adolescents cambodgiens.*' Doctoral thesis no. 99. Fac. royale de Médecine, Phnom Penh. mimeo. 82 pp.

CHENG, Tê-k'un. (1959). *Prehistoric China.* I. Heffer and Sons, Cambridge. 250 pp.

CHONG, Y.H. (1969). *Food and nutrition in Malaysia.* Bulletin no. 14, Institute for Medical Research, Kuala Lumpur. 16 pp.

—————, LOURDENADIN, S., THEAN, P.K., LIM, R. *and* LOPEZ, C.G. (1968). 'Nutritional status during pregnancy.' *Far East Med. J.* 4, 214—9.

CHOW, B.F., BLACKWELL, R.Q., BLACKWELL, B.N., SHERWIN, R.W., HSUEH, A.M. *and* LEE, C.J. (1966). 'Studies on the progeny of underfed mothers.' *Proc. 7th International Congress of Nutrition,* Hamburg. 4, 3—7. Verlag Friedr. Vieweg und Sohn, Braunschweig.

————— , Blackwell R. *and* SHERWIN, R.W. (1968). 'Nutrition and development.' *Borden Review of Nutrition Res.* 29, 25—39.

————— *and* LEE, C.J. (1964). 'Effect of dietary restriction of pregnant rats on body weight gain of the offspring.' *J. Nutrition* 82, 10—18.

CHURCHILL, J.A., NEFF, J.W. *and* CALDWELL, D.F. (1966). 'Birth weight and intelligence.' *Obstet. Gynecol.* 28, 425—29.

CLARK, C. *and* HASWELL, M.R. (1967). *The economics of subsistence agriculture.* (3rd ed.). Macmillan, London. 245 pp.

CLARK, T.W. (1966). Personal communication cited in C.S. Coon and E.E. Hunt, p. 204.

CLARKSON, J.D. (1968). *The cultural ecology of a Chinese village: Cameron Highlands, Malaysia.* Department of Geography Research Paper no. 114. University of Chicago. 174 pp.

COCKRILL, W.R. (1966) 'A key animal for a hungry world.' *New Scientist* 12 May, 370—2.

COEDES, G. (1964). *Les états hindouisés d'Indochine et d'Indonésie.* (2nd ed.) Editions E. de Boccard, Paris. 494 pp.

————— (1967). *The making of South-East Asia.* University of California Press, Berkeley and Los Angeles. 268 pp.

COLWELL, E.J., WELSH, J.D., BOONE, S.C. *and* LEGTERS, L.J. (1971). 'Intestinal parasitism in residents of the Mekong Delta of Vietnam.' *Southeast Asian J. Trop. Med. Public Health* 2, 25—8.

COOLEY, F.L. (1967). 'Allang: a village on Ambon Island.' In *Villages in Indonesia* (ed. Koentjaraningrat), pp 129–156. Cornell University Press, Ithaca.

COON, C.S. (1959). 'Race and ecology in man.' *Cold Spring Harbor Symposia on Quantitative Biology* 24, 153–9.

———— *with* HUNT, E.E. Jr. (1966). *The living races of man.* Jonathan Cape, London. 344 pp.

COOPER, J.P. (1970). 'Potential production and energy conversion in temperate and tropical grasses.' *Herbage Abst.* 40, 1–15.

CRAVIOTO, J., BIRCH, H.G., DE LICARDIE, E., ROSALES, L. *and* VEGA, L. (1969). 'The ecology of growth and development in a Mexican preindustrial community. Report I. Method and findings from birth to one month of age.' *Social Res. in Child Development* 34, (5), 76 pp.

CRAVIOTO, J., DE LICARDIE, E., and BIRCH, H.G. (1966). 'Nutrition, growth and neurointegrative development: an experimental and ecologic study.' *Pediatrics* 38, 319–72.

————, GAONA, C.E., and BIRCH, H.G. (1967). 'Early malnutrition and auditory-visual integration in school-age children.' *J. Special Education* 2, 75–82.

————, PINERO, C., ARROYO, M. and ALCADE, E. (1969). 'Mental performance of school children who suffered malnutrition in early age.' *Swedish Nutrition Foundation Symposia* vii, 85–91.

CRESTA, M. (1968). 'International tables on amino acid content and protein quality of foods.' *Nutrition Newsletter* 6(2), 14–19.

————, PERISSE, J. and AUTRET, M. (1969). 'Study of the correlations between biological and chemical measurements of food quality.' *Nutrition Newsletter* 7, (2), 1–15.

CROOKE-FRY, P. (1965). 'The nutritive value of the diets of Hong Kong children.' *J. Trop. Pediat.* March, 100–104.

————, LEVERTON, R.M. *and* SUNA, G. (1967). 'Growth of Hong Kong children.' *Amer. J. Clin. Nutrition* 20, 954–59.

CROSS, J.H., GUNAWAN, S., GABA, A., WATTEN, R.H., *and* SULIANTI, J. (1970). 'Survey for human intestinal and blood parasites in Bojolali, Central Java, Indonesia.' *Southeast Asian J. Trop. Med. Pub. Health* 1, 354–60.

CULLUMBINE, H. (1951). 'A national nutritional survey in Ceylon.' *Ceylon J. Med. Sci.* 8, 17–50.

CUNNINGHAM, C.E. (1967). 'An Atoni village of west Timor.' In *Villages in Indonesia* (ed. Koentjaraningrat), pp. 63–89. Cornell University Press, Ithaca.

DALRYMPLE, D.G. (1971). *Imports and plantings of high-yielding varieties of wheat and rice in the less developed nations.* Foreign Economic Development Service, U.S.D.A., Washington. 43 pp.

DANI, A.H. (1960). *Prehistory and protohistory of eastern India.* Mukhopadhyay, Calcutta. 248 pp.

DAVIDSON, Sir S. *and* PASSMORE, R. (1966). *Human nutrition and dietetics.* (3rd ed.). Livingstone, Edinburgh and London. 864 pp.

DAVIS, A.E. *and* BOLIN, T.D. (1967). 'Lactose intolerance in Asians.' *Nature, Lond.* 216, 1244–5.

DE GARINE, I. (1969). 'Food, nutrition and urbanization.' *Nutrition Newsletter* 7(1), 1–19.

DE LANGEN, C.D. (1934). 'The general state of health of the inhabitants.' *Landbouw.* 10(4 and 5), 399–416.

DE SILVA, C.C. (1956). 'Present state of child health in Ceylon.' *Pediatrics* 18, 999–1012.

———— *and* BAPTIST, N.G. (1969). *Tropical nutritional disorders of infants and children.* Thomas, Springfield, Illinois. 226 pp.

———— *and* FERNANDO, R.P. (1966). 'Anaemias of Ceylonese children.' *Israel J. Med. Sci.* 2, 499–505.

DEYOUNG, J.E. (1955). *Village life in modern Thailand.* California University Press, Berkeley and Los Angeles. 225 pp.

DEAN, R.F.A. (1961). 'Kwashiorkor in Malaya. The clinical evidence I.' *J. Trop. Pediat.* 7, 3–15. 'II', *J. Trop. Pediat.* 7, 39–48.

DEEVEY, E.S. (1960). 'The human population.' *Sci. American* 203, 194–204.

DELVERT, J. (1961). *Le paysan cambodgien.* Mouton, Paris and The Hague. 740 pp.

DEMETRIO, Father F., S.J. (1969). Pre-publication extracts from *A dictionary of Philippine folk beliefs and customs.* Philippine Folklore and Folklife Centre, Xavier University, Cagayan de Oro.

DENTAN, R.K. (1968). *The Semai: A non-violent people of Malaya.* Holt, Rinehart and Winston. New York, Toronto, London. 110 pp.

DEOSTHALE, Y.G., SURYANARAYANA RAO, K. *and* MOHAN, V.S. (1969) 'Nutritive value of some varieties of wheat.' *J. Nutrition Dietetics* 6, 182–6.

DEVADAS, R.P., ANANDAM, K. *and* BHANUMATHI, L. (1967). 'Effects of school lunch with Indian Multi-purpose Food, skim milk powder or their combination on the nutritional status of children.' *J. Nutrition Dietetics* 4, 1–5.

———— *and* EASWARAN, P.P. (1967). 'Influence of socio-economic factors on the nutritional status and food intake of pre-school children in a rural community.' *J. Nutrition Dietetics* 4, 155–60.

———— *and* PREMA, L. (1965). 'The nutritional status of nursing mothers and infants in an applied nutrition area in Madras State.' *J. Nutrition Dietetics* 2, 149–53.

————, SHENBAGAVALLI, P.N. *and* VIJAYALAKSHMI, R. (1970). 'The impact of an A.N.P. on the nutritional status of selected expectant women.' *J. Nutrition Dietetics* 7, 293–6.

————, USHA, T.M., SHANKARI, L., RAJALAKSHMI, R.S., PATRATH, G. *and* BABTIWALA, M. (1965). 'Diet and nutrition survey of a village community in south India.' *J. Nutrition Dietetics* 2, 83–87.

DEVAKUL, A.S., CHANTACHUM, Y., BOONYANANTHA, C., EGORAMAIPHOL, S. *and* VIRAVAN, C. (1971). 'Gastrointestinal protein loss in patients with hookworm infection.' *J. Med. Assoc. Thailand* 54, 28.

DIAMOND, N. (1969). *K'un Shen: a Taiwan village.* Holt, Rinehart and Winston, New York, Toronto, London. 110 pp.

DICKERSON, J.W.T., *and* JOHN, P.M. (1969). 'The effect of protein-calorie malnutrition on the composition of the human femur.' *Brit. J. Nutrition* 23, 917–24.

DOBBY, E.H.G. (1960). *Southeast Asia.* (7th ed.) University of London Press, London. 415 pp.

DONNITHORNE, A. (1970). *China's grain: output, procurement, transfers and trade.* Chinese University of Hong Kong. 36 pp.

DONOSO, G., MILLER, D.S. *and* PAYNE, P.R. (1964). 'The efficiency of utilization of limiting amino acids: some sulphur and nitrogen balances.' *Proc. Nutrition Soc.* 23, xiii–xiv.

DORAISWAMY, T.R., DANIEL, V.A., RAJALAKSHMI, D., SWAMINATHAN, M. and PARPIA, H.A.B. (1971). 'Effect of supplementing a poor diet based on rice and wheat consumed by school children with vitamins, minerals, lysine and protein-rich food, on their growth and nutritional status.' *Nutrition Repert. Internat.* 3, 67–78.

————, RAO, S.V., SWAMINATHAN, M. *and* PARPIA, H.A.B. (1968). 'Effect of supplementation of poor kaffir corn diet with L-lysine on N retention and growth of school children.' *J. Nutrition Dietetics* 5, 191–6.

————, SINGH, N. *and* DANIEL, V.A. (1969). 'Effects of supplementing ragi (*Eleusine coracana*) diets with lysine or leaf protein on the growth and nitrogen metabolism of children.' *Brit. J. Nutrition* 23, 731–3.

DUBE, L. (1956). 'Diet, health and disease in a north Indian village.' manuscript. Department of Anthropology, Cornell University, Ithaca.

DUBE, S.C. (1958). *India's changing villages.* Routledge and Kegan Paul, London. 260 pp.

DUGGAL, K.K. (1970). 'India: too many people, too few jobs.' *World Hunger* 11, (4), 9–10.

EASTWOOD, G.C. (1971). *Report to the Government of Thailand on nutrition education training programs.* T.A. Report no. 2934, F.A.O., Rome. 37 pp.

EICHENWALD, H.F. and CROOKE-FRY, P. (1969). 'Nutrition and learning.' *Science* 163, 644–48.

EL-MARAGHI, N.R.H. and STEWART, R.J.C. (1963). 'Interaction of protein and calcium on the growth and composition of bones in rats.' *Proc. Nutrition Soc.* 22, xxx–xxxi.

EL RAWI, I. (1961). *Biochemical nutrition problems in Indonesia: Report to Government.* E.T.A.P. Report no. 1329. F.A.O., Rome. 28 pp.

EMBREE, J.F. (1939). *A Japanese village: Suye Mura.* University of Chicago Press, 354 pp.

FEWSTER, W.J. (1970). 'Communicating home economics information: reaching and teaching women by radio.' *Nutrition Newsletter* 8, (1), 23–34.

FIELD, C.E. (1971). 'A child rearing study in Hong Kong.' *Bull. Hong Kong Medical Assoc.* 23, 29–38.
———— *and* BABER, F.M. (1973) *Growing up in Hong Kong.* Hong Kong University Press, 178 pp.

FIELD, R.M. (1969). 'A note on the population of Communist China.' *China Quarterly* 38, 158–63.

FIRTH, Rosemary. (1966). *Housekeeping among Malay peasants.* University of London Press, London. 244 pp.

FISHER, C.A. (1969). Review of *Saraphi. Royal Central Asian J.* 56, p. 64.

FLATZ, G. *and* SAENGUDOM, C. (1969). 'Lactose tolerance in Asians: a family study.' *Nature, Lond.* 224, 915–16.

———— *and* SANGUANBHOKHAI, T. (1969). 'Lactose intolerance in Thailand.' *Nature, Lond.* 221, 758–9.

FLOWERS, W.S. (1948). 'Causes of blindness in China.' *Chinese Med. J.* 66, 38–46.

FONSECA, A. (1968). 'A computerized estimate of need-based wage.' *The Statesman,* New Delhi and Calcutta. 23 October.

FOOD AND AGRICULTURE ORGANIZATION (F.A.O.). (1957). *Second Committee on Calorie Requirements.* Nutritional Studies no. 15. Rome. 67 pp.

F.A.O. (1959). *Report of the F.A.O./C.C.T.A. technical meeting on legumes in agriculture and human nutrition in Africa. Bukavu, Belgian Congo, 1958.* FAO Meeting Report no. 1958/22. Rome. 92 pp.

———— (1962). *Joint F.A.O./W.H.O. Expert Committee on Nutrition. 6th Report.* F.A.O. Nutrition Meetings Report Series no. 32. Rome. 65 pp.

———— (1965). *Protein requirements: report of a Joint F.A.O./W.H.O. Expert Group.* F.A.O. Nutrition Meetings Report Series no. 37. Rome. 71 pp.

———— (1967a). *Joint F.A.O./W.H.O. Expert Committee on Nutrition.* F.A.O. Nutrition Meetings Report Series no. 42. Rome. 114 pp.

———— (1967b). *Report of a Joint F.A.O./W.H.O. Seminar on the Planning and Evaluation of Applied Nutrition Programs in Asia and the Far East. New Delhi, 1966.* Nutrition Special Reports no. 5. mimeo. Rome. 62 pp.

———— (1968). *Report of the interdivisional Working Party on high-yielding varieties of basic food crops.* mimeo. Rome. 12 plus 12 pp. annexes.

———— (1969a). Joint F.A.O./W.H.O. Expert Group on Vitamin and Mineral Requirements. Summary of recommendations. *Nutrition Newsletter* 7, (3), 42–4.

———— (1969b). *Food composition tables – annotated bibliography.* Nutrition Information Documents Series no. 1. Rome. 168 pp.

———— (1969c). *Report of the Joint U.N.D.P./F.A.O. Mission on the review of the agricultural work of the Mekong Committee, with special reference to the agricultural research, demonstration and training programmes.* offset. Rome. 89 pp.

———— (1969d). Personal communication from Director, Statistics Division.

———— (1970a). *Amino-acid content of foods and biological data on proteins.* Rome. 285 pp.

———— (1970b). *Requirements of ascorbic acid, vitamin D, vitamin B_{12}, folate and iron.* Report of a Joint F.A.O./W.H.O. Expert Group. F.A.O. Nutrition Meetings Report Series no. 47. F.A.O., Rome. 75 pp.

———— (1970c). *Review of food consumption surveys. Vol. 1A. Household food consumption by economic groups.* F.A.O., Rome. 139 pp.

———— (1970d). *Rural youth food and nutrition project.* mimeo. F.A.O., Rome. 30 pp.

————(1971a). Food and nutrition education in the primary school. FAO Nutritional Studies no. 25. FAO, Rome. 107 pp.

———— (1971b). *Joint F.A.O./W.H.O. Expert Committee on Nutrition. Eighth Report.* F.A.O. Nutrition Meetings Report Series No. 49. Rome. 104 pp.

F.A.O. NUTRITION DIVISION (1966). *Soybean acceptability and consumer adoptability in relation to food habits in different parts of the world.* Paper for International Conference on Soybean Foods, Peoria. mimeo. F.A.O., Rome. 8 pp.

———— (1969). 'Meeting of the Protein Advisory Group, Ad Hoc Working Group on Feeding the Pre-school Child. Summary.' *Nutrition Newsletter* 7 (4), 50–52.

F.A.O. NUTRITION DIVISION, PLANT PRODUCTION AND PROTECTION DIVISION *and* ECONOMIC ANALYSIS DIVISION. (1967). 'Soybean: production, cultivation, economics of supply, processing and marketing.' *P.A.G. Bulletin* 7, 25–44.

FOSTER, G.M. (1969). *Applied anthropology.* Little and Brown. Boston. 238 pp.

FOY, H., KONDI, A. and SARMA, B. (1958). 'Anaemias of the tropics. India and Ceylon.' *J. Trop. Med. Hyg.* 61, 27–49.

FRANCOIS, P. (1969a). 'Nutrimetric study on dietary disparities.' *Nutrition Newsletter* 7, (3), 10–33.

———— (1969b). 'Effects of income projection on the protein structure of the diet.' *Nutrition Newsletter* 7, (4), 1–15.

———— (1970). 'Food consumption surveys – study on a general formula for the estimation of per caput, household and group consumption.' *Nutrition Newsletter* 8(4). 10–26.

FRASER, T.M. Jr. (1960). *Rusembilan: a Malay fishing village.* Cornell University Press, Ithaca. 281 pp.

———— (1966). *Fishermen of south Thailand.* Holt, Rinehart and Winston, New York, Toronto, London. 110 pp.

———— (1968a). *Culture and change in India: the Barpali experiment.* University of Massachusetts Press, Amherst. 460 pp.

———— (1968b). *Personal communication.*

FREEDMAN, M. (1954). *A report on some aspects of food, health and society in Indonesia.* mimeo. W.H.O., Geneva. 144 pp.

———— (1965). *Lineage organization in southeastern China.* (2nd ed.). University of London Press, London. 154 pp.

———— (1966). *Chinese lineage and society: Fukien and Kwangtung.* University of London Press, London, 207 pp.

FREEMAN, J.D. (1955). *Iban agriculture.* H.M.S.O., London. 148 pp.

FRENZEL, B. (1968). 'The Pleistocene vegetation of northern Eurasia.' *Science* 161, 637–49.

FRESNOZA, F. (1969). *Rural teacher training. Consolidated final report on the Thailand-UNESCO project.* UNESCO Paris. mimeo. 141 pp.

FRIEND, C.J., HEARD, C.R.C., PLATT, B.S., STEWART, R.J.C. *and* TURNER, M.R. (1961). 'The effect of dietary protein deficiency on transport of vitamin A in the blood and its storage in the liver.' *Brit. J. Nutrition* 15, 231–400.

FUKUI, T., FUKUI, H., SASAKI, T. *and* MURAKAMI, T. (1961). 'Lysine supply to children of school age.' *Tokushima J. Exp. Med.* 8, 1–14.

FUKUTAKE, T. (1967). *Asian rural society: China, India, Japan.* University of Washington Press, Seattle and London. 207 pp.

GALBRAITH, J.K. (1970). *Asahi Evening News,* Tokyo. 1 September. *Times,* London, 2 September.

GALLIN, B. (1966). *Hsin Hsing, Taiwan: A Chinese village in change.* University of California Press, Berkeley and Los Angeles. 324 pp.

GEDDES, W.R. (1954). *The Land Dayaks of Sarawak.* H.M.S.O., London. 113 pp.

GEERTZ, C. (1967). 'Tihingan: a Balinese village.' In *Villages in Indonesia* (ed. Koentjaraningrat). pp. 210–43. Cornell University Press, Ithaea.

———— (1968). *Agricultural involution: the processes of ecological change in Indonesia.* University of California Press, Berkeley and Los Angeles. 176 pp.

GEERTZ, H. (1961). *The Javanese family.* Free Press of Glencoe Inc., 176 pp.

GENEST, A.A., SARWONO, D. and GYORGY, P. (1967). 'Vitamin A blood serum levels and electroretinogram in 5- to 14-years age group in Indonesia and Thailand. A preliminary report.' *Amer. J. Clin. Nutrition* 20, 1275–79

GERHOLD, C. (1965). 'Food habits in a Lao village.' mimeo. U.S.A.I.D. 16 pp.

GETZ, H.R., LONG, E.R. *and* HENDERSON, H.J. (1951). 'A study of the relation of nutrition to the development of tuberculosis.' *Amer. Rev. Tuberc.* 64, 381–93.

GILL, P.S., PRASAD, B.G. *and* SHRIVASTAVA, R.N. (1968). 'Nutritional status of primary schoolchildren in a rural area of Lucknow.' *Indian J. Pediat.* 35, 314–26.

GIOK, L.T., ROSE, C.S. *and* GYORGY, P. (1967). 'Influence of early malnutrition on some aspects of the health of school-age children.' *Amer. J. Clin. Nutrition* 20, 1280–89.

GOETHALS, P.R. (1967). 'Rarak: a swidden village of west Sumbawa.' In *Villages in Indonesia* (ed. Koentjaraningrat). pp. 30–62. Cornell University Press, Ithaca.

———— (1969). Personal communication.

GOPALAN, C. (1968). 'Kwashiorkor and marasmus: evolution and distinguishing features.' In *Calorie deficiencies and protein deficiencies* (ed. R.A. McCance and E.M. Widdowson). pp. 49–58. Churchill, London.

———— (1969a). 'Possible role for dietary leucine in the pathogenesis of pellagra.' *Lancet* i, 197–99.

———— (1969b). 'Studies on the pathogenesis of some nutritional deficiency states.' *Indian J. Med. Res.* 57, (8), 75–91.

GOSWAMI, P.C. (1967). *A study in rural change in Assam: Dispur. (A report on socio-economic resurvey of a village in Kamrup District).* Agro-Economic Research Centre for North East India, Jorhat, Assam. 165 pp.

GOTO, F., TAKEUCHI, A., SASAKI, H., TODA, T., MASUDA, H., KOZAWA, N., NIWA, S. *and* KATAYAMA, R. (1968). 'Study of the nutritional education in a remote rural district. I. Proteinaceous foods in Obara village, Aichi Prefecture.' *Jap. J. Nutrition* 26, 98–105.

————, YAMAGUCHI, Y., SASAKI, H., OSZAWA, N., TODA, T., MASUDA, H. and NIWA, S. (1969). 'Fundamental data for evaluation of the nutritional betterment in Obara Village, Aichi Prefecture.' *Japanese J. Nutrition* 27, 58–63.

GOUGH, K. (1955). 'The social structure of a Tanjore village.' In *India's villages* (ed. McKim Marriott). pp. 36–52. Chicago University Press.

GOVIL, K.K., MITRA, D. *and* PANT, K.C. (1953). 'Dietary habits of school boys in Uttar Pradesh.' *Indian Med. Gaz.* 88, p. 357.

————, PRASAD, B.G. *and* PANT, K.C. (1958). 'Results of diet surveys in Uttar Pradesh.' *Indian J. Pub. Health.* 2, (4) (no pp. nos.).

GREENBERG, B.C. *and* BRYAN, H.A. (1951). 'Methodology in the study of physical measurements of school children. I.' *Human Biology* 23, 1–20.

GRUENWALD, P., FUNAKAWA, H., MITANI, S., NISHIMURA, T., and TAKEUCHI, S. (1967). 'Influence of environmental factors on foetal growth in Japan.' *Lancet* i, (May 13), 1026.

GUPTA, S., PURI, R.K., INDIRA, O.C. *and* DATTA, S.P. (1968). 'Morbidity in children under 14 in south India.' *Indian Pediat.* 5, 485–97.

GUTHRIE, G.M. (1964). 'Impressions of Ifugao health and social activities.' mimeo. Pennsylvania State University, 68 pp.

GUTHRIE, H.A. (1964). 'Infant feeding practices in five community groups in the Philippines.' *J. Trop. Pediat.* 10, 65–73.

————, GUTHRIE, G.M. *and* TAYAG, A. (1969). 'Nutritional status and intellectual performance in a rural Philippines community.' *Philippine J. Nutrition* 22, 2–10.

———— *and* STONE, R. (1970). 'Dietary practices of young adult women in Manila.' *Philippine J. Nutrition* 23, 1–12.

GUZMAN, M.A., SCRIMSHAW, N.S., BRUCH, H.A. *and* GORDON, J.E. (1968). 'Nutrition and infection field study in Guatemalan villages, 1959–64. VII. Physical growth and development of pre-school children.' *Arch. Environ. Health* 17, 107–18.

GYORGY, P. *and* KLINE, O.L. (eds.). (1970). *Malnutrition is a problem of ecology.* Bibliotheca Nutritio et Dieta no. 14. Karger, Basel. 224 pp.

HALL, D.G.E. (1968). *A history of South-East Asia.* (3rd. ed.). Macmillan, London, Melbourne, Toronto. 1017 pp.

HALPERN, J.M. (1964). *Economy and society of Laos: a brief survey.* Yale Southeast Asia Studies, Monograph Series 5. Yale University Press, New Haven. 180 pp.

HALSTEAD, S.B. *and* VALYASEVI, A. (1967a). 'Studies of bladder stone disease in Thailand. I. Introduction and description of area studies.' *Amer. J. Clin. Nutrition* 20, 1312–19.

———— (1967b). 'III. Epidemiologic studies in Ubol Province.' *Amer. J. Clin. Nutrition* 20, 1329–39.

———— *and* UMPAIVIT, P. (1967). 'V. Dietary habits and disease prevalence.' *Amer. J. Clin. Nutrition* 20, 1352–61.

HANKS, J.R. (1963). *Maternity and its rituals in Bang Chan.* Cornell Thailand Project Interim Report Series 6. Data Paper no. 51. Southeast Asia Program. mimeo. Cornell University, Ithaca. 128 pp.

HARINASUTA, C., JETANASEN, S., IMPAND, P. *and* MAEGRAITH, B.G. (1970). 'Health problems and socio-economic development: investigations on the endemicity of the diseases occurring following the construction of dams in northeast Thailand.' *Southeast Asian J. Trop. Med. Public Health* 1, 530–52.

HARPER, R.J. (1968). *Melbourne Sun,* Australia. 12 September.

HARRISON, B. (1954). *South-east Asia: a short history.* Macmillan, London 268 pp.

HART, D.V. (1969). Bisayan Filipino and Malayan humoral pathologies: folk medicine ethnohistory in Southeast Asia. Data Paper no. 76. Southeast Asia Program. Cornell University, Ithaca. 96 pp.

HAUCK, H.M., RAJATASILPIN, A., INDRASUD, S., KITTIVEJA, C. *and* SUDSANEH, S. (1956). *Aspects of health, sanitation and nutritional status in a Siamese rice village: Studies in Bang Chan, 1952–54.* Southeast Asia Program. Data Paper 22. mimeo. Cornell University, Ithaca. 73 pp.

————, RAJATASILPIN, A., INDRASUD, S., CAMPBELL, M.B. *and* THORANGKUL, D. (1958). *Food habits and nutrient intakes in a Siamese rice village: studies in Bang Chan,* 1952–54. Southeast Asia Program Data Paper 29. mimeo. Cornell University, Ithaca. 129 pp.

HAW, K., YU, J.Y., LEE, K.Y., SUNG, N.E., TCHAI, B.S. *and* CHA, C.H. (1970). 'A report of nutrition survey 1969.' *Korean J. Nutrition* 3, 1–64.

HAYAMI, H., TAMURA, Y., CHIKARAISHI, S., SHIRAI, E. *and* OKABE, M. (1970). 'The table of surface area of Japanese peoples calculated by new formula.' *Jap. J. Nutrition* 28, 264–8.

HELBAEK, H. (1969). 'Plant collecting, dry-farming and irrigation agriculture in prehistoric Deh Luran.' In *Prehistory and human ecology of the Deh Luran Plain: an early village sequence from Khuzistan, Iran* (eds. F. Hole, K.V. Flannery, J.A. Neely). Museum of Anthropology Memoirs 1. 383–426. University of Michigan, Ann Arbor.

HENDRY, J. (1959). *The study of a Vietnamese rural community – economic activities.* mimeo. Vietnamese Advisory Group, Michigan State University.

HICKEY, G.C. (1964). *Village in Viet Nam.* Yale University Press, New Haven. 325 pp.

HIN, Tong Hor, (1967). *Des anémies infantiles au Cambodge.* Doctoral thesis no. 65. Faculté royale de médecine, Phnom Penh. 75 pp.

HITCHCOCK, J.T. (1966). *The Magars of Banyan Hill.* Holt, Rinehart and Winston, New York, Toronto, London. 115 pp.

———— (1968). Personal communication.

HO, J.H. *and* KIM, S.H. (1970). 'The protein-rich food mixtures for Korean infants.' *Korean J. Nutrition* 3, 95–9.

HO, Ping-ti. (1959). *Studies on the population of China.* Harvard East Asian Studies, Harvard University Press, Cambridge. 341 pp.

———— (1969). 'The loess and the origin of Chinese agriculture.' *Amer. Hist. Rev.* 75, 1–36.

HODSON, H.V. (1969). 'Can India and Pakistan survive?' *Royal Central Asian J.* 56, 259–71.

HOLMES, A.C. (1968). *Visual aids in nutrition education.* F.A.O., Rome. 154 pp.

HONG KONG INSTITUTE OF SOCIAL RESEARCH (1965). *Journal of the Hong Kong Institute of Social Research* I. 126 pp.

HONG, K.K. (1968). 'Contribution a l'etude de la malnutrition au Cambodge.' Doctoral thesis no. 97. Faculte royale de Medecine, Phnom Penh. 111 pp.

HOU, Chi-Ming. (1968). 'Sources of agricultural growth in Communist China.' *J. Asian Studies* 27, 721–37.

HSU, F.L.K. (1952). *Religion, science and human crisis.* Routledge and Kegan Paul, London. 142 pp.

HSU, S.C. (1964). 'Report on the nutrition program in Taiwan.' *Chinese Med. J.* 2, 71–94.

HUANG, Ping-wei. (1961). *The complex natural zonation of China.* U.S.S.R. Academy of Sciences Geographical Series 1, 25–39.

HUANG, Po-Chao, TUNG, Ta-cheng. (1968). 'Studies on acceptability, tolerance and nutritional value of corn-soybean mixture in infants and toddlers.' *J. Formosan Med. Assoc.* 67, 19–27.

——————, TUNG, Ta-cheng, LUE, Hung-chi, LEE, Chin-yun, *and* WEI, H. (1967). 'Feeding of infants with full-fat soya bean-rice foods.' *J. Trop. Pediat.* 13, 27–36.

HUANG, S.S. *and* BAYLESS, T.M. (1967). 'Lactose intolerance in healthy children.' *New England J. Medicine.* 276, 1283–87.

——————(1968). 'Milk and lactose intolerance in healthy orientals.' *Science* 160, 83–4.

HUARD, P. *and* WONG, M. (1968). *Chinese medicine.* Wiedenfeld and Nicolson, London. 256 pp.

HUDSON, A.B. *and* HUDSON, J.M. (1967). 'Telang: A Ma'anjan village of central Kalimantan.' In *Villages in Indonesia* (ed. Koentjaraningrat). pp. 90–114. Cornell University Press, Ithaca.

HUECK, O. (1952). 'Beriberi in Tungkun, south China.' *Ztschr. Tropenmed. Parasitol.* 4, 127–30.

HUGEN, Nguyen T. (1967). 'Contribution à l'étude de la croissance ponderale, staturale et ségmentaire de 2,500 écoliers des écoles primaires de la région Saigon-Cholon.' Doctoral thesis. 56 pp.

HUNTER, J.M. (1971). 'Geography, genetics and culture history: the case of lactose intolerance.' *Geogr. Rev.* 61, 605–608.

HUNTINGTON, E. (1907). *The pulse of Asia.* Houghton Mifflin Co., Boston. 415 pp.

—————— (1924). *Civilization and climate.* (3rd ed.) Yale University Press, New Haven/Oxford University Press, London. 453 pp. Reprinted Archon Books, Hamden, Conn/Lyon, Grant and Green, London, 1971.

HUTCHINSON, J. (1968). 'Closing discussion on the relative importance of calorie deficiencies and protein deficiencies.' In *Calorie deficiencies and protein deficiencies. Proc. Colloq. Cambridge. 1967.* (eds. R.A. McCance and E. Widdowson). Churchill, London. pp. 351–56.

—————— (1970). 'The evolutionary diversity of the pulses.' In *Plant breeding and nutrition: Proc. Nutrition Society, 212th scientific meeting, 1969.* pp. 1-80. Cambridge University Press, London.

HYTTEN, F.E. *and* LEITCH, I. (1964). *The physiology of human pregnancy.* Blackwell, Oxford. 463 pp.

INDIAN AGRICULTURAL RESEARCH INSTITUTE. (1970). *A new technology for dry land farming.* Delhi. 189 pp.

INDIAN COUNCIL OF MEDICAL RESEARCH. (1951). *Results of diet surveys in India 1935–48.* Special Report Series no. 20. 152 pp.

—————— (1953). *Results of diet surveys in India 1935–48.* Special Report Series no. 25. 67 pp.

——————(1959). *Tuberculosis in India: a sample survey, 1955–58.* 121 pp.

—————— (1964). *Diet Atlas of India.* Nutrition Research Laboratories, Hyderabad. Special Report Series no. 48. 83 pp.

—————— (1967). *Annual report 1966–67.* 173 pp.

—————— (1968). *Growth and physical development of Indian infants and children. All-India Part 1-A.* Statistics Division, Delhi. 20 pp. plus 16 tables.

——————(1969). *Annual report for the year 1968–69.* 196 pp.

INDIA, GOVERNMENT of (1928). *Royal Commission on Agriculture in India (presided over by Lord Linlithgow). Abridged report.* Government Central Press, Bombay. 101 pp.

INDIAN INSTITUTE OF MANAGEMENT. (1967). *The protein emergency.* Ahmedabad. (no pagination).

INDIA, NATIONAL INSTITUTE OF NUTRITION. (1969). *Annual report.*

——— (1970) *Annual report.*

INDIA, NUTRITION SOCIETY of. (1967). Symposium on population problems and food resources of southeast Asia. *Proc. Nutr. Soc. India* 1. 77 pp.

INDONESIAN INSTITUTE OF SCIENCES (1968). *Report of Workshop on Food (with U.S. National Academy of Sciences), Djakarta. I. Overall findings and recommendations.* 34 pp. 2. *Report of the Working Groups.* 154 pp. 3. *Keynote addresses, list of participants, background papers.* 116 pp.

INSULL, W., OISO, T., *and* TSUCHIYA, K. (1968). 'Diet and nutritional status of Japanese.' *Amer. J. Clin. Nutrition* 21, 753–7.

INTENGAN, C. (1966). 'Programs for combatting malnutrition in the pre-school child in the Philippines.' In *Pre-school child malnutrition* (ed. U.S. National Academy of Sciences). pp. 112–22. Publication no. 1282.

——— *and* FOOD AND NUTRITION RESEARCH CENTER, PHILIPPINES. (1970). 'Recommended dietary allowances for Filipinos – 1970 revision.' *Philippine J. Nutrition* 23, (2), 1–17.

——— *and* MARFORI, C.G. (1971). 'The protein quality of the Filipino diet.' *Philippine J. Nutrition* 24, 37–43.

INTERDEPARTMENTAL COMMITTEE ON NUTRITION FOR NATIONAL DEFENSE (I.C.N.N.D.). (1960). *Republic of Vietnam: Nutrition survey.* National Institutes of Health, Bethesda, Md. 257 pp.

I.C.N.N.D. (1963a). *Manual for nutrition surveys.* National Institutes of Health, Bethesda, Md.

——— (1963b). *Union of Burma: Nutrition survey.* National Institutes of Health, Bethesda, Md. 287 pp.

——— (1964). *Federation of Malaya: Nutrition survey.* National Institutes of Health, Bethesda, Md. 355 pp.

INTERNATIONAL RICE RESEARCH INSTITUTE (IRRI). (1972). *Annual report for 1971.* Los Banos, Philippines. 238 pp.

IRANI, S.E. (1969). 'Low birth weight babies. A follow-up study of 100 cases.' *Pediat. Clins. India* 4, 339–50.

ISHIKAWA, S. (1967). *Economic development in Asian perspective.* Kinokuniya Bookstore, Tokyo.

JANLEKHA, K.O. (1955). *A study of the economy of a rice-growing village in central Thailand.* Division of Agricultural Economics, Ministry of Agriculture, Thailand. 192 pp.

——— (1968). *Saraphi: a survey of socio-economic conditions in a rural community in north-east Thailand.* Geographical Publications Ltd., Bude, Cornwall. 63 pp.

JAPAN, CENTER FOR SOUTHEAST ASIAN STUDIES, KYOTO UNIVERSITY. (1968). *Medical problems in southeast Asia.* Symposium Series 14. 125 pp.

JAPAN, ESSENTIAL AMINO ACIDS ASSOCIATION. (1966). *Report on the feeding experiment of lysine-enriched bread to school-age children.* mimeo. 23 pp.

JAPAN, MINISTRY OF AGRICULTURE AND FORESTS. (1968). *Farm household economy survey.* Agricultural development series. (in Japanese)

JAPAN, MINISTRY OF HEALTH AND WELFARE. (1969). *Nutrient intakes for Japanese people.* Nutrition Section, Ministry of Health and Welfare, Tokyo. 59 pp. (in Japanese)

——— (1972). *Report of national nutrition survey made in 1971.* Nutrition Section, Ministry of Health and Welfare, Tokyo. 61 pp. (in Japanese).

JAPAN TIMES. (1970a). 'Life in a Red Chinese Commune.' 7 August.

——— (1970b). 'Survey bares nutrition standards for Japanese.' 17 October.

JASPAN, M.A. (1967). 'Tolerance and rejection of cultural impediments to economic growth: the south Sumatran case.' *Bull. Indon. Econ. Studies* no. 7, 38–59.

JAY, R.R. (1956). 'Local government in rural central Java.' *Far Eastern Quarterly* 15, 215–28.

JELLIFFE, D.B. (1966). *Assessment of the nutritional status of the community.* W.H.O. Monograph Series no. 53, Geneva. 271 pp.

———— (1968a). *Infant nutrition in the tropics and subtropics.* W.H.O. Monograph Series no. 29 (2nd ed.). Geneva. 335 pp.

———— (1968b). *Child nutrition in developing countries.* U.S. Government Printing Office, Public Health Service Publication no. 1822. 200 pp.

———— and JELLIFFE, E.F.P. (1969). 'The arm circumference as a public health index of protein-calorie malnutrition of early childhood. 20. Current conclusions.' *J. Trop. Pediat.* 15, 253–60.

JOCANO, F.L. (1969). *Growing up in a Philippine barrio.* Holt, Rinehart and Winston, New York, Toronto, London. 121 pp.

JOLLIFFE, N. *and* TUNG, T.C. (1959). 'Nutrition status survey of the civilian population of Formosa.' *Metabolism* 5, 309–27.

JYOTHI, K.K., DHAKSHAYANI, R., SWAMINATHAN, M.C. *and* VENKATACHALAM, P.S. (1963). 'A study of the socio-economic diet and nutritional status of a rural community near Hyderabad.' *Trop. geogr. Med.* 15, 403–10.

KALAB, M. (1968). 'Study of a Cambodian village.' *Geographical J.* 134, 521–37.

———— (1969). 'Notes on Cambodian diet.' (personal communication).

KAMBARA, T. (1970). 'Studies on growth and nutritional intake of school children in Kagawa Prefecture. 2. Regional differences of nutritional intake.' *Shikoku Acta Med.* 26, 15–30.

KAN, S.P., SINGH, M., CHEAH, J.S. *and* SIAK, C.L. (1971). 'Survey of helminthic infections in Singapore.' *Southeast Asian J. Trop. Med. Public Health* 2, 190–195.

KANAWATI, A.A. *and* McLAREN, D.S. (1970). 'Assessment of marginal malnutrition.' *Nature. Lond.* 228, 573–74.

KANEDA, H. (1967). *Long-term changes in food consumption patterns in Japan, 1878–1964.* Economic Growth Center, Yale University, Discussion paper no. 21. mimeo. Yale University, New Haven, 51 pp.

KAR, B. (1968). *Nutrition research profile – India.* U.S. Agency for International Development, New Delhi. 201 pp.

KHAING, Mi Mi. (1962). *Burmese family.* Indiana University Press, Bloomington. 200 pp.

KHAN, M.H. (1969). 'Some aspects of food consumption and its long-term perspective in Pakistan, 1961–1986.' *J. Agric. Econ.* 20, 133–42.

KIM, D.J. (1968). *Final report of the studies of basal metabolism and energy expenditure of Koreans in daily life and work.* College of Medicine, Ewha Woman's University, Seoul. mimeo. 6 pp. plus 12 tables.

KLERKS, J.V. (1959). *Final report on nutrition in Thailand.* W.H.O. mimeo. Geneva. 28 pp.

KORN, J. (1971). 'Indigestible food aid.' *Ceres* 4 (1), 62–3.

KRINKS, P.A. (1970). 'Peasant colonization in Mindanao.' *J. Trop. Geography* 30, 38–47.

KRISHNAMOORTHY, R. (1966). 'Angular stomatitis and xerosis incidence among schoolchildren of Madurai City.' *Antiseptic* 63, 919–26.

KRISHNANDHI, S. (1969). 'The economic development of Indonesia's sea fishing industry.' *Bull. Indon. Econ. Studies* 5, 49–71.

KROEBER, A.L. (1952). 'The societies of primitive man.' In *The nature of culture* (ed. A.L. Kroeber). pp. 219–25. Chicago University Press.

KUNSTADTER, P. (ed.). (1967). *Southeast Asian tribes, minorities and nations.* Princeton University Press. (2 vols.) 902 pp.

———— (1968). Personal communication.

———— (1969). 'Fertility, mortality and migration of hill and valley populations in northwestern Thailand.' mimeo. University of Washington, Seattle. 16 pp.

KWON, E., KIM, T.R., CHA, C.H., YUN, D.R., KO, U.R., *and* PARK, H.J. (1967). *A study in urban slum population.* College of Medicine and School of Public Health, Seoul National University. 278 pp.

LALA, V.R. *and* DESAI, A.B. (1970). 'Feeding of newborns and infants (cultural aspects).' *Pediat. Clins. India* 5, 191–7.

———— *and* REDDY, V. (1970). 'Absorption of beta-carotene from green leafy vegetables in under-nourished children.' *Amer. J. Clin. Nutrition* 23, 110–13.

LAN DINH, Nguyen. (1966). 'La malnutrition en calories et protéines.' *Bull. Syndicat des Médecins du Vietnam* 19, 29–44.

LATHAM, M. (1972). *Planning and evaluation of Applied Nutrition Programmes.* FAO Nutritional Studies no. 26. FAO, Rome. 115 pp.

LEACH, E.R. (1950). *Social science research in Sarawak.* H.M.S.O., London. 93 pp.

————(1961). *Pul Eliya: a village in Ceylon.* Cambridge University Press, London. 344 pp.

LEBAR, F.M., HICKEY, G.C. *and* MUSGRAVE, J.K. (1964). *Ethnic groups of mainland southeast Asia.* Yale University Press, New Haven. 288 pp.

LEE, C.C. (1948). 'Birth weights of full-term infants in west China.' *Chinese Med. J.* 66, 153–55.

LEE, Chong-Sik and KIM, Nam-Sik. (1970). 'Control and administrative mechanisms in the North Korean countryside.' *J. Asian Studies* 29, 309–26.

LEE, E. (1970). 'Nutritional problems in Malaysia.' *Canadian Nutrition Notes* 26, 1–5.

LEE, K.Y., BANG, S. and YUN, D.J. (1963). 'Dietary survey of weanling infants in South Korea.' *J. Amer. Dietet. Assoc.* 43, 457–61.

LEE, R.B. *and* DE VORE, I. (eds). (1968). *Man the Hunter.* Aldine, Chicago. 416 pp.

LEE, Yong Leng. (1970). *Population and settlement in Sarawak.* Asia Pacific Press, Singapore. 257 pp.

LEHMAN, F.K. (1963). *The structure of Chin society: a tribal people in Burma adapted to a non-western civilization.* University of Illinois Press, Urbana. 244 pp.

LEWIS, O. (1955). 'Peasant culture in India and Mexico: a comparative analysis.' In *Village India* (ed. M. Marriott). 145–70. Chicago University Press.

LEY, C.H. (1967). 'Muruts of Sabah.' In *Southeast Asian tribes, minorities and nations.* (ed. P. Kunstadter). Princeton University Press.

LIANG, P.H., HIE, T.T., JAN, O.H. *and* GIOK, L.T. (1967). 'Evaluation of mental development in relation to early malnutrition.' *Amer. J. Clin. Nutrition* 20, 1290–4.

LIE, K.J., KWO, E.H. and OWYANG, C.K. (1971). 'Soil-transmitted helminths in rural infants and children near Kuala Lumpur.' *Southeast Asian J. Trop. Med. Public Health* 2, 196–200.

LÖRSTAD, M.H. (1971). 'Recommended intake and its relation to nutrient deficiency.' *Nutrition News-letter* 9(1), 18–31.

LOURDENADIN, S. (1964). 'Pattern of anaemia and its effects on pregnant women in Malaya.' *Med. J. Malaya* 19, 87–93.

————(1969). 'Hazards of child birth in West Malaysia.' *Med. J. Malaya* 23, 239–43.

LOW, H.B. (1937). 'The standard of living.' In *Land utilization in China* (ed. J. Lossing Buck). pp. 437–72. Shanghai, Commercial Press. Reprinted Paragon Book Reprint Co., New York. (1964).

LUCAS, J.W. (1969). 'Food production in the year 2000 A.D.' *Plant Foods Human Nutrition* 1, 265–67.

McARTHUR, M. (1962). 'Assignment Report, Malaya 12.' W.H.O. mimeo. Geneva. 137 pp.

McCANCE, R.A. and WIDDOWSON, E.M. (eds). (1968). *Calorie deficiencies and protein deficiencies. Proc. Colloq. Cambridge, 1967.* Churchill, London. 386 pp.

McGILLIVRAY, W.A. (1968). 'Lactose intolerance.' *Nature, Lond.* 219, 615.

MacINTOSH, R.G. (1968). *Report to the Government of Ceylon on the Applied Nutrition and Agricultural Extension Project.* C.E.P. Report No. 49. mimeo. F.A.O., Rome. 7 pp.

McKAY, D.A. (1969). 'The arm circumference as a public health index of protein-calorie malnutrition of early childhood. 10. Experience with the mid-arm circumference as a nutritional indicator in field surveys in Malaysia.' *J. Trop. Pediat.* 15, 213–16.

————— *and* WADE, T.L. (1970). 'Nutrition, environment and health in the Iban longhouse.' *Southeast Asian J. Trop. Med. Public Health* 1, 68–77.

MACKINDER, H.J. (1904). 'The geographical pivot of history.' *Geogr. J.* 23, 421–37.

McLAREN, D.S. (1968). 'Vitamin deficiencies complicating the severer forms of protein-calorie malnutrition, with special reference to vitamin A.' In *Calorie deficiencies and protein deficiencies* (eds. R.A. McCance and E.M. Widdowson). 191–99. Churchill, London.

MacLEAN, J.D. *and* KAMATH, K.R. (1970). 'Infantile scurvy in Malaysia.' *Med. J. Malaya* 24, 200–7.

MADALGI, S.S. (1967). 'Foodgrains demand projections 1964–65 to 1975–76.' *Reserve Bank of India Bulletin.* mimeo. 22 pp.

————— (1968). 'Hunger in rural India.' *Economic and Political Weekly,* Annual number. pp. 61–68.

MAHADEVAN, I. (1961). 'Belief systems in food of the Telugu-speaking people of the Telengana region.' *Ind. J. Soc. Work.* 21, 387–96.

————— (1962). 'Social factors in some nutritional deficiency diseases.' *Indian J. Soc. Work.* 22, 41–51.

MAHAR', M. (1969). Personal communication.

MAKALIWE, W.H. (1969). 'An economic survey of south Sulawesi.' *Bull. Indon. Econ. Studies.* 5, (2), 17–36.

MALAVIYA, M.B., SEN GUPTA, L.M.F., SRIVASTAVA, M.D. *and* PRASAD, B.G. (n.d.). 'Nutrition status of primary school children in the area of the Rural Health Training Centre, Sarojini Nagar.' 20 pp.

MALENBAUM, W. (1959). 'India and China: contrasts in development performance.' *American Econ. Rev.* 49:284–309.

MALLORY, W.H. (1926). *China: land of famine.* American Geographical Society, Special Publication no. 6. 199 pp.

MALONEY, C. (1970). 'The beginnings of civilization in south India.' *J. Asian Studies* 29, 603–616.

MANNING, C. (1971). 'The timber boom.' *Bull. Indon. Econ. Studies* 7(3), 30–60.

MAQSOOD, S.A. (1961). 'Problems and some solutions. Pakistan.' In *The place of science and technology in the campaign against malnutrition.* (Symposium). Reviewed in *Proc. Nutrition Soc.* 20, 105–108.

MARETZKI, T.W. (1968). Personal communication.

————— and MARETZKI, H. (1966). *Taira: an Okinawan village.* Wiley, New York, London, Sydney. 176 pp.

MARKS, J., REINER, M.L. *and* AHMAD, K. (1965). *Nutrition manual for East Pakistan.* Ministry of Health, Labour and Social Welfare, Dacca. 56 pp.

MARRIOTT, M. (ed). (1955). *Village India.* Chicago University Press. 269 pp.

MARZAN, A.M., TANTENGCO, V.O. and CAVILES, A.P. (1971). 'Nutritional anaemias among Filipinos during pregnancy.' *Southeast Asian J. Trop. Med. Public Health* 2, 564–74.

MATAWARAN, A.J. *and* GERVASIO, C.C. (1971). 'Average heights and weights of Filipinos.' *Philippine J. Nutrition* 24, 74–92.

MATSUDA, H., KOKAWA, I., MOKUBO, J., MIZUI, M., MATSUURA, K., FURUKAWA, S., OSUMI, M. and MIZUTA, K. (1968). 'Survey of infant care clinics in Kotoson, Tokushima Prefecture.' *Shikoku Acta Med.* 24, 221–9.

MATSUDAIRA, T. (1969). 'Nutrition status of housewives living in the rural mountain district of Kyoto City.' *Japanese J. Nutrition* 27, 153–9.

MATTHEWS, J.M. (1966). 'Hoabinhian in Indochina.' *Asian Perspectives* 9, 86–95.

MAXWELL, W.E. (1967). *Thai medical students and rural health service.* Institute of Advanced Projects, East-West Center, Hawaii. mimeo. 104 pp.

MAYNARD, L.A. *and* SWEN, Wenyuh. (1937). 'Nutrition.' In *Land utilization in China* (ed. J.L. Buck). pp. 400–436. Shanghai, Commercial Press. Reprinted Paragon Book Reprint Co., New York. (1964.)

MEADOWS D.H., MEADOWS D.L., RANDERS, J. *and* BEHRENS, W.W. III. (1972). *The limits to growth.* Earth Island; London. 205 pp.

MELLOR, J.W., WEAVER, T.F., LELE, U.J. *and* SIMON, S.R. (1968). *Developing rural India — Plan and practice.* Cornell University Press, Ithaca. 411 pp.

MEREDITH, H.V. (1968). 'Body size of contemporary groups of pre-school children studied in different parts of the world.' *Child Development* 39, 336–77.

——— (1969a). 'Body size of contemporary youth in different parts of the world.' *Monogr. Soc. Res. Child Development* 34, no. 7, 120 pp.

——— (1969b). 'Body size of contemporary groups of 8-year old children studied in different parts of the world.' *Monogr. Soc. Res. Child Development* 34 no. 1, 93 pp.

——— (1970a). 'Body weight at birth of viable human infants: a worldwide comparative treatise.' *Human Biology* 42, 217–64.

——— (1970b). 'Body size of contemporary groups of one-year old infants studied in different parts of the world.' *Child Development* 41, 551–600.

MILLIS, J. (1957). 'Growth of pre-school Malay infants in Singapore.' *Med. J. Malaya* 12, 416–22.

———(1958a). 'Growth of pre-school Chinese and southern Indian children in Singapore.' *Med. J. Malaya* 12, 531–39.

——— (1958b). 'Modifications in food selection observed by Malay women during pregnancy and after confinement.' *Med. J. Malaya* 13, 139–44.

———(1958c). 'Infant feeding among Malays.' *Med. J. Malaya* 13, 145–52.

MILNER, M. (1969). *Protein enriched cereal foods for world needs.* Amer. Assoc. Cereal Chemists, St. Paul, Minnesota, 343 pp.

MINTURN, L. *and* HITCHCOCK, J.T. (1966). *The Rajputs of Khalapur, India.* Wiley, New York, London, Sydney. 158 pp.

MITRA, K. (1941). 'Dietary and physique of mining population in Jharia coal fields (Bihar).' *Indian J. Med. Res.* 29:143–56.

MIZUI, M., KOCHI, T., KATO, M., ISHIKAWA, K., HAMAGUCHI, M. and KUROBE, M. (1968). 'Statistical observations of obesity, malnutrition and small stature of school children in Tokushima Prefecture.' *Shikoku Acta Med.* 24, 65–73.

MO, Sumi. (1966). 'A study of food taboos in agricultural villages in Korea.' *J. Korean Home Economics Assoc.* 5, 15–21.

MOERMAN, M. (1968). *Agricultural change and peasant choice in a Thai village.* California University Press, Berkeley and Los Angeles. 227 pp.

MONCKEBERG, F. (1971). 'Malnutrition and socioeconomic development.' P.A.G. Bulletin no. 11, pp. 9–17.

MONTAGU, A, (1972) 'Sociogenic brain damage.' *Amer. Anthropol.* 74, 1045–61.

MORRIS, H.S. (1953). *Report on a Melanau sago producing community in Sarawak.* H.M.S.O., London. 176 pp.

MYRDAL, G. (1968). *Asian drama: an inquiry into the poverty of nations.* N.Y. Twentieth Century Fund, New York. 3 vols. 2284 pp.

MYRDAL, J. (1966). *Report from a Chinese village.* Signet, New York. 397 pp.

NAGAMINE, S., ISOBE, S., ICHINOSE, Y., KAGA, A. *and* UZUKA, M. (1963). 'The nutritional status of the low income families. (Report 3). Families in the secluded villages.' *Ann. Department National Nutrition Inst.* 42, p. 44.

NAGARAJAN, V. (1969). 'Lathyrism.' *Indian J. Med. Res.* 57, (8), 92–101.

NAIR, K. (1961). *Blossoms in the dust.* Praeger, New York. 201 pp.

NAISMITH, D.J. (1962). 'The role of dietary fat in the utilization of protein. II. The essential fatty acids.' *J. Nutrition* 77, 381–386.

——— (1964). 'The role of the essential fatty acids in the aetiology of kwashiorkor.' *Proc. Nutrition Soc.* 23, viii–ix.

——— and QURESHI, R.V. (1962). 'The role of dietary fat in the utilization of protein. I. Quality and and quantity of fat.' *J. Nutrition* 77, 373–80.

NAPITUPULU, B. (1968). 'Hunger in Indonesia.' *Bull. Indon. Econ. Studies* No. 9, 60–70.

NARAIN, R., GASSER, A., JAMBUNATHAN, M.V. *and* SUBRAMANIUM, M. (1963). 'Tuberculosis prevalence survey in Tumkur district.' *Bull. World Health Organiz.* 29, 641–64.

NARUSE, A. (1969). 'Studies on growth and nutritional intake of school children in Ehime Prefecture. 2. Regional differences in nutritional intake.' *Shikoku Acta Med.* 25, 467–90.

NASH, M. (1965). *The golden road to modernity.* Wiley, New York, London, Sydney. 333 pp.

———— (1966). *Primitive and peasant economic systems.* Chandler, San Francisco. 166 pp.

NEEDHAM, J. *and* LU, G.D. (1962). 'Hygiene and preventive medicine in ancient China.' *J. Hist. Med.* 17, 429–78.

NETRASIRI, A. *and* NETRASIRI, C. (1955). 'Kwashiorkor in Bangkok – an analytical study of 54 cases.' *J. Trop. Pediat.* 1, 148–55.

NIELSEN, I. (1965). *Report on assistance to the Applied Nutrition Project, Ubol, Thailand.* mimeo. F.A.O., Rome. 17 pp.

NIKI, K. (1968). 'Experiment of lysine-supplemented bread and its effect on physical development of school children.' *Shikoku Acta Med.* 24, 233–49.

NISHIDONO, N. (1970). 'On the nutrient allowance of pregnant women in Japan.
1. Monthly changes in the basal metabolism and metabolic functions in pregnancy.
2. Caloric allowance of pregnant women.' *Shikoku Acta Med.* 26, 216–25 and 226–31.

NOGUCHI, M. *and* NONOMURA, Y. (1970). 'The nutritional survey on eating habits in mountain area in Gifu Prefecture. Survey in Ichigatani, Yamato Village, Gujyo District.' *J. Japanese Soc. Food Nutrition* 23, 146–53.

NORBECK, E. (1967). *Changing Japan.* Holt, Rinehart and Winston. New York, Toronto, London. 82 pp.

NOUTH-SAVOUEN. (1966). 'Contribution à l'étude de la croissance physique des enfants cambodgiens de la naissance à 14 ans.' Doctoral thesis no. 48. Faculté royale de médecine, Phnom Penh. 112 pp.

NURGE, E. (1957). 'Infant feeding in the village of Guinhangdan, Leyte, Philippines.' *J. Trop. Pediat.* 3, 89–96.

———— (1965). *Life in a Leyte village.* University of Washington Press, Seattle. 157 pp.

NYDEGGER, W.F. *and* NYDEGGER, C. (1966). *Tarong: an Ilocos barrio in the Philippines.* Wiley, New York, London, Sydney. 180 pp.

OBEYESEKERE, G. (1963). 'Pregnancy cravings (dola-duka) in relation to social structure and personality in a Sinhalese village.' *Amer. Anthropol.* 65, 323–42.

———— (1968). 'Theodicy, sin and salvation in a sociology of Buddhism.' In *Dialectic in practical religion* (ed. E.R. Leach), 7–40. Cambridge University Press, London.

———— (1969). 'The ritual drama of the Sanni demons: collective representatives of disease in Ceylon.' *Comparative Studies Society and Hist.* 11, 174–216.

OBEYESEKERE, I. (1966). 'Malnutrition among Ceylonese adults.' *Amer. J. Clin. Nutrition* 18, 38–45.

———— (1968). 'Idiopathic cardiomegaly in Ceylon. Congestive cardiac failure, cardiomegaly, hepatomegaly and portal fibrosis associated with malnutrition.' *Brit. Heart J.* 30, 226–35.

OJHA, P.D. (1970). 'A configuration of Indian poverty.' *Reserve Bank of India Bulletin* 24, 16–27.

OLNESS, K.N. (1968). Personal communication.

OOMEN, H.A.P.C. (1963). 'Report on survey of xerophthalmia and keratomalacia caused by hypovitaminosis A. South and East Asia.' mimeo. W.H.O., Geneva. 84 pp.

ORLEANS, L.A. (1969). 'Propheteering: the population of Communist China'. *Current Scene, Hong Kong* 7, (24), 13–19.

ORR, K.G. (1967). 'Patterns of consumption in the Lao household.' mimeo. U.S.A.I.D. Vientiane. 110 pp.

PAKISTAN, GOVERNMENT OF. (1966). *Pakistan: nutrition survey of East Pakistan.* Ministry of Health, Government of Pakistan/University of Dacca/National Institutes of Health, U.S. Department of Health, Education and Welfare. Bethesda, Md. 426 pp.

PAKISTAN MEDICAL JOURNAL (1968). 'Editorial on availability of doctors.'*Pakistan Med. J.* 17, 355.

PARTADIREDJA, A. (1970). 'Economic survey of south Kalimantan.' *Bull. Indon. Econ. Studies* 6(2), 46—65.

PASCUAL, C.E. (1971). 'Proposed four-year nutrition program.' *Philippine J. Nutrition* 24, 103—109.

PASRICHA, S. (1958). 'Survey of dietary intake in a group of poor, pregnant and lactating women.' *Indian J. Med. Res.* 46, 605—9.

————— (1966). *Menus for low cost balanced diets and school lunch programmes, suitable for north India.* Nutrition Research Laboratories, Indian Council of Medical Research, Hyderabad. 30 pp.

PASSMORE, R. (1964). 'An assessment of the report of the Second Committee on Calorie Requirements.' mimeo. F.A.O., Rome. 18 pp.

PATWARDHAN, V.N. (1960). *Dietary allowance for Indians: calories and proteins.* Special Report Series no. 35. Indian Council of Medical Research, New Delhi.

—————, FARID, Z., DARBY, W.J., WOODRUFF, C. and FINCH, C.A. (1969). 'Symposium on nutritional anaemias.' *Amer. J. Clin. Nutrition.* 22, 495—517.

PAYUMO, E.M., LEGASPI, G.R.A. and APOLINARIO, K. (1972). 'Developments of drum-dried weaning foods based on indigenous sources. III. Coco cereal weaning flakes based on coconut skim milk solids.' *Philippine J. Nutrition* 25, 95—112.

PEDROSO, F.A. and GANDARA, F.A. (1958). 'Study of child development in the provinces of Macao.' *Ann. Inst. Med. Trop.* 15, 941—45, 947—75 and 977—1004.

PELZER, K.J. (1945). *Pioneer settlement in the Asiatic tropics.* Special Publication No. 29, American Geographical Society of New York. 288 pp.

————— (1968). 'Man's role in changing the landscape of southeast Asia.' *J. Asian Studies* 27, 269—79.

PENNY, D.H. (1966). 'The economics of peasant agriculture: the Indonesian case.' *Bull. Indon. Econ. Studies* No. 5, 22—44.

————— (1968). 'Hunger in Indonesia: comments.' *Bull. Indon. Econ. Studies* No. 9, 73—4.

————— and THALIB, D. (1969). 'Survey of recent developments — introduction.' *Bull. Indon. Econ. Studies* 5(1), 1—33.

PEREIRA, S.M., BEGUM, A., JESUDIAN, G. *and* SUNDARARAJ, R. (1969). 'Lysine supplemented wheat and growth of pre-school children.' *Amer. J. Clin. Nutrition* 22, 606—11.

PERILLO-DIA, M. (1968). 'An evaluation of the dietary adequacy of the food intake of selected female adolescents of the high school department of the University of the Southern Philippines, Cebu City.' *Philippine J. Nutrition* 21, 216—26.

PERISSE, J., SIZARET, F. *and* FRANCOIS, P. (1969). 'The effect of income on the structure of the diet.' *Nutrition Newsletter* 7 (3), 1—9.

PHILIPPINES, FOOD AND NUTRITION RESEARCH CENTER (F.N.R.C.). (1962). *Nutrition survey of Metropolitan Manila.* National Science Development Board, Manila. 79 pp.

PHILIPPINES, F.N.R.C. (1963a). *Nutrition survey of Ilocos Mountain Province region.* National Science Development Board, Manila. 88 pp.

————— (1963b). *Nutrition survey of the Cagayan Valley-Batanes region.* National Science Development Board, Manila. 89 pp.

————— (1965). *Nutrition survey of Southern Tagalog region.* National Science Development Board, Manila. 88 pp.

————— (1968). *Nutrition survey of Western Visayas region.* National Science Development Board, Manila. 104 pp.

————— (1969). *Nutrition survey of Eastern Visayas region.* National Science Development Board, Manila. 101 pp.

————— (in press). *Nutrition survey of north-eastern Mindanao.*

————— (in press). *Nutrition survey of south-western Mindanao.*

PHILLIPS, E.D. (1965). *The Royal Hordes: nomad peoples of the Steppes.* Thames and Hudson, London. 144 pp.

PHILLIPS, H.M. (1963). 'Social research and the problems of rural life in south-east Asia.' In *Social research and problems of rural development in south-east Asia.* (ed. V.Q. Thuc and K.F. Walker). pp. 27–51. U.N.E.S.C.O., Paris.

PILAC, L.M., ABDON, I.C. *and* MANDAP, E.P. (1971). 'Oxalic acid content and its relation to the calcium present in some Philippine plant foods.' *Philippine J. Nutrition* 24, 21–36.

PIRENNE, J. (1961) 'Un probleme-clef pour la chronologie de l'Orient: la date du "Périplé de la Mer Ery-thrée".' *J. Asiatique* 249, 441–59.

PLATT, H.S., STEWART, R.J.C. *and* PLATT, B.S. (1963). 'Transverse trabeculae in the bones of malnourished children.' *Proc. Nutrition Soc.* 22, xxix–xxx.

POLSON, R.A. (1966). 'The impact of change on the villagers of the Philippines.' *Indian Soc. Bull.* 3, 191–9.

——— *and* PAL, A.P. (n.d.). *Social change in the Dumaguete trade area: Philippines. 1951–58.* Cornell International Agricultural Development Mimeograph no. 4. Ithaca. 106 pp.

POLUNIN, I. (1960). 'The effects of shifting agriculture on human health and disease.' In *Symposium on the impact of man on humid tropics vegetation* (ed. Administrafion of Territory of Papua and New Guinea and UNESCO Science Co-operation Office for South-East Asia). 388–93. UNESCO Djakarta.

POSTMUS, S. *and* VAN VEEN, A.G. (1949). 'Dietary surveys in Java and east Indonesia.' *Chron. Nat.* 105, (10), 229–36; (11) 261–68; (12), 317–23.

PROTEIN ADVISORY GROUP. (1969). 'Recent trends on prevalence of protein-calorie malnutrition.' Document 1.2.1/1. mimeo. 14 pp. United Nations, New York.

——— (1970a). *Lives in peril: protein and the child.* F.A.O., Rome. 52 pp.

——— (1970b). 'Statement on amino acid fortification of foods.' United Nations, New York mimeo. 20 pp.

——— (1970c). 'P.A.G. Ad Hoc Working Group on Feeding the Pre-School Child.' *P.A.G. Bulletin* 10, p. 31.

——— (1971). 'Relationship of protein-calorie malnutrition in early childhood and its possible effects on mental development, learning and behaviour.' *P.A.G. Bulletin* 12, 4–5.

QUIOGUE, E.S. (1966a). 'Food consumption and supply in Philippines.' *Philippine J. Nutrition* 19, 173–93.

——— (1966b). 'Nutritional evaluation of 64 households. Diets in four barrios in Mountain Province.' *Philippine J. Nutrition.* 19, 272–93.

———, VILLAVIEJA, G.M. RAMOS, V., ALEJO, L.G., ROXAS, B.V., SALAMAT, L.A., KUIZON, D., BAYAN, A.A., MATAWARAN, A.J. *and* GERVASIO, C.C. (1969). 'Summary results of the eight regional nutrition surveys conducted in the Philippines by the Food and Nutrition Research Center.' *Philippine J. Nutrition* 22, 61–101.

RADHARUKMANI, A. *and* DEVADAS, R.P. (1964). 'The school lunch programmes.' *J. Nutrition Dietet.* 1, 66–71.

RAHEJA, P.C. (1965). 'Influence of climatic changes on vegetation of the arid zone in India.' *Ann. Arid Zone* 4, 64–73.

RAHMAN, M.F., IKRAMUL, H.M.Y., *and* MAQSOOD, A.S. (1968). 'Some observations on the state of nutrition of Lahore school children.' *Pakistan J. Med. Res.* 7, 124–33.

RAHMAN, M.H. (1968a). 'Present situation of nutritional status of infants and preschool children in Pakistan.' In *C.E.N.T.O. Conference on combating malnutrition in preschool children.* pp. 61–74. C.E.N.T.O., Ankara.

——— (1968b). 'Review of the present country programme in the field of nutrition in Pakistan.' In *C.E.N.T.O. Conference on combating malnutrition in preschool children.* pp. 89–94. C.E.N.T.O., Ankara.

RAJ, K.N. (1967). *India, Pakistan and China: economic growth and outlook.* Allied Publishers, New Delhi. 100 pp.

RAJALAKSHMI, R. (n.d.). 'Biochemistry of mental disorders with special reference to dietary factors.' Working Paper to W.H.O. Expert Committee on Biochemistry of Mental Disorders. University of Baroda, mimeo. 19 pp.

———— (1969). *Applied nutrition.* University of Baroda. 384 pp.

————, GOVINDARAJAN, K.R. and RAMAKRISHNAN, C.V. (1965). 'Effect of dietary protein content on visual discrimination learning and brain biochemistry in the albino rat.' *J. Neurochemistry* 12, 261–71.

———— *and* NANAVATY, K. (n.d.). 'Results of diet and nutrition surveys in and around Baroda.' mimeo. University of Baroda. 23 pp.

———— and RAMAKRISHNAN, C.V. (n.d.). 'Formulation and evaluation of low cost balanced meals.' mimeo. Biochemistry Department, University of Baroda. 15 pp. plus 49 tables.

————*and* RAMAKRISHNAN (1969). 'Dietary and nutrient allowances for Indians.' *Plant Foods Human Nutrition* 1, 163–91.

RAJASURIYA, K., NAGARATNAM, N., SOMASUNDERAM, M. *and* FERNANDO, C.F.O. (1960). 'Nutritional megaloblastic anaemias of Ceylon.' *J. Trop. Med. Hyg.* 63, 275–86.

RAMALINGASWAMI, V. (1956). *Summary report on nutritional situation in Thailand.* W.H.O. mimeo. 16 pp.

RAMASASTRI, B.V. *and* MOHAN, V.S. (1969). 'The nutritive value of foods.' *Indian. J. Med. Res.* 57, (8) 1–15.

RAO, B.R.H., KLONTZ, C.E. RAO, P.S.S., BEGUM, A. *and* DUMM, M.E. (1961). 'Nutrition status survey of the rural population of Sholavaram.' *Indian J. Med. Res.* 49, 316–29.

RAO, H.D. *and* BALASUBRAMANIAN, S.C. (1966). 'Socio-cultural aspects of infant-feeding practices in a Telengana village.' *Trop. Geogr. Med.* 18, 353–60.

RAO, K.S. (1962). 'Malnutrition in south India.' In *Malnutrition and food habits.* (eds. A. Burgess and R.F.A. Dean). pp. 29–36. Macmillan. New York.

————, SWAMINATHAN, M.C., SWARUP, S. *and* PATWARDHAN, V.N. (1959). 'Protein malnutrition in south India.' *Bull. World Health Organiz.* 20, 603–39.

RAO, N.B.S. (1969). 'Studies on nutrient requirements of Indians.' *Indian J. Med. Res.* 57 (8), 16–35.

RAWLINSON, H.G. (1937). 'India in European literature and thought.' In *The legacy of India* (ed. G.T. Garratt). pp. 1–37. Oxford at the Clarendon Press, Oxford.

REDDY, V. (1969). 'Vitamin A deficiency in children.' *Indian J. Med. Res.* 57 (8), 54–62.

REDFIELD, R. *and* SINGER, M. (1955). Foreword. In *Village India* (eds. Redfield and Singer). vii–xvi. Chicago University Press.

REH, E. (1963). 'Report to the Government of Brunei on the organization of food consumption surveys.' F.A.O. E.P.T.A. Report no. 1718. mimeo. Rome. 17 pp.

RITCHIE, J.A.S. (1967). *Learning better nutrition.* F.A.O., Rome. 264 pp.

ROBSON, R.K. (1972). *Malnutrition. Its causation and control.* 2 vols. Gordon and Breach, London. 660 pp.

ROMANI, J.H. (1956). 'The Philippines barrio.' *Far Eastern Quarterly* 15, 229–37.

ROXAS, B.V., DOMINGUEZ, A.A. *and* KUIZON, M.D. (1970). 'The nutritional re-evaluation of the Bayambang A.N.P.' *Philippine J. Nutrition* 23, 67–71.

ROY, J.K. *and* ROY, R.K. (1962). 'Diets of some Indian tribes.' *Indian J. Med. Res.* 50, 905–15.

———— and ROY, B.C. (1969). 'Food sources, dietary habits and nutrition intake of the Nicobarese of the Great Nicobar.' *Indian J. Med. Res.* 57, 58–64.

ROY, R.N. (1968). 'Tuberculosis in Sabah.' *Med. J. Malaya* 22, 204–16.

RUKMONO, B., NAUMAR, S.A. and TALOGO, R.W. (1971). 'Infantile diarrhoea in a population of low socio-economic group.' *Southeast Asian J. Trop. Med. Public Health* 2, 249–55.

RUTT, Father R. (1964). *Korean works and days.* Tuttle, Rutland, Vermont and Tokyo. 231 pp.

SAIKIA, P.D. (1968). *Changes in Mikir society: a case study of Kanther Terang village, Mikir Hills, Assam.*

Studies in Rural Change, Assam Series. Agro-Economic Research Centre for North-east India, Jorhat. 82 pp.

SAKSENA, R.N. (1962). *Social economy of a polyandrous people* (2nd ed.). Asia Publishing Co., London. 143 pp.

SANDOSHAM, A.A. (1970). 'Malaria in rural Malaya.' *Med. J. Malaya* 24, 221–6.

SANGAL, P.M. (1971). 'Forest food of the tribal populations of Andaman and Nicobar Islands.' *Ind. For.* 97, 640–50.

SANKALIA, H.D. (1962). *Prehistory and protohistory in India and Pakistan.* University of Bombay Press. 315 pp.

SAXENA, S. and GARG, O.P. (1968). 'Study of methods used for child rearing in Bikaner.' *Indian J. Pediat.* 35, 342–9.

SCHURMANN, F. and SCHELL, O. (eds.). (1968). *China readings 3: Communist China.* Pelican. Penguin Books, Harmondsworth. 647 pp.

SCHWEITZER, C.J. and RIES, S.K. (1969). 'Protein content of seed: increased expressions of growth and yield.' *Science* 165, 73–5.

SCRIMSHAW, N.S. (1969). 'Early malnutrition and central nervous system function.' *Protein Advisory Group Bull.* 8, 20–28.

———, TAYLOR, C.E. *and* GORDON, J.E. (1968). *Interaction of nutrition and infection.* W.H.O. Monograph Series no. 57. Geneva. 329 pp.

SETH, S.K. (1963). 'A review of evidence concerning changes of climate in India during the Protohistorical and Historical periods.' In *Change of climate, with special reference to the arid zones.* pp. 443-452. Arid Zone Research Series XX. UNESCO, Paris.

SHAH, P.M. and UDANI, P.M. (1968). 'Medical examination of rural school children in Palghar Taluk.' *Indian Pediat.* 5, 343–61.

SHARAT, S., KHANDUJA, P.C., AGARWAL, K.N., SAHA, M.M., GUPTA, S. and BHARDWAJ, O.P. (1970). 'Skeletal growth in school children.' *Indian Pediat.* 7, 98–108.

SHEN, T.H. (1957). *Agricultural resources of China.* (2nd ed.). Cornell University Press, Ithaca/Oxford University Press. 425 pp.

SHIROLE, D.B. and PHADKE, M.V. (1970). 'Anthropometric study of·1000 new-born babies.' *Indian Pediat.* 7, 219–20.

SHU, E.H. (1963). *Developmental history of medicine in China.* Wah Young Co., Seattle. 285 pp.

SHWAY YOE. (1882). *The Burman, his life and notions.* (reprinted 1963). Norton, New York. 609 pp.

SINGARIMBUN, N. (1967). 'Kutagamber: a village of the Karo.' In *Villages in Indonesia* (ed. Koentjaraningrat). pp. 115–28. Cornell University Press, Ithaca.

——— (1968). Personal communication.

SINITSYN, V.M. (1959). *Central Asia* (in Russian). Moscow.

SKINNER, G.W. (1964–65). 'Marketing and social structure in rural China.' *J. Asian Studies* 24, 3–43; 195–228; and 363–399.

SLIMMING, J. (1958). *Temiar jungle.* John Murray, London. 176 pp.

SMITH, L.P. (1969). Personal communication.

SNYDER, C. (1970). 'Malthus versus Marx.' *Far Eastern Economic Review* 69:52:28–32.

SOBHAN, R. (1968). *Basic democracies: works programme and rural development in East Pakistan.* Oxford University Press/Pakistan Bureau of Economic Research, Dacca. 328 pp.

SOLHEIM, W.G. (1967). 'Southeast Asia and the West.' *Science* 157, 896–902.

SOONG, F.S. (1972). 'Some beliefs and practices affecting the health of the aborigines (Orang Asli) of Bukit Lanjan, West Malaysia.' *Southeast Asian J. Trop. Med. Public Health* 3, 267–76.

SPENCER, J.E. (1966). *Shifting cultivation in southeast Asia.* University of California Publications in Geography, Los Angeles. 247 pp.

———— *and* THOMAS, W.L. (1971). *Asia, east by south: a cultural geography.* (2nd ed.) Wiley, New York, London, Sydney, Toronto. 669 pp.

SPIRO, M.E. (1966). 'Buddhism and economic action in Burma.' *Amer. Anthropol.* 68, 1163–73.

————(1968). 'Religion, personality and behaviour in Burma.' *Amer. Anthropol.* 70, 359–63.

SRIKANTIA, S.G. (1969). 'Protein-calorie malnutrition in Indian children.' *Indian J. Med. Res.* 57 (8), 36–53.

SRINIVAS, M.N. (ed.) (1960). *India's villages* (2nd ed.). Asia Publishing Co., London. 222 pp.

———— (1961). *Sociological aspects of Indian diet.* Paper to Freedom from Hunger Campaign Symposium, New Delhi. 3 pp.

———— (1966). *Social change in modern India.* California University Press, Berkeley and Los Angeles/ Cambridge University Press. 194 pp.

SRINIVASA RAO, P. and RAMASASTRI, B.V. (1969). 'The nutritive value of some indica, japonica and hybrid varieties of rice.' *J. Nutrition Dietetics* 6, 204–8.

SRINIVASAN, N. (1956). 'Village government in India.' *Far Eastern Quarterly* 15, 201–14.

STANTON, W.R. and WALLBRIDGE, A. (1969). 'Fermented food processes.' *Process Biochem.* April. 7 pp.

STEINER, K. (1956). 'The Japanese village and its government.' *Far Eastern Quarterly* 15, 185–200.

SUKHATME, P.V. (1966). 'Malthus bicentenary discussion on fertility, mortality and world food supplies; the world's food supplies.' *J. Roy. Statistical Soc. Series A, (Gen.)* 129, 222–43.

———— (1970). 'Incidence of protein deficiency in relation to different diets in India.' *Brit. J. Nutrition* 24, 477–487.

SUNDARARAJ, R., BEGUM, A., JESUDIAN, G. and PEREIRA, S.M. (1969). 'Seasonal variation in the diets of pre-school children in a village (North Arcot District.)' *Indian J. Med. Res.* 57, 249–59.

———— *and* PEREIRA, S.M. (1971). 'A diet survey in a village of North Arcot.' *J. Nutrition Dietet.* 8, 9–12.

SUTEDJO. (1968). 'Nutritional problems in Indonesia.' *Paediat. Indonesiana* 8, 255–59.

———— (1970). 'Health problems for children and youth in Indonesian national development planning.' *Paediat. Indonesiana* 10, 109–13.

SWAMINATHAN, M. (1970). 'Protein requirements – a critical evaluation of the F.A.O./W.H.O. Expert Group recommendations.' *Nutrition Rep. Internat.* 2, 153–71.

————, RAO, S.V. and DANIEL, V.A. (1969). 'Relationship between free plasma amino acids, limiting essential amino acids in dietary proteins and protein nutriture of the individual.' *J. Nutrition Dietet.* 6, 49–60.

SWAMINATHAN, M.C., APTE, S.V. and RAO, K.S. (1960). 'Nutrition of people of Ankola Taluk, north Kanara.' *Indian J. Med. Res.* 48, 762–64.

————, SUSHEELA, T.P. and THIMMAYAMMA, B.V.S. (1970). 'Field prophylactic trial with a single annual oral massive dose of vitamin A.' *Amer. J. Clin. Nutrition* 23, 119–22.

TAIWAN, JOINT COMMISSION FOR RURAL RECONSTRUCTION. (1968a). Discussions (1968b). *Twentieth anniversary report 1948–68.* Taipei.

TAKAGI, K., MASUDA, T. and KIDA, N. (1970). 'A report on the food intake of farmers in single and double crop districts before the introduction of power cultivators.' *J. Sci. Labour* 46, 593–625.

TAMARI, Y., MORI, E. and SHIRAI. (1969). 'On the calorie allowances of lactating women and infants.' *Shikoku Acta Med.* 25, 797–801.

TANTENGCO, V.O., SALVOSA, C.B., DE CASTRO, C.R. and PANTAS, F. (1971). 'Serum and red cell folate activity in Filipino school children with hookworm anaemia.' *Southeast Asian J. Trop. Med. Public Health* 2, 210–221.

TERRA, G.J.A. (1961). 'Food patterns in Indonesia.' *Proc. 3rd International Congress of Dietetics* London. 6 pp.

TEWARI, R.N., JAIN, P.C. and PRASAD, B.G. (1969). 'A medico-social study of pulmonary tuberculosis in Mati village, Lucknow.' *Indian J. Med. Res.* 59, 283–88.

THAMAN, O.P. and MANCHANDA, S.S. (1968). 'Child rearing practices in Punjab.' *Indian J. Pediat.* 35, 334–41.

THANANGKUL, O. *and* WHITAKER, J.A. (1966). 'Childhood thiamine deficiency in northern Thailand.' *Amer. J. Clin. Nutrition* 18, 275–77.

————, WHITAKER, J.A. and FORT, E.G. (1966). 'Malnutrition in northern Thailand.' *Amer. J. Clin. Nutrition* 18, 379–89.

THOMSEN, B. (1966). *Report on assistance to the Applied Nutrition Project, Ubol, Thailand.* mimeo. F.A.O., Rome. 15 pp.

THOMSON, F.A. (1960). *Child nutrition: a survey in Parit District of Perak, Federation of Malaya.* Bull. Inst. Med. Res. Malaya 10. 73 pp.

————, RUIZ, E. and BAKAR, M. (1964). 'Vitamin A and protein deficiency in Malayan children.' *Trans. Roy. Soc. Trop. Med. Hyg.* 58. 425–31.

THUC, V.Q. (1963). 'The rural problem in the countries of south-east Asia. 'In *Social research and problems of rural development in south-east Asia.* (eds. V.Q. Thuc and K.F. Walker). pp. 61–73. U.N.E.S.C.O., Paris.

THURNHAM, D.I., MIGASENA, P. and VUDHIVAI, N. (1971). 'Angular stomatitis and biochemical aribo-flavinosis in village pre-school children in northeast Thailand.' *Southeast Asian J. Trop. Med. Public Health* 2, 259–60.

———— *and* SUPAWAN, V. (1971). 'A longitudinal study on dietary and social influences on riboflavin status in pre-school children in northern Thailand.' *Southern Asian J. Trop. Med. Public Health* 2, 552–63.

TIE, L.T., LIAN, O.K., ONG, T.W.L. and ROSE, C.S. (1967). 'Health, development and nutritional survey of pre-school children in Indonesia.' *Amer. J. Clin. Nutrition* 20, 1260–66.

———— (1968). 'Health, development and nutritional survey of pre-school children in central Java.' *Paediat. Indonesiana* 8, 203–14.

TIGLAO, T.V. (1964). *Health practices in a rural community.* Community Development Research Council, University of Philippines, Quezon City. 232 pp.

TINKER, H. (1969). 'Continuity and change in Asian societies.' *Modern Asian Studies* 3, 97–116.

TODA, Y. and MORI, H. (1967). "Research on public health of Lombok Island in Indonesia. Vital statistics, physical fitness, nutrition, blood groups and habits of Sasak Tribe.' *Kobe J. Med. Sci.* 13, 139–55.

TONG, W.F., CHU, Y.E. and LI, H.W. (1970). 'Variations in protein and amino acid contents among genetic stock of rice.' *Bot. Bull. Acad. Sin. Taipei.* 11, 55–60.

TOPLEY, M. (1970). 'Chinese traditional ideas and treatment of disease: two examples from Hongkong.' *Man* 5, 421–37.

———— (1973). (Survey of child rearing practices and beliefs about illness in Hong Kong) (in preparation).

TOVERUD, K.U., STEARNS, G., and MACY, I.G. (1950). *Maternal nutrition and child health: an interpretative review.* Bull. Nat. Res. Coun. no. 123. Washington.

TRIBAL RESEARCH CENTRE (1969). *Proc. First Symposium of the Tribal Research Centre.* Chiang Mai, Thailand. 117 pp.

TRIESTMAN, J.M. (1970). 'Problems in contemporary Asian archaeology.' *J. Asian Studies* 29, 363–71.

———— (1972). *The prehistory of China, an archaeological exploration.* The Natural History Press, Double-day, Garden City. 143 pp.

TROPICAL MEDICINE AND MALARIA. (1968). 8th International Congress: *Health problems in pre-school children.* Iran. (reviewed) *J. Trop. Pediat.* 14, 214–60.

TULPULE, P.G. (1969). 'Aflatoxicosis.' *Indian J. Med. Res.* 57 (8), 102–114.

UHLIG, H. (1969). *Hill tribes and rice farmers in the Himalayas and south-east Asia.* Institute Brit. Geographers, Trans. and Papers no. 47. 23 pp.

———— (1970). 'Die agrarlandschaften des Chenab-tals in Jammu and Kaschmir.' In *Beiträge zur Geographie der Tropen und Subtropen. Festschrift für Herbert Wilhelmy.* Heft 34, pp. 309—23. Geographical Institute, University of *Tübingen.*

UCKO, J. and DIMBLEBY, G.W. (eds). (1969). *The domestication and exploitation of plants and animals.* Duckworth, London. 581 pp.

UNG PEANG (1966). *La xérophthalmie au Cambodge.* Doctoral thesis no. 59. Faculté royale de médecine, Phnom Penh. 118 pp.

UNG TENG (1967). *Les aliments usuels au Cambodge.* Doctoral thesis no. 75. Faculté royale de médecine. Phnom Penh. 154 pp.

UNGKU Omar-Ahmad and RAMANATHAN, K. (1968). Oral carcinoma. *Med. J. Malaya* 22, 172—81.

UNITED NATIONS EDUCATIONAL, SCIENTIFIC AND CULTURAL ORGANIZATION. *Manuals on adult and youth education:* (1959). I. *Filmstrips: use, evaluation and production;* (1961). II. *Literacy primers: construction, evaluation and use;* (1964). III. *Simple reading material for adults: its preparation and use;* (1966a). IV. *Planning and organization of adult literacy programmes in Africa;* (1966b). V. *School teaching and the education of adults.* Paris.

UNESCO (1963). *Social research and problems of rural development in south-east Asia.* (eds. V.Q. Thuc and K.F. Walker). Paris. 268 pp.

———— (1965). *Handbook for social research in urban areas.* Paris. 214 pp.

UNITED STATES AGENCY FOR INTERNATIONAL DEVELOPMENT (n.d.). A comprehensive national nutrition program for combating malnutrition in the Philippines. mimeo. 42 pp.

UNITED STATES CONSULATE IN HONG KONG. (1970). Personal discussions.

UNITED STATES NATIONAL ACADEMY OF SCIENCES (1943). *The problem of changing food habits.* Report of the Committee on Food Habits, 1941—43. National Research Council, Washington D.C. 177 pp.

———— (1961). *Proceedings of an international conference, Washington, August, 1960: Meeting protein needs of infants and pre-school children.* National Research Council, publication no. 843. Washington. 569 pp.

———— (1966). *Proceedings of an international conference on prevention of malnutrition in the pre-school child, Washington, December, 1964. Pre-school child malnutrition: primary deterrent to human progress.* National Research Council, publication no. 1282. Washington. 355 pp.

———— (1968). *Recommended dietary allowances: a report of the Food and Nutrition Board.* National Research Council, Washington. 101 pp.

USUTANI, S., KIMURA, S., KIMURA, H., NISHIDONO, Y., MORI, K. *and* SUZUKI, J. (1971). 'Labour and health of the farmers growing vegetables in a vinyl-house. 5. A nutritional survey of the farmers in Tokushima Prefecture'. *Jap. J. Nutrition* 29, 26—35.

UTOMO, K. (1967). 'Villages of unplanned resettlers in the Subdistrict Kaliredjo, Central Lampung.' In *Villages in Indonesia* (ed. Koentjaraningrat). pp. 281—98. Cornell University Press, Ithaca.

VALDECANAS, O. (1972), 'Beliefs and practices in food and nutrition of some rural women.' *Philippine J. Nutrition* 25, 43—52.

VALYASEVI, A., HALSTEAD, S.B., PANTUWATANA, S. and TANKAYUL, C. (1967). 'IV. Dietary habits, nutritional intake and infant feeding practices among residents of a hypo- and hyper-endemic area. *Amer. J. Clin. Nutrition* 20, 1340—51.

VAN VEEN, A.G. (1970) *Report to the Government of Indonesia: food and nutrition policy in relation to the food needs.* Nutrition Consultants' Reports Series no. 14 F.A.O., Rome. 45 pp.

VENKATACHALAM, P.S. and REBELLO, L.M. (1966). *Nutrition for mother and child.* Indian Council of Medical Research Special Report Series no. 41. Nutrition Research Laboratories, Hyderabad. 53 pp.

VON EICKSTEDT, E.F. (1944). *Rassen dynamik von Ostasien: China und Japan, Tai und Kmer, von der Urzeit bis Heute.* Walter de Gruyter, Berlin. 648 pp.

WALIA, B.N.S., and KAUL, K.K. (1970). 'The three faces of malnutrition. A comparative study of marasmus and nutritional oedema including kwashiorkor.' *Pediat. Clins. India* 5, 117—21.

WANG, Y.C. (1947). 'Dietary survey in Lichung.' *Chinese J. Nutrition* 2, 21–32.

WATERLOW, J.C. (1968). 'Observations on mechanism of adaptation to low protein intakes.' *Lancet* ii, 1091–97.

———— *and* STEPHEN, J.M.L. (1969). 'Enzymes and the assessment of protein nutrition.' *Proc. Nutrition Soc.* 28, 234–42.

WATSON, W. (1969). 'Early animal domestication in China'; 'Early cereal cultivation in China.' In *The domestication and exploitation of plants and animals* (ed. P.J. Ucko and G.W. Dimblely). pp. 393–5 and 397–402. Duckworth, London.

WENMOHS, J.R. (1967). 'Agriculture in mainland China – 1967.' *Current Scene, Hong Kong.* 6(21), 1–12.

WEST BENGAL, CENTRAL COMBINED NUTRITION LABORATORY (1968). *Report on nutrition work done in the State of West Bengal, 1967.* mimeo. Calcutta. 12 pp.

WEST BENGAL, DEPARTMENT OF ANIMAL HUSBANDRY, DARJEELING/KALIMPONG. (1969). Personal discussions.

WHARTON, C.R. (1965). *Research on agricultural development in southeast Asia.* Monograph no. 1 for the Research Program of the Agricultural Development Council. New York. 62 pp.

———— (1969a). 'The green revolution.' *Foreign Affairs* 47, 464.

———— (1969b). *Subsistence agriculture and economic development.* Aldine, Chicago. 482 pp.

WHEATLEY, P. (1965). 'A note on the extension of milking practices into southeast Asia during the first millenium A.D.' *Anthropos* 60, 577–90.

WHITEHEAD, R.G. (1969). 'Assessment of nutritional status in protein-malnourished children.' *Proc. Nutrition Soc.* 28, 1–16.

WHITING, J.W.M., CHILD, I.L. and LAMBERT, W.W. (1966). *Field guide for a study of socialization.* Wiley. New York, Sydney, London. 176 pp.

WHYTE, R.O. (1963). 'The significance of climatic change for natural vegetation and agriculture'. In *Change of climate with special reference to the arid zones.* pp. 381–6. Arid Zone Research Series XX, UNESCO, Paris.

———— (1968a). *Land, livestock and human nutrition in India.* Praeger, New York and London. 309 pp.

———— (1968b). *Grasslands of the monsoon.* Faber and Faber, London/Praeger, New York. 325 pp.

———— (1972a). *Rural nutrition in China.* Oxford University Press in Asia, Hong Kong. 54 pp.

———— (1972b). 'The Gramineae, wild and cultivated, of monsoonal and equatorial Asia. I. South-East Asia. *Asian Perspectives* 15:

———— and MATHUR, M.L. (1966). 'The buffalo in India.' *Indian Dairyman* 18, 161–80.

———— (1968). *The planning of milk production in India.* Orient Longmans, New Delhi. 221 pp.

————, NILSSON-LEISSNER, G. and TRUMBLE H.C. (1953). *Legumes in agriculture.* F.A.O. Agricultural Study no. 21. Rome. 367 pp.

WIENS, H.J. (1954). *China's march to the tropics.* Shoe String Press, Handon, Conn. 441 pp.

WILLIAMS, C.N. *and* JOSEPH, K.T. (1970). *Climate, soil and crop production in the humid tropics.* Oxford University Press, Kuala Lumpur and Singapore. 177 pp.

WILLIAMS, T.R. (1965). *The Dusun: A North Borneo society.* Holt, Rinehart and Winston, New York, Toronto, London. 100 pp.

WILSON, C.S. (1970a). 'Food beliefs and practices of Malay fishermen.' Department of Nutritional Sciences, University of California, Berkeley. mimeo. 21 pp.

———— (1970b). 'Food beliefs and practices of Malay fishermen: an ethnographic study of diet on the east coast of Malaya.' Doctoral dissertation in nutrition. University of California, Berkeley.

———— (1971). 'Cultural effects on the diet of east coast Malay fishermen.' *Bull. Public Health Soc.* 5, 26–8.

———— and ANDERSON, J.N. (1968). 'Socioeconomic status and nutrient intakes in a Philippine village.' *Fed. Proc.* 27, 680.

WILSON, P.J. (1967). *A Malay village and Malaysia.* Yale University, New Haven. 171 pp.

WINICK, M. (1968). 'Nutrition and cell growth.' *Nutrition Rev.* 26, 195—7.

———— (1969a). 'Cellular growth of the placenta as an indicator of abnormal fetal growth.' In *Diagnosis and treatment of fetal disorders* (ed. K. Adamsons). pp. 83—101. Springer Verlag, New York.

————(1969b). 'Malnutrition and brain development.' *J. Pediat.* 74, 667—9.

————(1969c). 'Food, time and cellular growth of brain.' *New York State J. Med.* 69, 302—4.

———— FISH, I. and ROSSO, P. (1968). 'Cellular recovery in rat tissues after a brief period of neonatal malnutrition.' *J. Nutrition* 95, 623—26.

———— and NOBLE, A. (1966). 'Quantitative changes in ribonucleic acids and protein during normal growth of rat placenta.' *Nature, London.* 212, 34—5;

———— and ROSSO, P. (1969a). 'The effect of severe early malnutrition on cellular growth of human brain.' *Pediat. Res.* 3, 181—84.

———— *and* ———— (1969b). 'Head circumference and cellular growth of the brain in normal and marasmic children.' *J. Pediat.* 74, 774—8.

WOLF, E.R. (1966). *Peasants.* Prentice Hall. Englewood Cliffs, N.J. 116 pp.

WOLFF, R.J. (1962). 'Food habits in Malaya.' University of California. mimeo. 25 pp.

WOODRUFF, A.W. (1968). 'Anaemia associated with protein-calorie malnutrition.' In *Calorie deficiencies and protein deficiencies.* (Eds. R.A. McCance and E.M. Widdowson). pp. 165—70. Churchill, London.

WORLD HEALTH ORGANIZATION (1962). *Calcium requirements.* W.H.O. Technical Report Series no. 230. 54 pp.

———— (1963). *Expert Committee on Medical Assessment of Nutritional Status.* W.H.O. Technical Report Series. No. 258. Geneva. 67 pp.

———— (1965a). *Nutrition in pregnancy and lactation: Report of a W.H.O. Expert Committee.* W.H.O. Technical Report Series no. 302. Geneva. 54 pp.

———— (1965b). *Nutrition and infection: Report of a W.H.O. Expert Committee.* W.H.O. Technical Report Series no. 314. Geneva. 30 pp.

———— (1967). *Requirements of vitamin A, thiamine, riboflavine and niacin. Report of a Joint F.A.O./ W.H.O. Expert Group.* W.H.O., Geneva. 86 pp.

————(1968a). *Nutritional anaemias.* W.H.O. Technical Report Series no. 405. Geneva. 37 pp.

———— (1968b). 'Nutrition in maternal and child health, with special reference to the Western Pacific.' *J. Trop. Pediat.* 14, 149—95.

————(1969). *The health aspects of food and nutrition.* W.H.O., Western Pacific Regional Office, Manila. 380 pp.

WORTH, R.M. *and* SHAH, N.K. (1969). *Nepal health survey, 1965-1966.* University of Hawaii Press, Honolulu. 158 pp.

YAKTIN, U.S. and McLAREN, D.S. (1970). 'The behavioural development of infants recovering from severe malnutrition.' *J. Mental Deficiency Res.* 14, 25—32.

YANG, C.K. (1959). *A Chinese village in early Communist transition.* Technology Press, Mass. 284 pp.

YANG, M.C. (1945). *A Chinese village: Taitou, Shantung Province.* Routledge and Kegan Paul, London. 275 pp.

YANG, T.H. (1966). *Report to the Government of the Republic of Korea on development of nutrition projects.* F.A.O. U.N.D.P. Report no. T.A. 2236. mimeo. Rome. 21 pp.

———— (1970). *Report to the Government of the Republic of Korea on the Applied Nutrition Program.* T.A. Report no. 2841. F.A.O., Rome. 62 pp.

YONEDA, S., OMI, K., OE, M., KISHI, M., YAMANASHI, N., SAKO, T., YUMURA, Y., SANO, T., OTSUKA, T. and TOMIDA, T. (1966). 'The nutrient research for pregnant women in Tokushima Prefecture, Japan.' *Japan J. Nutrition* 24, 59—63.

YONSEI UNIVERSITY. (1967—68). *A study on the food intake and nutritional status of elementary school-*

children and their family in urban and rural Korea. College of Home Economics and College of Medicine, Yonsei University, Korea. 150 pp.

YOON, J.J. and KIM, I.D. (1970). 'Study on weaning pattern and nutritional status of infants and toddlers in Korea.' *Korean J. Nutrition* 3, 65–80.

YOSHIMURA, H., YOSHIOKA, T. and FUKUSHIGE, M. (1969). 'Studies on the optimum protein requirements.' *J. Japanese Soc. Food Nutrition* 21, 32–42.

YOUNG, K.S. (1968). *Household consumption patterns of food grains in Suwon. Field survey 1966–67.* Department of Agricultural Economics, College of Agriculture, Seoul National University. mimeo. Seoul. 75 pp.

ZEUNER, F.E. (1963). *A history of domesticated animals.* Hutchinson, London. 560 pp.